Peptides as Drugs

Edited by
Bernd Groner

Further Reading

Sewald, N., Jakubke, H.-D.

Peptides: Chemistry and Biology

2009
ISBN: 978-3-527-31867-4

Jakubke, H.-D., Sewald, N.

Peptides from A to Z

A Concise Encyclopedia

2008
ISBN: 978-3-527-31722-6

Mannhold, R. (ed.)

Molecular Drug Properties

Measurement and Prediction

Volume 37 of Series "Methods and Pinciples in Medicinal Chemistry" edited by Mannhold, R., Kubinyi, H., Folkers, G.

2008
ISBN: 978-3-527-31755-4

Van de Waterbeemd, H. Testa, B. (eds.)

Drug Bioavailability

Estimation of Solubility, Permeability, Absorption and Bioavailability

Volume 40 of Series "Methods and Pinciples in Medicinal Chemistry" edited by Mannhold, R., Kubinyi, H., Folkers, G.

2009
ISBN: 978-3-527-32051-6

Ottow, E., Weinmann, H. (eds.)

Nuclear Receptors as Drug Targets

Volume 39 of Series "Methods and Pinciples in Medicinal Chemistry" edited by Mannhold, R., Kubinyi, H., Folkers, G.

2008
ISBN: 978-3-527-31872-8

Rognan, D. (ed.)

Ligand Design for G Protein-coupled Receptors

Volume 30 of Series "Methods and Pinciples in Medicinal Chemistry" edited by Mannhold, R., Kubinyi, H., Folkers, G.

2006
ISBN: 978-3-527-31284-9

Bertau, M., Mosekilde, E., Westerhoff, H. V.

Biosimulation in Drug Development

2008
ISBN: 978-3-527-31699-1

Fischer, J., Ganellin, C. R. (eds.)

Analogue-based Drug Discovery

2006
ISBN: 978-3-527-31257-3

Peptides as Drugs

Discovery and Development

Edited by
Bernd Groner

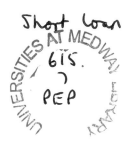

**WILEY-
VCH**

WILEY-VCH Verlag GmbH & Co. KGaA

The Editor

Prof. Dr. Bernd Groner
Georg-Speyer-Haus
Paul-Ehrlich-Straße 42 -44
60596 Frankfurt
Germany

Cover
The cover shows a cartoon illustration of two
protein strands (in blue and yellow
respectively) whose interaction is
competitively inhibited by a peptide (in red).

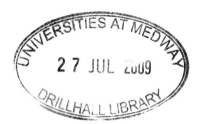

Library of Congress Card No.:
applied for

British Library Cataloguing-in-Publication Data
A catalogue record for this book is available from
the British Library.

**Bibliographic information published by
the Deutsche Nationalbibliothek**
The Deutsche Nationalbibliothek lists this
publication in the Deutsche Nationalbibliografie;
detailed bibliographic data are available on the
Internet at <http://dnb.d-nb.de>.

© 2009 WILEY-VCH Verlag GmbH & Co. KGaA,
Weinheim

Composition   SNP Best-set Typesetter Ltd.,
Hong Kong

Printing   Strauss GmbH, Mörlenbach

Bookbinding   Litges & Dopf GmbH, Heppenheim

Cover Design   Adam Design, Weinheim

Printed in the Federal Republic of Germany
Printed on acid-free paper

ISBN 978-3-527-32205-3

Contents

Peptides as Drugs. Discovery and Development. Edited by Bernd Groner
Copyright © 2009 WILEY-VCH Verlag GmbH & Co. KGaA, Weinheim
ISBN: 978-3-527-32205-3

Preface

The biological revolution of the past three decades has provided spectacular insights into the structure and function of macromolecules, cells and organisms, has changed our appreciation of the material basis of life, and has also provided the tools for targeted interferences with cellular processes. The technological advances which made this progress possible are based on, for example, molecular cloning, DNA sequencing, and the genetic manipulations of cells and organisms, and these methods have always preceded – or at least have accompanied – major conceptual advances.

Today, these successes in individual areas of biology are being extrapolated, and highly ambitious system biology projects have been initiated which will attempt to describe how the function of individual genes and the entirety of their interactions result in quantitative phenotypes of particular cells or organisms. The efforts to gain insights into quantitative behaviors are still restricted to simple model organisms and a few well-defined signal transduction pathways. Genetic manipulations are used to study information transmission through signaling systems, and to interpret them in the light of the resulting phenotypes. Interdisciplinary collaborations aim at identifying and predicting responses, and formulating new hypotheses concerning system functions.

Despite this remarkable progress in almost all areas of biology, reasonable predictions about gene functions in the organismal context remain very difficult. Whilst it is possible to annotate genes, and to recognize particular functional domains or subcellular localization signals, the cell-type specificity of expression, the regulation of expression, and the contribution of individual genes to particular phenotypic manifestations remain to be determined on an empirical basis. This has important implications for the development and use of drugs because, even if a drug can be developed to target a molecule that plays a central role in a particular pathological process, the adverse side effects of such a drug might still be unpredictable.

In life, if problems are very complex and the methods to approach them are still not fully developed, then there is a temptation to say "It can't be done". The Human Genome Project and targeted homologous recombination in embryonal stem cells are two such examples. But, in hindsight, advances in technologies tend to make the skeptic appear timid. Whilst the need to develop new drugs, to exploit additional drug targets and to meet medical needs is undisputed, many hurdles persist which

Peptides as Drugs. Discovery and Development. Edited by Bernd Groner
Copyright © 2009 WILEY-VCH Verlag GmbH & Co. KGaA, Weinheim
ISBN: 978-3-527-32205-3

might deter the use of a bold approach. One criterion which is most important for the decision makers is that of *oral bioavailability*. The design of small-molecular-weight compounds takes into consideration the "rule-of-five" ("Lipinski's rule of drug-likeness"), and this has had a profound influence on the thinking of medicinal chemists. Biologically active small molecules and drugs are many optimization steps apart, and sometimes even incompatible. Their pharmacokinetic properties clearly must be considered at an early stage in the development process, but this can also can stifle innovation. "Drug-likeness" and "druggability" represent two most valuable concepts, and the majority of the successful small-molecular-weight compounds are seen to adhere to certain rules which, if applied dogmatically, may tend to eliminate many possible target structures, even from only a theoretical consideration. It should be borne in mind that these rules are not absolute, and do not extend to biological substances – for example, in recent years monoclonal antibodies have become not only clinically successful but also commercially viable. Future drug discoveries will undoubtedly include more unconventional approaches, particularly in those cases where small-molecular-weight compounds with ideally defined properties have not yet been identified.

The versatility of protein functions and the power of peptides might represent a good starting point for considering some new options. Proteins are often composed of multiple functional domains which can operate independently of each other. Indeed, their autonomous functions are often based on the formation of distinct structures and conformations which are independent from any accompanying domains. Such domains can vary from 25 to 500 amino acids, and be stabilized with the help of metal ions or disulfide bridges. They also often embody functional units and act autonomously and, for this reason, can be taken out of context and recombined with other functional domains to yield new proteins with novel properties. Such characteristics of peptides can be exploited for practical purposes, notably the design of highly specific ligands and inhibitors. Peptide ligands may function as either agonists or antagonists, and in turn can influence protein conformations, protein interactions, or their DNA-binding properties. Upon the identification of a useful target structure, peptides recognizing this structure can be assembled into carriers or scaffolds and delivered as therapeutic proteins.

The design and production of *Peptides as Drugs* appears at first sight much like many of the seemingly insurmountable problems associated with novel approaches. Yet, this volume shows not only that such problems are currently being addressed, but also that many important contributions have in fact already been elucidated. It is inevitable that, in the foreseeable future, peptides will find their way into the drug repertoire, at which point "It can't be done" will be replaced by "It has been done". And, perhaps unsurprisingly, when this new class of drugs reaches the clinic and helps to improve existing therapies, then everybody will be convinced it was "... a good idea to begin with".

May 2009   *Bernd Groner*

List of Contributors

Yvonne Becker
Georg Speyer Haus
Institute for Biomedical Research
Paul Ehrlich Straße 42
60596 Frankfurt am Main
Germany

Corina Borghouts
Georg Speyer Haus
Institute for Biomedical Research
Paul Ehrlich Straße 42
60596 Frankfurt am Main
Germany

Ursula Dietrich
Georg Speyer Haus
Institute for Biomedical Research
Paul Ehrlich Straße 42
60596 Frankfurt am Main
Germany

Susanne Dymalla
German Cancer Research
   Center
Molecular Therapy of Virus-
   Associated Cancers (F065)
Im Neuenheimer Feld 242
69120 Heidelberg
Germany

Lisa Egerer
Georg Speyer Haus
Institute for Biomedical Research
Paul Ehrlich Straße 42
60596 Frankfurt am Main
Germany

Elo Eriste
University of Tartu
Institute of Technology
Nooruse 1
50411 Tartu
Estonia

Manuel Grez
Georg Speyer Haus
Institute for Biomedical Research
Paul Ehrlich Straße 42
60596 Frankfurt am Main
Germany

Bernd Groner
Georg Speyer Haus
Institute for Biomedical Research
Paul Ehrlich Straße 42
60596 Frankfurt am Main
Germany

Peptides as Drugs Edited by Bernd Groner
© 2008 WILEY-VCH Verlag GmbH & Co. KGaA, Weinheim
ISBN: 978-3-527-32205-3

Joachim Grötzinger
Christian-Albrechts-University
Kiel
Institute of Biochemistry
Olshausenstraße 40
24098 Kiel
Germany

Mats Hansen
Stockholm University
Department of Neurochemistry
Svante Arrheniusv. 21A
10691 Stockholm
Sweden
University of Tartu
Institute of Technology
Nooruse 1
50411 Tartu
Estonia

Felix Hoppe-Seyler
German Cancer Research Center
Molecular Therapy of Virus-
  Associated Cancers (F065)
Im Neuenheimer Feld 242
69120 Heidelberg
Germany

Karin Hoppe-Seyler
German Cancer Research Center
Molecular Therapy of Virus-
  Associated Cancers (F065)
Im Neuenheimer Feld 242
69120 Heidelberg
Germany

Anne Hubert
Georg Speyer Haus
Institute for Biomedical Research
Paul Ehrlich Straße 42
60596 Frankfurt am Main
Germany

Joachim Koch
Georg Speyer Haus
Institute for Biomedical Research
Paul Ehrlich Straße 42
60596 Frankfurt am Main
Germany

Dorothee von Laer
Georg Speyer Haus
Institute for Biomedical Research
Paul Ehrlich Straße 42
60596 Frankfurt am Main
Germany

Ülo Langel
Stockholm University
Department of Neurochemistry
Svante Arrheniusv. 21A
10691 Stockholm
Sweden
University of Tartu
Institute of Technology
Nooruse 1
50411 Tartu
Estonia

Markus A. Moosmeier
German Cancer Research Center
Molecular Therapy of Virus-Associated
  Cancers (F065)
Im Neuenheimer Feld 242
69120 Heidelberg
Germany

Véronique Orian-Rousseau
Forschungszentrum Karlsruhe
Institute of Technology and Genetics
P.O. Box 3640
76021 Karlsruhe
Germany

Helmut Ponta
Forschungszentrum Karlsruhe
Institute of Technology and
    Genetics
P.O. Box 3640
76021 Karlsruhe
Germany

Stefan Rose-John
Christian-Albrechts-University
    Kiel
Institute of Biochemistry
Olshausenstraße 40
24098 Kiel
Germany

Jürgen Scheller
Christian-Albrechts-University
    Kiel
Institute of Biochemistry
Olshausenstraße 40
24098 Kiel
Germany

Mike Schutkowski
JPT Peptide Technologies GmbH
Volmerstrasse 5
12489 Berlin
Germany

Alexandra Thiele
Max-Planck Research Unit for
    Enzymology of Protein Folding
Weinbergweg 22
06120 Halle
Germany

Astrid Weiss
Georg Speyer Haus
Institute for Biomedical Research
Paul Ehrlich Straße 42
60596 Frankfurt am Main
Germany

Christian Wichmann
Georg Speyer Haus
Institute for Biomedical Research
Paul Ehrlich Straße 42
60596 Frankfurt am Main
Germany

1
Peptides as Drugs: Discovery and Development

Bernd Groner

> *"The necessity to exploit new drug targets and the suitability of peptides as drugs."*

1.1
Discovery of New Potential Drug Targets and the Limitations of Druggability

Complex networks of interacting proteins constitute the signaling pathways which mediate the intracellular propagation of biological information. Signals can originate from the cell surface and be relayed to sites in the cell where a biological response is triggered. The recognition of receptors by specific ligands is usually the initiating event which regulates cellular homeostasis, but also causes cellular responses such as proliferation, migration, angiogenesis, immune responses and cell death. The transient assembly of higher-order protein complexes, mediated by specific protein interaction domains and often regulated by secondary protein modifications, underlies the signaling mechanisms. In many instances platform proteins, for example, bring together enzymes and substrates and, in turn, recruit negative regulators which assure the transient nature of the signaling processes. The high complexity of these interactions makes them susceptible to disturbances arising from mutations in participating components, and the deregulation of specific protein–protein interactions has been recognized as the cause of diverse diseases. Conversely, the aberrant interaction of proteins is often a hallmark of diseased cells, and the inhibition of interactions required either to initiate or to maintain a particular disease state provides challenging opportunities for targeted therapies.

The importance of specific protein interactions has not only been recognized for diseases which originate from mutations in endogenous genes, but also extends to exogenous causes of disease and pathogenic microorganisms. Today, many disease-causing organisms and diseases are starting to be understood in molecular detail [1], with almost 600 microbial genomes having already been sequenced and 1800 others currently under investigation. This has led to the

Peptides as Drugs. Discovery and Development. Edited by Bernd Groner
Copyright © 2009 WILEY-VCH Verlag GmbH & Co. KGaA, Weinheim
ISBN: 978-3-527-32205-3

identification of virulence genes, metabolic pathways and cell-surface proteins as new targets for antimicrobial drug development and candidate vaccines. New directions are primarily set by technologies aimed at the elucidation of global gene expression patterns, and these high-throughput molecular profiling techniques have accelerated the discovery of drug targets. Genomics, transcriptomics and proteomics not only play a decisive role in the investigation of infectious diseases, but also are becoming increasingly important in the understanding of multigenic human diseases such as diabetes, heart diseases and cancer [2]. However, the task to integrate such global and descriptive analyses into manageable models has only just begun, and the large and unwieldy datasets available not only still preclude the rational prediction of gene functions in an organismal context, but also hamper predictions about the benefits and side effects of targeted drugs.

The present limitations concerning the evaluation and interpretation of datasets collected from global gene expression patterns are not deterring progress, however. Today, large-scale efforts are under way to gain insights into whole genome alterations that distinguish cancer cells from their normal counterparts [3, 4]. Cancer cells exhibit multiple genetic alterations in their DNA sequences, in the number of individual genes, and in their epigenetic DNA and histone modifications. These alterations cause both the activation and inhibition of biological events, interpretable in the context of the pathophysiology of cancer cells [5]. The comparison of the human genome which is present in normal, healthy cells with that present in breast, colon, pancreatic cancer cells and glioblastomas, has shown that hundreds of genes can be present in mutated forms. Although about 60 genes have been found to be altered in individual tumors, the mutations varied when individual tumors were compared. Initially, it seems difficult to distinguish molecular alterations which are causal and drive tumor-related phenotypes, such as cell proliferation, cell death, metabolism, metastasis, angiogenesis or immune evasion, and those which are correlative and do not contribute to tumor formation. Nevertheless, consistent patterns could be identified. The most important mutations affect a limited number of cellular signaling pathways. The suggestion is that, interference with these pathways – but not necessarily the targeting of mutated gene products – might represent the most promising approach to therapy [3].

Elucidation of the functions of many of mutated gene products supports the overriding importance of deregulated pathways. Both, oncogenes and tumor suppressor genes control crucial points in the cell cycle, transitions from a resting stage (G_0 or G_1) to a replicating phase (S), inhibit cell growth, and stimulate cell death when induced by cellular stress [6]. The cells continuously respond to 'prods' emanating from external and internal signals. The oncogene and tumor suppressor gene products are usually components of signaling cascades and are integrated in networks of protein interactions. These protein interactions are most frequently regulated through post-translational modifications [7]. Proteins such as histones, p53, RNA polymerase II, tubulin, Cdc25C and tyrosine kinases can be modified at multiple sites through phosphorylation, acetylation, methylation, ubiquitination, sumoylation, and citrullination. These modifications can act in a combinatorial fashion and constitute regulatory programs. Covalent modifications can modulate protein interaction domains and coordinate intermolecular and intra-molecular signaling.

The multitude of molecules functionally involved in cancer formation and pro-gression provides a rich source of potential points of interference, although the exploitation of these possibilities is still in its initial stages. The heterogeneity of tumor cells, mirrored in the large variety of mutations found, makes it difficult to define the most promising drug targets. Such targets should comprise molecules which are functionally crucial for cancer cells, and at least temporarily dispensable for normal cells. As the mutations found in tumor cells are not random, and the functional consequences are usually manifested in deregulated signaling path-ways, the targeted inhibition of components encoded by oncogenes or components activated by oncogene products, has attracted much attention. Tumor cells do encode proteins, on which they are totally dependent – that is, the downregulation or functional inhibition of such components causes tumor cell death. The inactiva-tion of such a component in normal cells is often tolerated and has led to the concept of "tumor cell oncogene addiction" [8]. Such proteins appear as appealing drug targets, and the development of inhibitors of oncogenic kinases – such as members of the EGF receptor family, BCR-ABL, PDGF receptor or c-KIT – has led to most impressive clinical advances. Other kinase inhibitors have been approved or are currently under development [9, 10]. Since components of oncogenic path-ways, however, are not always necessarily kinases, pharmacological problems must also be addressed.

The theoretical considerations of pharmacologists were applied to information gained from sequencing of the human genome, and resulted in an estimate of a relatively small number of molecular drug targets [11]. The term "druggable genome" was coined with the intent to delimit the subset of molecular targets for which orally available, commercial drugs could be developed. The majority of cur-rently used drugs are directed towards classical druggable targets such as enzymes, G-protein coupled receptors (GPCRs), carriers and nuclear hormone receptors (NHRs) and ion channels [12]. The term "druggable" refers to targets which exhibit protein folds capable of interacting with drug-like chemical compounds. These compounds recognize the substrate-binding pockets of proteins, and it is for this reason that enzymes have mainly been used as therapeutic drug targets. Typically, they provided the prerequisites to develop rapid, sensitive screening assays and the detection of low-molecular-weight inhibitors that blocked the active site. Many of the inhibitors are derivatives of substrates – analogues which serve as starting points for the development of specific drugs. Such compounds are then further modified to exhibit a defined set of properties which lend them satisfactory phar-macokinetics [13]. However, in the case of proteins which interact with other proteins – rather than with small substrate molecules – a lack of binding pockets means that this approach is not generally applicable. Proteins which do not exhibit structural features that allow the derivation of such small-molecular-weight binders are considered by pharmacologists as unlikely to be modulated in their function through pharmaceutical intervention [14, 15].

Since many of the molecules that play crucial roles in disease processes as diverse as infectious diseases, diabetes, heart diseases and cancer cannot easily be modulated by small-molecular-weight inhibitors which recognize particular binding pockets, it is becoming mandatory to design and exploit molecules that do not necessarily fit the description of classical drug classes. Biological molecules and structures – such as peptides, recombinant proteins, antibodies, therapeutic genes or even whole cells – have the potential to fill part of this gap and thus blur the current distinction between "druggable" and "nondruggable" target molecules.

1.2
Protein Interaction Domains Are at the Core of Signaling Pathways

Modular interactions among proteins are at the heart of protein functions and cellular organization. Biological signaling requires that protein complexes are formed and activated at the right time and in the right place, and that their formation is both reversible and transient. The strength and duration of a signal may be critical for the effects of hormones, cytokines and growth factors, and a large number of specific protein interaction domains are known which mediate this machinery [16]. Since many proteins thus exert their biological activity through interactions with other proteins, an interference with such interactions would represent an attractive option. Moreover, those molecules capable of preventing these interactions could become a new class of drugs.

The structural diversity of the possible protein interfaces involved pose chances and challenges [17]. The *chances* are presented by the diversity of the interactions and the possibility for subtle perturbations. However, there exist also a number of potential problems, stemming from the dimensions of the targeted structures and from the relative inexperience in dealing with them. The main features of these difficulties have recently been identified [18], and range from structural to cell biological aspects. Protein interfaces and their interactions are not easily inhibited by low-molecular-weight compounds, and the search for specific inhibitors might therefore require new strategies. Intracellular protein concentrations are very high, estimated at $100\,\text{mg\,ml}^{-1}$, while protein complexes may comprise identical subunits or different subunits. Oligomers can be formed in conjunction with protein synthesis, and result in so-called "obligate complexes"; alternatively, later on in the life of the protein they may form nonobligate complexes. Protein complexes exhibit different stabilities, and can be regulated through secondary modifications of the participating components [7]. In addition, complex formation and stability can be modulated by effector molecules or changes in their relative ratios and localization.

Protein complexes are held together by their contact interfaces. The size of the subunit interfaces is large, and ranges from approximately 300 to $4800\,\text{Å}^2$ [19]. The structure of participating proteins can undergo conformational changes when they form large interfaces [20]. Recognition patches are essential for binding, and usually one per interface has been found. Therefore, the design of inhibitors of protein–protein interactions, especially with small organic molecules, is a difficult and challenging – but not impossible – task. The principal of selective interference of protein–protein interactions with small synthetic molecules is actively being explored [21, 22]. Recently, transcription factors have received attention as suitable target structures, because they can be considered as end points of signal transduction pathways, and many of them also require dimerization in order to assume DNA binding activities. The dimerization domains and the DNA-binding domains of transcription factors, such as the hypoxia-inducible factor (HIF)-1, c-Myc and signal transducer and activator of transcription (STAT) 3, are currently being investigated, while drug-like small molecules are being sought which might potently and selectively inhibit these functional domains.

1.3
Peptides as Inhibitors of Protein Interactions

Proteins and peptides offer alternatives as interfering agents when the inhibition of protein–protein interactions is being considered. If protein interfaces mediate the contact between two proteins, then a compound mimicking the properties of one of the interfaces should act as a competitive inhibitor and prevent interaction of the binding partners. Peptides derived from such protein–protein interaction sites could possibly serve as antagonists. Proteins usually interact through interfaces which comprise proline, isoleucine, tyrosine, tryptophan, asparagine and arginine residues, and using this information peptides have been identified which act as agonists or antagonists of, for example, cell-surface receptors [23].

The use of peptides as specific inhibitors of protein–protein interactions might circumvent a number of problems which have been associated with small-molecular-weight compounds considered for the same purpose. Although, the large surface areas involved in protein–protein interactions may be dissected into much smaller contact points, and only a small number of amino acids might actually be critical for the specificity of the interactions, the general rules are still difficult to derive [24]. A straightforward approach for the discovery of peptides which might serve as potential antagonists is an exploitation of the complementary surfaces of naturally occurring binding partners. These peptides could function as competitive inhibitors, masking an interaction site and making it inaccessible for the binding of the protein from which it has been derived. These peptides themselves could serve as potential drugs, if problems such as affinity, stability, delivery and specificity can be managed. Alternatively, information about the structure of the crucial amino acids that constitute the contact site could be used as a basis to design mimetics; indeed, this strategy has been used to develop peptide ligand mimetics for integrin receptors [25].

The vast complexity of random peptide libraries provides another possibility to identify specific peptide ligands. Peptides can be selected to fit any macromolecular surface and thus may act for example as ligands for functional domains of proteins. If the functional domain is appropriately chosen, the peptide aptamers may bind to protein targets and be able to interfere with the target function. Although the mechanism of action can be based on the masking of a binding domain for an interaction partner, it can also result from conformational changes induced as a consequence of the ligand–target interaction. Peptide aptamers are comprised of a variable peptide region of 8 to 20 amino acids in length, displayed in a scaffold protein, and have been selected for multiple targets. The isolation and use of peptide aptamers as inhibitors of individual signaling components represents an excellent starting point for highly selective and unconventional drugs, and also a new challenge for drug development [26–28].

The use of proteins and peptides as competitive inhibitors for any functional domain of a given target protein is most attractive, and would increase the subtlety of targeted interference considerably. Despite the conceptual appeal to develop protein antagonists as therapeutic agents, there are many technical and biological hurdles which must first be overcome. The affinity between a peptide ligand and a target domain can depend on multiple parameters, and may need to be optimized by mutational analysis and array procedures. The form in which a protein–protein interaction is integrated into a particular high-molecular-weight complex *in vivo* is difficult to predict. The complexity of a multiprotein assembly, such as a ribosome or a transcription complex, entails a large number of interactions, and the consequences of a single interruption could be compensated by other interactions. Kinetic parameters, the intracellular localization and accessibility of the target structure, and the immunogenicity and stability of the construct into which the peptide is integrated, are all determinants of the potential therapeutic usefulness.

The discovery and development of peptide-based drugs have both rational and empirical aspects. Random screening procedures can be used to identify ligands for known functional domains of target proteins in high-complexity libraries. These screens can be complemented by structural, computational or biochemical information to identify ligands for targets for which natural interaction partners are known. Biotechnology will then allow the supply of such ligands with the additional functional domains that are required if they are to be used as drugs. Integration into scaffold proteins, the provision of a protein transduction domain, as well as favorable properties for recombinant expression and protein purification, are all required if the peptide itself is to be used as an effector. Ironically, many of these issues are reminiscent of the "rocky road" which monoclonal antibodies had to take before they became a commercial success.

However, the development of peptides into tools for diagnostic purposes and drugs, based on their fantastic specificity of target recognition and their versatility of mechanisms by which they can exert interference with protein functions, offers enormous promise. While peptides as drugs is a concept that still involves considerable challenge, encouragement may be gleaned from the wise words of the visionary Arthur C. Clarke (1917–2008), who admitted that "...we do not have all the answers, but we have plenty of questions certainly worth thinking about; and when the technology is finally sufficiently advanced it is indistinguishable from magic".

References

1 Kaushik, D.K. and Sehgal, D. (2008) Developing antibacterial vaccines in genomics and proteomics era. *Scand. J. Immunol.*, **67** (6), 544–52.

2 Chen, Y., Zhu, J. *et al.* (2008) Variations in DNA elucidate molecular networks that cause disease. *Nature*, **452** (7186), 429–35.

3 Jones, S., Zhang, X., Parsons, D.W. *et al.* (2008) Core signaling pathways in human pancreatic cancers revealed by global genomic analyses. *Science*, **321** (5897), 1801–6.

4 Parsons, D.W., Jones, S., Zhang, X. *et al.* (2008) An integrated genomic analysis of human glioblastoma multiforme. *Science*, **321** (5897), 1807–12.

5 Greenman, C., Stephens, P. *et al.* (2007) Patterns of somatic mutation in human cancer genomes. *Nature*, **446** (7132), 153–8.

6 Vogelstein, B. and Kinzler, K.W. (2004) Cancer genes and the pathways they control. *Nat. Med.*, **10** (8), 789–99.

7 Seet, B.T., Dikic, I. *et al.* (2006) Reading protein modifications with interaction domains. *Nat. Rev. Mol. Cell. Biol.*, **7** (7), 473–83.

8 Sharma, S.V. and Settleman, J. (2007) Oncogene addiction: setting the stage for molecularly targeted cancer therapy. *Genes Dev.*, **21** (24), 3214–31.

9 Collins, I. and Workman, P. (2006) New approaches to molecular cancer therapeutics. *Nat. Chem. Biol.*, **2** (12), 689–700.

10 Sharma, S.V., Bell, D.W. *et al.* (2007) Epidermal growth factor receptor mutations in lung cancer. *Nat. Rev. Cancer*, **7** (3), 169–81.

11 Hopkins, A.L. and Groom, C.R. (2002) The druggable genome. *Nat. Rev. Drug Discov.*, **1** (9), 727–30.

12 Betz, U.A., Farquhar, R. *et al.* (2005) Genomics: success or failure to deliver drug targets? *Curr. Opin. Chem. Biol.*, **9** (4), 387–91.

13 Keller, T.H., Pichota, A. *et al.* (2006) A practical view of 'druggability'. *Curr. Opin. Chem. Biol.*, **10** (4), 357–61.

14 Imming, P., Sinning, C. *et al.* (2006) Drugs, their targets and the nature and number of drug targets. *Nat. Rev. Drug Discov.*, **5** (10), 821–34.

15 Russ, A.P. and Lampel, S. (2005) The druggable genome: an update. *Drug. Discov. Today*, **10** (23-24), 1607–10.

16 Pawson, T. (2004) Specificity in signal transduction: from phosphotyrosine-SH2 domain interactions to complex cellular systems. *Cell*, **116** (2), 191–203.

17 Li, S., Armstrong, C.M. *et al.* (2004) A map of the interactome network of the metazoan *C. elegans*. *Science*, **303** (5657), 540–3.

18 Chene, P. (2006) Drugs targeting protein–protein interactions. *ChemMedChem*, **1** (4), 400–11.

19 Pal, A., Chakrabarti, P. *et al.* (2007) Peptide segments in protein–protein interfaces. *J. Biosci.*, **32** (1), 101–11.

20 Wodak, S.J. and Janin, J. (2002) Structural basis of macromolecular recognition. *Adv. Protein Chem.*, **61**, 9–73.

21 Berg, T. (2008) Inhibition of transcription factors with small organic molecules. *Curr. Opin. Chem. Biol.*, **12** (4), 464–71.

22 White, A.W., Westwell, A.D. *et al.* (2008) Protein-protein interactions as targets for small-molecule therapeutics in cancer. *Expert. Rev. Mol. Med.*, **10**, e8.

23 Jones, D.S., Silverman, A.P. *et al.* (2008) Developing therapeutic proteins by engineering ligand–receptor interactions. *Trends Biotechnol.*, **26** (9), 498–505.

24 Lo Conte, L., Chothia, C. *et al.* (1999) The atomic structure of protein–protein recognition sites. *J. Mol. Biol.*, **285** (5), 2177–98.

25 Sillerud, L.O. and Larson, R.S. (2005) Design and structure of peptide and peptidomimetic antagonists of protein-protein interaction. *Curr. Protein Pept. Sci.*, **6** (2), 151–69.

26 Baines, I.C. and Colas, P. (2006) Peptide aptamers as guides for small-molecule drug discovery. *Drug Discov. Today*, **11** (7-8), 334–41.

27 Borghouts, C., Kunz, C. *et al.*
(2005) Current strategies for the
development of peptide-based
anti-cancer therapeutics. *J. Pept. Sci.*,
11 (11), 713–26.

28 Borghouts, C., Kunz, C. *et al.* (2008)
Peptide aptamer libraries. *Comb.
Chem. High Throughput Screen.*, **11** (2),
135–45.

2
Mimics of Growth Factors and Cytokines

Jürgen Scheller, Joachim Grötzinger, and Stefan Rose-John

2.1
Introduction

Growth hormones and cytokines are important mediators of many cellular functions, including the regulation of regenerative processes and coordination of the immune system. Consequently, as these molecules have therapeutic value, strategies are being developed to modulate their functions. In general, proteins can be altered by either an ordered approach based on structural information, or by a random approach based on high-throughput techniques involving error-prone polymerase chain reactions and phage display. These methods can be used to design proteins with enhanced or neutralizing biological activities. All of these proteins are ligands, and mediate their biological effects through binding to specific epitopes of cognate receptors. These epitopes are often the starting point for the design process. Cytokines have been designed with the aim of increasing the affinity to their receptors; alternatively, cytokine variants have been created which still bind to their specific receptors but do not trigger cellular signaling. Such designer cytokines can be used to block specific cytokine actions and are called *cytokine receptor antagonists*. With the help of phage display techniques, peptides have been generated which exhibit cytokine activity. Interestingly, such mimetic peptides do not show sequence similarities with their naturally occurring functional homologues, and might be used as lead structures to design and develop nonpeptidic molecules with specific cytokine activities.

2.2
The Cytokines

In 1990, Fernando Bazan produced two seminal reports in which he suggested that the known cytokines share a common protein fold [1, 2]. Based on theoretical considerations, Bazan categorized these proteins into the superfamily of "four helical" cytokines. In this fold, the four helices are arranged in an up-up-down-

down topology, which demands that the three loops connecting the helices are long-short-long. This superfamily is further subdivided into the long-chain, the short-chain cytokines and the interferon/interleukin-10 families. The latter family contains an additional helix in one of the crossover connections. Signal transduction of all these cytokines is initiated by the assembly of multi-subunit receptor complexes on the cell surface. Subfamilies of cytokines have been defined based on the fact that certain signal transducing subunits are shared by their cognate receptors. One such receptor subunits is gp130, which is shared by the interleukin-6 (IL-6) -type cytokines [IL-6, IL-11, CNTF (ciliary neurotrophic factor), CT-1 (cardiotrophin-1), CLC (cardiotrophin-1 like cytokine), LIF (leukemia inhibitory factor), OSM (oncostatin M)], IL-27 and IL-31 as part of the signal transducing complex. Similarly, the β-subunit of the IL-3 receptor is shared by IL-3, IL-5, granulocyte macrophage colony-stimulating factor (GM-CSF) receptors. The IL-2γ receptor is a common subunit for the IL-2, IL-4, IL-7, and IL-15 receptors [3]. The three-dimensional (3-D) structures of these cytokines have been solved by crystallography or NMR and have confirmed Bazan's landmark prediction.

Another option by which these cytokines may be grouped into subfamilies is the number of different receptors that are engaged in the functional signal transducing receptor complex; this is tantamount to the number of interaction epitopes present on the corresponding cytokine. As an example, growth hormone (GH), erythropoietin (EPO) or IL-4 have two ligand–receptor interaction sites, whereas cytokines such as CNTF, IL-11, IL-15 and IL-6 have three sites [4–6], designated I, II and III (Figure 2.1). The presence of a different number of epitopes, and their relative orientation to each other, raises questions as to what extent these epitopes might be exchanged between different cytokines, thereby changing their receptor repertoire and specificity.

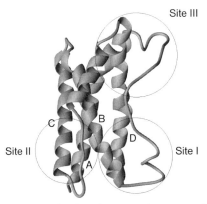

Figure 2.1 The three-dimensional structure of interleukin-6 (IL-6). The four long helices are marked A–D, while the receptor interaction sites with the IL-6R and the two gp130 proteins are labeled I, II and III, respectively.

2.2.1
The Receptors

Cytokine receptors are type I membrane proteins; they span the cellular membrane, such that their amino terminus resides at the extracellular and their carboxy terminus at the intracellular side. The extracellular part interacts with the ligand, the binding of which initiates an intracellular signaling cascade. The extracellular parts of these receptors show a modular architecture, consisting of a different number of domains of approximately 100 residues, each with a fibronectin type III-like fold. Two of these consecutive domains are called the cytokine binding domain (CBD), and are characterized by four conserved cysteines in the first domain and a Trp-Ser-X-Trp-Ser motif in the second domain (Figure 2.2).

The cytokine receptors can be divided into two classes with respect to their complexity. For the remainder of this chapter, receptors such as GHR (growth hormone receptor), EpoR (erythropoietin receptor) and IL-4R–which contain only domains in the extracellular region that are involved in ligand binding–will be referred to as "simple" receptors. Receptors such as gp130 and G-CSFR–which contain additional domains apparently not involved in ligand binding–will be designated "complex" receptors.

Some of these receptors exist also as nonmembrane-bound, soluble molecules; these either entirely lack a transmembrane region or they are generated as soluble proteins due to translation from alternative spliced mRNAs or by proteolytic shedding processes. As an example: the IL-6 receptor exists as a membrane-bound receptor as well as a soluble protein [7]. The soluble form is either generated by

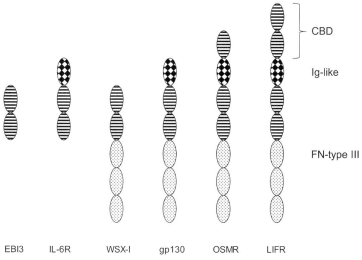

EBI3   IL-6R   WSX-I   gp130   OSMR   LIFR

Figure 2.2 Receptors of the IL-6-type cytokines. The modular composition of the receptors of the IL-6-type family of cytokines. Representative receptors of each modular architecture are given.

alternative splicing or by a proteolytic cleavage of the membrane-bound form by proteases belonging to the ADAM family [8]. These soluble receptors are still able to bind their ligands and to induce signal transduction on cells lacking the IL-6 receptor by binding to the signal transducer gp130. This process has been referred to as "trans-signaling" [7].

2.2.2
"Simple" Receptors

The class of "simple" receptors can be further subdivided into two groups, which either homodimerize or heterodimerize upon ligand binding. Examples of ligands for these receptors are GH or IL-4, respectively, and they differ in the mode of interaction with their receptors [9, 10]. One GH molecule binds two receptor molecules via two contact epitopes designated sites I and II (Figure 2.3).

Remarkably, the two receptors use identical amino-acid residues to bind the two different epitopes of the cytokine [4, 9, 10]. However, the two interaction sites differ in their free energy of binding. One paradigmatic conclusion derived from these studies was that cytokines generally are recognized by their cognate receptors at sites equivalent to sites I and II of GH [4, 9]. A detailed analysis of the interaction epitopes suggested a common design. Yet, by using an alanine scan, in which all residues in the interaction area have been mutated to alanine, the contribution of each amino-acid residue to the binding energy has been determined [4, 9]. Hydrophobic residues, the aliphatic parts of polar side chains and parts of the backbone are involved in the most important interactions. This hydrophobic core is sur-

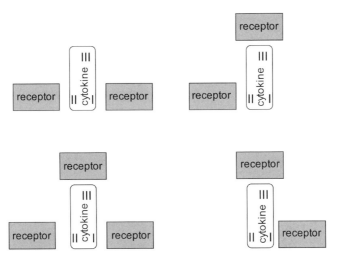

Figure 2.3 The four combinations of three (I, II and III) distinct receptor interaction sites on cytokines. Interaction via site I/site II (top left). Interaction via site II/site III (top right). Interaction via site I/site II/site III (bottom left). Interaction via site I/site III (bottom right). The cytokine is shown in white, the receptors in gray.

rounded by a region consisting of polar and charged amino-acid residues which only slightly contribute to the binding energy, but are involved in the specific recognition of the two molecules [9]. In contrast to this architecture, the IL-4/IL-4R interaction epitopes have been described as "avocado clusters", where a nucleus is also enveloped by an oily shell [5]. Instead of having a hydrophobic core, the central interaction is mediated by charged side chains or amino-acid residues capable of forming hydrogen bonds. This central area is surrounded by a shell of hydrophobic amino acids [5]. The specific mode of interaction GH and IL-4 with their receptors has similar consequences, as they are thought to cause dimerization of the receptor chains by bringing the intracellular parts in close proximity, thereby initiating the signaling cascade. Therefore, it appeared that dimerization was needed and was sufficient for the onset of signal transduction.

There are some refinements to this model. For example, it has been shown that dimerization is needed but not sufficient for the biological function of some homodimeric receptors, and that they exist as preformed dimers on the cell surface. In the case of the EpoR, there is crystallographic evidence for preformed dimers of this receptor. Distinct dimeric configurations exist for this receptor in the absence of ligand, whether complexed with Epo or with agonistic or antagonistic peptides [11, 12]. The presence of a ligand and its agonist or antagonist activity resulted in different distances and orientations of the receptor domain close to the membrane, and thus different signaling properties [11].

The observation of preformed dimers in the absence of ligand was complemented by data which suggested that dimerization occurs via epitopes that are also involved in ligand binding [11]. Therefore, ligand binding to these receptors might be regarded as a competition event in which the ligand binding replaces the inherent receptor dimerization and thereby changes their relative orientation. This concept would suggest that mutations in the ligand-binding epitope of the receptor would not only affect ligand binding, but also inhibit the formation of preformed dimers, which might be a prerequisite for efficient signal initiation.

2.2.3
"Complex" Receptors

The "complex" receptors consist of more components than are needed for ligand binding, and can therefore be subdivided into two parts–one responsible for ligand binding and the other involved in transmitting the signal into the cell. One paradigmatic conclusion derived from the studies of the GH/GHR complex was that, in general, the cytokines are recognized by their cognate receptors at sites equivalent to site I and site II of GH.

This paradigm does not hold true for IL-6-type cytokines and their "complex" receptors gp130, LIF-R (leukemia inhibitory factor receptor), and OSM-R (oncostatin--M receptor). The existence of three distinct receptor binding epitopes has been clearly demonstrated for IL-6, IL-11 and CNTF. In analogy to GHR, that occupies site I (end of AB-loop, C-terminal D-helix) and site II (A/C-helix) of the GH, the cognate alpha-receptor is located at site I and the common signal transducer gp130 at site II of these cytokines. A third β-receptor binding epitope (site III) is not present on GH, and is occupied by a second gp130 molecule (IL-6, IL-11) or serves as a specific LIF-R binding site on CNTF [13–15]. Site III consists of the COOH-terminal A-helix, the NH_2-terminal AB-loop, the BC-loop with adjacent amino-acid residues, the COOH-terminal CD-loop and the NH_2-terminal D-helix [13, 14]. Based on mutagenesis studies in combination with molecular modeling studies, it has been shown that sites I and II of the IL-6-type cytokines interact exclusively with the corresponding CBD of the involved receptors, whereas site III utilizes the Ig-like domain of the "complex" receptors. These results have been recently confirmed by determination of the structure of the hexameric complex of two IL-6, two IL-6R and two gp130 molecules [16]. Thus, the "complex" receptors have two distinct binding regions. While these data are mostly derived from biochemical studies, they have been confirmed by the X-ray structure of the viral IL-6 molecule in complex with two gp130 molecules [17]. In this complex, the CBD of one gp130 molecule is bound to the ligand via its CBD to site II, while the second gp130 molecule uses its Ig-like domain to bind to site III of the viral IL-6 [17–19].

Since one gp130 molecule has two distinct binding sites, two gp130 molecules are able to bind two ligands in a symmetrical arrangement, as seen in the X-ray structure [17]. Yet, most interestingly, only one of these two symmetrical binding sites per gp130 molecule is needed to induce signal transduction. This has been shown by Pflanz *et al.*, who used two mutants of gp130 that either lacked the Ig-like domain or contained a distinct mutation within the CBD. Both mutants alone were unable to induce IL-6 signal transduction [20], but after cotransfection of both inactive cDNAs coding for the mutant gp130 receptors, the IL-6 bioactivity was restored. Since the combination of the two gp130-mutant proteins is able to bind only one IL-6/IL-6R complex, it can be concluded that the formation of a tetrameric complex, consisting of one IL-6, one IL-6R and two gp130 molecules, is sufficient for biological activity. The same authors also showed that the two epitopes cooperate sequentially upon IL-6-induced receptor activation, and combining the two mutations restores the high affinity of ligand binding [20].

The question remains – How can two intact binding epitopes cooperate within two different molecules? One attractive explanation might be the formation of preformed dimers, in analogy to the situation of the EpoR. In this receptor, the same epitopes are responsible for dimerization and for ligand binding. In the case of gp130, the Ig-like domain of one gp130 could interact with the CBD of the second, and *vice versa*. Therefore, mutations in the CBD or removal of the Ig-like domain would affect both interaction sites and thereby prevent dimerization, whereas a combination of the two mutated gp130 molecules would still allow the formation of dimers by a combination of the two intact epitopes present in each molecule. In the case of the heterodimeric receptor complex gp130/OSM-R, it has been shown that this complex exists as a preformed dimer on the cell surface by coimmunoprecipitation experiments [21]. As these cells were not transfected with the corresponding cDNAs, and do not overexpress the receptor molecules, the observed dimers are most likely not experimental artifacts. Furthermore, mutations within the CBM of gp130 abrogate signaling by IL-6, but not by LIF or OSM [22, 23]. In the case of IL-6, these mutations might be able to interfere with the formation of a symmetric preformed dimeric gp130, but not within the preformed asymmetric gp130/LIF-R or gp130/OSM-R.

In contrast to the "simple" receptors, the "complex" receptors have more then one epitope for interaction with the ligand. Moreover, to make the situation even more "complex", they also have domains that are not involved in ligand binding. The signal transducing subunits of the IL-6-type family of cytokines – namely gp130, LIF-R and OSM-R – contain three membrane-proximal fibronectin type III domains (see Figure 2.2), an architecture that is also seen in the G-CSFR. Mutational studies on soluble and membrane-bound gp130 have shed light on the functional role of these domains, with deletion and substitution mutants having been derived to study their contribution to signal transduction [24, 25].

The deletion of any of these domains in the soluble protein had no impact on the binding characteristics [25]. When membrane-bound mutant receptors were studied, the results were contradictory. Not all of the mutant proteins were able to initiate signal transduction but, surprisingly, some of them were no longer able to bind the ligand. Deletions of the fourth and sixth domains led to a complete loss of binding, whereas deletion of the fifth domain resulted in the retention of some residual binding [25]. Therefore, these domains seem to be necessary to position the upper domains in a specific way that enables these domains to bind the ligand.

Taken together, the results described above show that the three membrane-proximal domains play a pivotal role in the transmission of signals, and that dimerization is needed – but is not sufficient – for receptor activation and the initiation of signaling [26]. The paradigm of the GH/(GHR)2 complex is not valid for all cytokines, and in particular not for IL-6-type cytokines, as it represents only one out of four possible combinations of three sites: site I/site II, site II/site III, site I/site II/site III and site I/site III (Figure 2.3). Whereas, three of these four combinations have been found to date, there is as yet no example of a cytokine using the combination of site I/site III.

2.3
Defining Receptor Recognition Sites in Cytokines Using Chimeric Proteins

The first structure–function analysis of the cytokine IL-6 made use of truncation studies at both the NH_2-terminus [27] and the COOH-terminus [28, 29], and allowed the definition of residues important for the biological activities of the cytokine. A total of 28 amino acids could be removed from the NH_2-terminus without loss of activity, whereas the removal of only three amino acids from the COOH-terminus resulted in an inactive cytokine variant [28, 29].

While murine IL-6 does not act on human cells, human IL-6 is active on both, human and murine cells [30]. It was speculated that this species specificity could be exploited to define domains within the IL-6 protein responsible for receptor–ligand interactions, and for this purpose regions in the human IL-6 protein were substituted with the corresponding murine sequences. An investigation was then undertaken to determine which of the introduced sequences would provide the

(a)

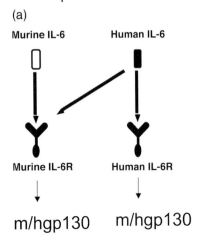

(b)

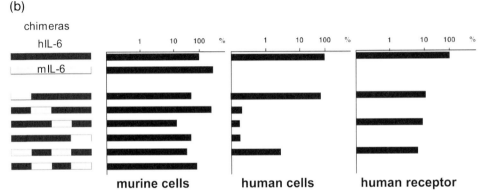

Figure 2.4 Species specificity of human and murine IL-6 and activity of chimeric human/ mouse IL-6 proteins. (a) Human IL-6 is active on murine and human cells, whereas mouse IL-6 only acts on murine but not on human cells; (b) Chimeric human/mouse IL-6 proteins were constructed and their activity was tested on murine cells (B9) and human cells (HepG2). Additionally, binding of the proteins to the human IL-6R was measured. It can be seen that all chimeric proteins are active on murine cells, whereas selective activity is found on human cells, leading to the identification of receptor-interacting epitopes.

chimeric molecule with the murine cytokine properties – that is, being inactive on human cells. The construction of the chimeras was based on the secondary structure boundaries as predicted by the 4-helical cytokine model of Bazan [1]. The advantage of this approach was that it was expected that all human/mouse IL-6 chimeric proteins – when properly folded – should show biological activity on murine cells [31]. The details of this study are summarized in Figure 2.4.

The results confirmed the importance of amino-acid residues at the NH_2-and COOH-termini of the IL-6 protein, and also indicated an unexpected involvement of sequences within the loop between helix A and helix B in the species specificity of IL-6 and in the receptor interactions [31]. In a subsequent study, when the loop was subdivided between helix A and B, it was found that the amino acids at the beginning of the AB loop were important for signaling, but the residues at the end of the AB loop were involved in binding the IL-6R [13, 32]. These data were complemented by information from the laboratory of Lucien Aarden, who analyzed the binding epitopes of neutralizing monoclonal antibodies against human IL-6 [33]. These studies resulted in the identification of monoclonal antibodies, which prevented IL-6 binding to the receptor, and of those which prevented signaling but not binding. The results of these experiments led to the notion that different regions of the IL-6 protein interacted with different receptor subunits, namely with the IL-6R and with gp130 [34]. This provided the basis for the construction of the first IL-6 receptor antagonists, which could bind to the IL-6R but were unable to stimulate gp130-mediated signaling [35, 36]. At the same time, the group of Ciliberto, using homology modeling of the IL-6/IL-6R complex and the information gained from the X-ray structure of the GH/GHR complex, identified a second interaction site of IL-6 with gp130. This site was analogous to site II of the GH/GHR complex [37]; subsequently, when Ciliberto and coworkers derived site II mutants to construct IL-6R antagonists, these molecules bound to the IL-6R but failed to stimulate gp130 signaling [15].

2.4
Receptor Recognition Sites are Organized as Exchangeable Modules

The analysis of chimeric proteins led to the identification of a site of receptor interaction within the IL-6 protein which was completely novel. Unlike the definition of site II, which was deduced from the analogy with the GH/GHR complex, a prediction of site III was not possible, because an informative 3-D structure of a cytokine/cytokine receptor complex was not available. Only years later was the existence of site III directly confirmed by solution of the structure of the complex of vIL-6 with the extracellular portion of gp130, using X-ray crystallography [17].

A similar approach was used to investigate a different question. IL-6 is known to interact with two molecules of gp130 at sites II and III, whereas CNTF interacts with gp130 at site II and the related receptor protein LIF-R at site III. The aim was to determine whether the information required for the formation of this heterodimeric complex of CNTF with gp130 and LIF-R was encoded within the CNTF protein. Taking into consideration the conserved four-helical bundle structure of most cytokines, it was reasoned that the receptor recognition sites of cytokines might have evolved as autonomous modules, which should possibly be exchangeable between different cytokines. A comparison of the homology-based IL-6 model and the X-ray structure of CNTF [6, 38] prompted definition of the boundaries of the potential LIF-R binding epitope of CNTF. This was shown to comprise residues of the C-terminal A-helix, the N-terminal AB-loop, the BC-loop, the C-terminal CD-loop, and the N-terminal D-helix (Figure 2.5). The transfer of this putative LIF-R binding module from CNTF to IL-6 resulted in a chimeric IL-6/CNTF protein that bound to IL-6R and signaled via a heterodimer of gp130 and LIF-R. Effectively, this module swap created a new cytokine with LIF-like – but IL-6R-

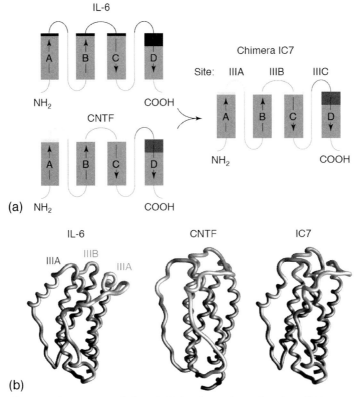

Figure 2.5 Construction of chimeric IL-6 and ciliary neurotrophic factor (CNTF) proteins. (a) Epitope shuffle of receptor-binding sites of IL-6-and CNTF. The typical four-helix bundle fold of IL-6, the CNTF and chimera IC7, with the characteristic up-up-down-down orientation of the α-helices is shown. Consequently, two long loops (AB and CD) and one short loop (BC) connect the helices. The exchanged epitopes are marked in black (IL-6) or shaded (CNTF); (b) Ribbon models of IL-6, CNTF and the chimera IC7. The structures of IL-6 and CNTF were generated from coordinates downloaded from the Protein Databank (PDB; accession numbers 1IL-6 and 1CNT).

dependent–activity on cells expressing gp130, IL-6R and LIF-R. On a more general basis, these results indicated that cytokines are organized as a set of modules, making specific contacts to different receptors [14, 39].

One surprising finding in this study was the observation that the chimeric molecule IC5–which carried the C-terminal A-helix, the N-terminal AB loop, the C-terminal CD-loop, and the N-terminal D-helix from CNTF grafted onto the IL-6 protein–differed in its activity on cells expressing gp130, IL-6R and LIF-R by a factor of 100 from the chimera IC7 which, in addition, contained the BC-loop of CNTF. The chimeric IC7 protein, when applied to cells expressing gp130, IL-6R and LIF-R, was as active as human LIF [14]. An overview of this study is depicted in Figure 2.2. In the structure of vIL-6 bound to gp130, the BC-loop is not involved in establishing contact between the cytokine and gp130 at site III [17], and therefore does not yield an explanation for the involvement of site III in the geometry of this receptor interaction site.

Recent investigations have focused on an elucidation of the mechanism by which vIL-6 binds to gp130, without need of the IL-6R [40]. When the chimeric proteins of human IL-6 and vIL-6 were constructed and tested for IL-6R-independent gp130 binding and activation, it transpired that only chimeric proteins which contained the C-terminal A helix, the N-terminal AB loop, the BC loop, the C-terminal CD-loop and the N terminal D-helix of vIL-6 grafted onto the human IL-6 protein, had the desired property of contacting and activating gp130 without the help of IL-6R [108]. These results led to speculation regarding the functional role of the BC-loop in establishment of the contact between the site III of IL-6-type cytokines and gp130. It is possible that a receptor-induced, intramolecular conformational change within the cytokine protein leads to an as-yet unrecognized contact between the BC-loop and gp130 (or the LIF-R), and the establishment of a new functional binding contact at site III.

2.5
The Concept of Fusing the Cytokine to the Soluble Receptor: Hyper-IL-6

IL-6 can stimulate cells, which express gp130 but not IL-6R, when the naturally occurring sIL-6R is present–a paradigm referred to as "trans-signaling" [41, 42]. An analysis was conducted of the concentrations required for the stimulation of cells lacking the IL-6R with the complex of IL-6/sIL-6R. For full stimulation, the concentrations required were considerably higher than predicted from the affinity of IL-6 to the IL-6R, which was in the range of $1\,nM$ [43]. It was speculated that the efficacy to form a complex of IL-6, sIL-6R and gp130 on the cell surface could be largely enhanced by converting the IL-6/sIL-6R complex into a single polypeptide. For this, flexible peptide linkers were used that were long enough to bridge the distance between the C-terminus of the sIL-6R and the N-terminus of IL-6. The design was deduced from a 3-D model of the complex of IL-6 bound to the sIL-6R [44]. The resultant fusion protein of IL-6 and sIL-6R–referred to as "Hyper-IL-6"–was 100 to 1000 times more effective in stimulating IL-6R-lacking cells than was the combination of native IL-6 and sIL-6R [43]. This may reflect the higher affinity of the IL-6/sIL-6R complex to gp130, which is in the low picomolar range [45]. The structure of the fusion protein Hyper-IL-6 is shown in Figure 2.6.

Use was then made of the Hyper-IL-6 protein to demonstrate the existence of the IL-6 trans-signaling machinery in hematopoietic stem cells [46], neural cells [47, 48], smooth muscle cells [49], endothelial cells [50] and embryonic stem cells (ESC)s [51, 52]. Furthermore, it could be shown that the administration of Hyper-IL-6 *in vivo* led to a more profound and longer-lasting stimulation of hepatocytes as compared to IL-6, possibly due to the fact that Hyper-IL-6 had a longer half-life and was internalized much less efficiently than IL-6 by itself [53].

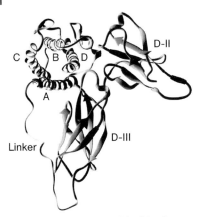

Figure 2.6 Molecular model of the fusion protein Hyper-IL-6. Hyper-IL-6 is a highly active designer cytokine consisting of IL-6 and soluble IL-6R. Depicted is a molecular model of the fusion protein of IL-6 and sIL-6R (Hyper-IL-6), consisting of IL-6 and sIL-6R fused by a flexible peptide linker. A, B, C, D denote the four helices of IL-6; D-II and D-III are the two cytokine-binding receptor domains of the sIL-6R which were used for construction of the fusion protein.

The concept of fusing a cytokine to the soluble receptor was further exploited in the construction of a CNTF/sCNTF-R fusion protein [54]. This was used to block glutamate-induced excitotoxicity on primary hippocampal neurons of the rat [55]. Other groups have used this concept to construct a fusion protein of IL-11 with the sIL-11R [56] and a fusion protein of the two components of IL-27, namely EBI3 and p28 [57]. Additional use of Hyper-IL-6-like fusion proteins was made by combining the fusion protein approach with the concept of IL-6R antagonists. It could be shown that a fusion protein of sIL-6R and an IL-6R antagonist with a defective site II or site III could be used to block the IL-6-induced proliferation of cells, and also the proliferation mediated by LIF, OSM and CNTF [58].

2.6
Antagonists Specifically Inhibiting IL-6 Trans-Signaling

A fusion protein consisting of the extracellular portion of gp130 covalently linked to the constant part of a human IgG_1 antibody (sgp130Fc) can act as a specific inhibitor of IL-6 trans-signaling. This molecule leaves the activity of IL-6 mediated by the membrane-bound IL-6R unaffected [59], a situation explained by the fact that human IL-6 does not exhibit a measurable affinity to gp130 in the absence of either membrane-bound or soluble IL-6R. Therefore, when cells are stimulated with IL-6 alone, the latter binds to the membrane-bound IL-6R and subsequently interacts with the membrane-bound gp130. The sgp130Fc protein apparently does not have access in this situation, and therefore fails to inhibit the activity of IL-6. In contrast, the IL-6/sIL-6R complex can bind with similar affinity to both the

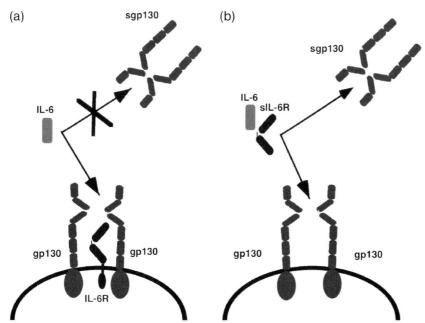

Figure 2.7 Scheme of the mechanism of IL-6 trans-signaling by soluble gp130. (a) IL-6 does not bind to sgp130 in the absence of soluble IL-6R. The sgp130 protein has no access to IL-6 complexed by membrane-bound IL-6R and two molecules of membrane-bound gp130; (b) The IL-6/sIL-6R complex can bind to both, membrane-bound and sgp130. Consequently, a molar excess of sgp130 leads to competitive inhibition of the IL-6/sIL-6R response.

membrane-bound and soluble gp130 receptor protein. Therefore, sgp130Fc is a specific inhibitor of IL-6 trans-signaling [59] (Figure 2.7).

The sgp130Fc protein has recently been used to define these signaling options in animal models of human diseases. The investigators sought to distinguish conventional IL-6 signaling via the membrane-bound IL-6R and IL-6 trans-signaling in gp130-dependent processes. Surprisingly, it was found that most – if not all – gp130-driven inflammatory diseases such as inflammatory bowel disease [60, 61], rheumatoid arthritis [62, 63], peritonitis [64] and inflammation-induced colon cancer [65, 66] were dependent upon the IL-6 trans-signaling mechanism. In corroborating these observations, a transgenic mouse with expression of the human sgp130Fc protein in the circulation, was largely protected in the gp130-mediated local inflammatory air pouch model. IL-6 trans-signaling is important for the trafficking of neutrophils and macrophages during the course of the inflammation [50, 67]. Therefore, the sgp130Fc protein is currently under development as a novel therapeutic drug for the treatment of chronic inflammatory diseases [68]. A scheme of the molecular mechanism by which the sgp130Fc protein specifically inhibits IL-6 trans-signaling, without affecting IL-6 classic signaling, is shown in Figure 2.7.

The analysis of the 3-D structure of gp130 in complex with IL-6 and sIL-6R suggested that the amino acid side chains in gp130 might be candidates for the generation of sgp130Fc variants with an increased binding affinity to the IL-6/

IL-6R complex. Thus, an optimized variant of sgp130Fc was produced which showed a higher stability and formed fewer aggregates upon purification. These proteins were tested for binding to the IL-6/IL-6R by using ELISA and surface plasmon resonance (SPR), for the inhibition of IL-6/sIL-6R-induced cell proliferation, and for the inhibition of induction of the acute-phase response. The resultant modified sgp130Fc variants proved to be 10- to 100-fold more effective in the specific inhibition of IL-6 trans-signaling [109].

2.7
In Vitro Evolution of Peptides and Proteins

Even today, evolutionary selection remains the most efficient method for generating cytokine/cytokine receptor variants with enhanced agonistic or antagonistic activity. Although rational design has made major progress, it is still not reliable enough to predict improved protein–protein interactions. Consequently, the development of *in vitro* recombinant DNA technology to randomize cytokine cDNA sequences has paved the way to generate cytokines/cytokine receptors with high specificity and affinity, selected from large libraries. Moreover, this is possible without any prior knowledge of the structure of the interaction sites, with large repertoires being generated by, for example, error-prone PCR, cassette mutagenesis, *Escherichia coli* mutator strains or DNA-shuffling [69]. DNA-shuffling is a combinatorial approach to the modification of proteins which utilizes the recombination of homologous genes. For this, individual genes are first cut down to fragments of 50–100 base pairs, after which the DNA is reassembled in a self-priming process, similar to PCR (Figure 2.8). The reassembled genes are then re-amplified using conventional PCR, cloned, and screened for the desired properties. The repertoires of randomly or semi-randomly mutated cytokines (from 10^9 to 10^{12}) can be displayed on the surface of phages, in cells, or in combination with RNA/DNA in certain display technologies [70]. Combinatorial libraries of peptides or proteins are generated in such a way that the genotype and phenotype of a single clone are directly coupled to each other (RNA/DNA and peptide/protein). The displayed peptides, or proteins with the desired properties, are then selected from populations containing tens of millions of individual clones and decoded by sequencing of the genotypic information (RNA/DNA) [71].

The binding of proteins/peptides to target structures can be achieved either in solution or by the immobilization of targets on plastic surfaces such as ELISA plates. Nonbinding proteins within the library are not detected, or are washed away and discarded. Finally, the binders are selected by using fluorescence-activated cell sorting (FACS), or they may be eluted from the surface-coupled antigen and re-amplified. Two to three subsequent rounds of screening led to a million-fold enrichment of specific binder populations, which were then ready for sequence analysis. Thereafter, the selected proteins could be expressed without phenotype/genotype fusion, purified, and further characterized (Figure 2.9).

DNA-Shuffling

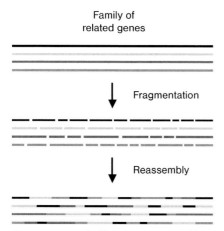

Figure 2.8 DNA-shuffling. To generate a library, genes were fragmented into various lengths and reassembled into full-length genes using a primerless PCR.

Selected peptides might be directly incorporated into cytokine or cytokine receptor proteins or into suitable scaffold proteins such as the complementary-determining regions (CDR) – these are loops of an antibody framework. This is exemplified by a peptide agonist of the thrombopoietin receptor that has been screened by phage display and then transferred to antibody fragments (Fabs) using rational protein design. In the newly generated agonistic thrombopoietin-mimicking Fabs, the CDRs were altered to present two copies of the peptide, which represents one approach to prolonging the *in vivo* half-life of a normally short-lived peptide [72, 73]. Alternatively, selected peptides might serve as lead structures for the development of nonpeptidic chemical compounds [74].

One major limitation of randomly mutated cytokine libraries is the limited or poor coverage of all possible combinations, which is exemplified by the following calculation. As one amino acid is coded by three nucleotides, the randomization of only seven amino acids requires randomization of 21 nucleotides, leading to 4^{21} (=4.4 $\times$ 10^{12}) different sequences. Good libraries consist of 10^9 to 10^{12} different clones; consequently, only relatively short peptide sequences can be used for randomization and screening, and only very limited combinations of amino-acid exchanges can be realized if a protein of, for example, 200 amino acids is used for randomization. Therefore, it is impossible to generate completely randomized cytokine or cytokine receptor libraries. If such an approach is chosen, only a limited number of variants can be established and screened. Consequently, even in evolutionary design the detailed structure–function analysis of cytokines and cytokine receptors is an important prerequisite to define the interaction epitopes, which in subsequent steps can be randomly modified for display techniques.

Screening

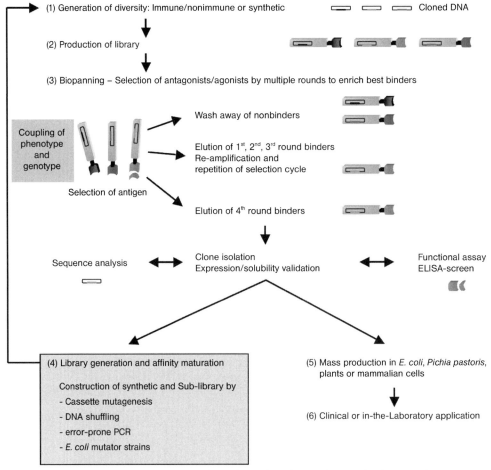

Figure 2.9 *In vitro* evolution of peptides and proteins. (1) To generate libraries, pools of randomized genes are cloned in a suitable vector, (2) followed by presentation of the library-proteins. (3) Biopanning, to enrich the best binders is carried out by multiple rounds of binding, washing away of non-binders and elution of specific binders. (4) Library generation and affinity maturation. (5) Selected binders can be produced in several hosts including *E. coli*, *Pichia pastoris*, plants or mammalian cells, (6) and used for clinical or in-the-laboratory applications.

2.7.1
Platforms for the Selection of High-Affinity Binders

The different selection strategies for *in vitro* evolution (Figure 2.9) all share key steps: (i) library construction (genomic diversity); (ii) coupling of genotype and phenotype; (iii) biopanning with selective pressure; and (iv) amplification of the

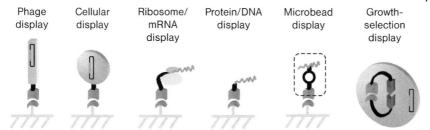

Figure 2.10 Display platforms for *in vitro* selection.

best binders. Phage display remains the most widely used method for *in vitro* evolution, and is applied to the selection of high-affinity human antibodies from nonimmune and synthetic libraries, including affinity maturation for picomolar affinity [single-chain antibodies (scFv), Fab fragment, single-domain antibodies (nanobodies)] (for a review, see Ref. [71]) (Figure 2.10).

Since the first description of phage display by G.P. Smith in 1985 [75], several additional systems have been established to display libraries of peptides or proteins on phage surfaces. With viral vectors, polyvalent display systems were developed, in which every phage cell-surface protein was fused to the presented peptide or protein. Polyvalent strategies harbor some disadvantages, because the function of the endogenous phage surface protein might be disturbed, and peptides or proteins with a lower affinity be preferentially selected due to avidity. The development of phagemid and helper phages enabled monovalent presentation in which both peptide-fused and nonfused phage surface proteins were present. Whereas several M13 phage surface proteins have been used (gp3, gp6, gp7, gp8 and gp9), fusions with gp3 via phagemids seemed to be the method of choice (for reviews, see Refs [76–78]).

Human single-chain Fv-antibodies selected from phage display libraries exhibit binding affinities (K_D) ranging from 10^{-6} to $10^{-9} M$. In the case of higher-affinity antibodies, alternative display platforms on prokaryotic and eukaryotic cells (e.g., *E. coli, Saccharomyces cerevisiae*, mammalian cells) have been used, which in addition provide the possibility to screen repertoires of cells by using flow cytometry [79–82]. Alternatively, ribosome display is well suited to select the highest-affinity binders [83].

When using the *E. coli* surface display, anchored periplasmic expression (APEx) allows the generation and screening of full-length IgG libraries on the bacteria [84]. APEx not only enables the generation of a large library size, but also overcomes the limitation of common phage display technology, where only partial antibody fragments such as ScFvs, Fabs and nanobodies could be expressed and screened. Full-length antibodies are secreted into the periplasm and captured by the synthetic inner membrane protein NlpA(1–6)-ZZ that binds to the Fc domain. The antibodies are accessible after permeabilization of the outer membrane, and may be detected using fluorescently labeled antigens and flow cytometry. In the *S. cerevisiae* yeast surface display, the peptides and proteins are fused to the α-agglutinin yeast adhesion receptor. On average, approximately 3×10^4 fusions per cell are presented, although this might lead to an intrinsic avidity and counteract the power of the system. Until now, the yeast-display method has yielded the highest affinity (48 fM) for any antibody. Although a eukaryotic display enables the presentation of complex and glycosylated proteins, one limitation of the system is the rather elaborate process of large library generation.

In ribosome display, the genotype–phenotype coupling is achieved by the ribosome. The library consists of mRNA molecules, and the protein is generated by *in vitro* translation, whereas the translation stops without releasing the protein and the mRNA [83]. Finally, ternary complexes of the ribosome, protein and mRNA are used for selection. In mRNA display the mRNA is covalently linked to the protein via the adaptor molecule puromycin [85, 86]. Both methods are carried out *in vitro*, thereby preventing the need for cell transformation.

A phenomenon known as the "affinity ceiling" was observed for antibodies produced by the mammalian immune system which display a maximal affinity of approximately $10^{-10} M$ [82]. Interestingly, the affinity of some proteins for their ligands may be much higher; for example, the affinity between avidin and biotin is $10^{-15} M$ [87]. The mammalian immune system is unable to select antibodies with a slower dissociation rate to an antigen relative to the intrinsic B-cell internalization rate of the antigen–antibody complex, which is in the range of 10–20 min [88, 89]. An effective limit of the off-rate constant was fixed at 10^{-3} to $10^{-4} M$. Antibodies with slower off-rates might arise but, due to a faster internalization of the receptor complex than dissociation of the antigen, they would not be selectable *in vivo* [88]. By using an *in vitro* affinity maturation, antibodies with antigen-binding affinities of $10^{-14} M$ have been selected using the yeast surface display [81]. Here, Boder *et al.* specifically screened for clones with very low dissociation rates, which led to the isolation of an antibody that bound the antigen almost irreversibly, with a decrease in the off-rate from 10^{-3} to $10^{-6} M$ and the on-rate from 4×10^{-7} to $3 \times 10^{-8} M$.

Affinity ceilings might exist for other ligand–receptor interactions, such as cytokine/cytokine receptors, because in general these complexes are internalized only minutes after ligand binding. It is tempting to speculate, that K_{on} and K_{off} rates haves evolved to induce fast and efficient binding (low K_{on}), but only a short duration of the interactions (high K_{off}) to ensure that the ligand does not dissociate until the complex is internalized. Interestingly, the dissociation constant of gp130 and its ligands IL-6/IL-6R is about 10^{-10}, with K_{on} being ca. 10^{-6} and K_{off} ca. 10^{-4} [109]; this is comparable to the dissociation rates for an antibody–antigen complex. It is likely that IL-6 binding to the receptor gp130 evolved in the same way so as to establish a rapid complex formation and maximal signaling, but only until the gp130/IL-6/IL-6R complex is internalized. The internalization rate of activated gp130 is 2.5 h, although the rate-limiting internalization of the IL-6R bound to IL-6 was only 15–30 min, and highly comparable to that of an antibody–lysozyme pair of ≤12 min [89–91]. Thus, the selection pressure affecting gp130/IL-6/IL-6R-complexes does not require a K_{off} rate $<10^{-4}$ to induce maximal IL-6 signaling. When considering the use of sgp130 as an inhibitor of IL-6/sIL-6R trans-signaling

(Figure 2.7), it might be easier to optimize K_{off} rather than K_{on} rates, since in nature the K_{off} rates have not been stringently selected for high affinity.

2.7.2
Agonists and Antagonists of Cytokines and Growth Hormones

The first monoclonal antibodies used in human therapeutic applications were of rodent origin, but caused strong endogenous antibody responses in patients. However, these responses could be circumvented by humanization of the rodent antibodies, such that the antibody consisted of a human framework but with a rodent CDR. Nonetheless, the humanized antibodies still had a 95% sequence homology with natural human antibodies [92]. The development of a human antibody phage display allowed a direct selection for obtaining specific antibodies of human origin. The first recombinant IgG antibody was developed in 2002 by Cambridge Antibody Technology (CAT; now MedImmune), and subsequently approved by the Federal Drug Administration (FDA) in the USA for the treatment of symptoms of rheumatoid arthritis. Adalimumab (Humira®) was selected as a single-chain Fv-fragment via phage display capable of blocking the inflammatory cytokine tumor necrosis factor-alpha (TNFα) [93]. Adalimumab was further developed by BASF and Abbott, and manufactured by Abbott under the trade name Humira®. In addition, single-chain Fv fragments have been described that are capable of binding and neutralizing the activity of human IL-1R [94], vascular endothelial growth factor (VEGF) [95], or human IL-6 [96].

Peptide agonists and antagonists have been identified for several cytokine and growth hormones and their receptors by the use of surface display. Prominent examples include peptide agonists of the thrombopoietin receptor [72] and EPO-receptor [97], as well as antagonistic peptides for endothelial growth factor receptor (EGFR) [98], TNFα [99], IL-1R [100], IL-5Rα [101] and IL-6R [102]. Agonistic peptides for interferon-β (IFN-β-signaling [103] have also been described. For the construction of IL-6 super-antagonists, IL-6 variants with an improved binding affinity to the IL-6R and impaired binding to gp130, were constructed. A better binding of IL-6 to the IL-6R, through the binding of site I, was achieved by the rational design of three amino acid substitutions within the D-helix. In order to obtain antagonistic properties, binding site II of IL-6 to gp130 was disturbed by introducing two critical mutations; the improved receptor-binding properties of this molecule resulted in a 10-fold more potent IL-6 antagonist [15].

To further improve the binding of IL-6 to the IL-6-R, mutations were introduced into the loop between helices A and B, which form part of the binding site I of IL-6 to IL-6R [104]. Four libraries with randomized stretches of four amino acids screened by phage display, and mutants with improved binding to the IL-6R (10- to 40-fold) were combined, and this resulted in a further increase in affinity of up to 70-fold. The combination of these mutations with the aforementioned mutations in binding sites I and II of IL-6 resulted in a further 10-fold increase in antagonistic potential [105]. Until now, however, only one report has been published on the affinity maturation of IL-6/IL-6R-complex to gp130 or ofgp130 to IL-6/IL-6R (Tenhumberg et al.).

LIF is a member of the IL-6 cytokine family which exerts its activity via binding to a heterodimer of gp130 and LIF-R, without the need for an alpha receptor. Therefore, the cytokine LIF contains only site II, the contact site to gp130, which comprises residues in the A-helix and C-helix and site III (contact site to the LIF-R) formed by the NH_2-terminal end of the D-helix and by residues within the A-B loop [106]. Fairlie *et al.* (2004) constructed six different libraries in which four to six amino acid residues around the interface of LIF and the LIF-R were randomized. Mutations in three of these six clusters resulted in proteins with a significantly increased affinity to the LIF-R, and the combination of these mutations resulted in agonistic LIF-muteins with a more than 1000-fold higher affinity when compared to the wild-type LIF [107]. The incorporation of two additional mutations in the interface of LIF to the receptor gp130 completely abrogated signaling and led to the generation of a super-antagonistic LIF-mutein [107].

2.8
Concluding Remarks

The presentation of peptides and proteins on display platforms such as phage, cells or ribosomes not only remains the current state-of-the-art method for the *in vitro* selection of superagonists and super-antagonists, but also represents an interesting *in vitro* alternative for identifying specific antibodies. Previously, engineered antibodies with affinities in the picomolar range could only be selected *in vitro*, due to the fact that an affinity ceiling of antibody selection existed *in vivo*. Currently, several *in vitro*-selected antibodies are undergoing clinical trials or have been approved for therapy. Constant progress in this field has also led to improvements of display technology with regards to the size and /or diversity of the library, and the selection strategy and development of affinity maturation. *In vitro* display platforms represent a powerful tool for selection of the highest-affinity binders, and in future might be used in combination to complement each other. A detailed knowledge of the architecture of cytokine receptor complexes, together with sophisticated techniques that not only allow screening of the binding properties of random peptides but also the evolution of ligands and receptors *in vitro* by gene shuffling, has provided a molecular toolbox of almost unlimited possibilities. Structure–function analyses of IL-6-type cytokines and their receptor complexes have shown that a detailed knowledge of the binding epitopes within the cytokine or cytokine receptor proteins can be used to develop designer proteins with novel functional properties. Cytokines with new receptor specificities might be used to stimulate hematopoietic stem cells or other cells types both *in vitro* and *in vivo*. Conversely, cytokine antagonists have been constructed which will undoubtedly prove to be useful for modifying the activity of the immune system not only in chronic inflammatory states but also in cancer.

References

1 Bazan, J.F. (1990) Haemopoietic receptors and helical cytokines. *Immunol. Today*, **11**, 350–4.

2 Bazan, J.F. (1990) Structural design and molecular evolution of a cytokine receptor superfamily. *Proc. Natl Acad. Sci. USA*, **87**, 6934–8.

3 Sprang, S.R. and Bazan, J.F. (1993) Cytokine structural taxonomy and mechanism of receptor engagement. *Curr. Opin. Struct. Biol.*, **3**, 815–27.

4 De Vos, A.M., Ultsch, M. and Kossiakoff, A.A. (1992) Human growth hormone and extracellular domain of its receptor: crystal structure and of the complex. *Science*, **255**, 306–12.

5 Hage, T., Sebald, W. and Reinemer, P. (1999) Crystal structure of the interleukin-4/receptor alpha chain complex reveals a mosaic binding interface. *Cell*, **97**, 271–81.

6 Grötzinger, J., Kernebeck, T., Kallen, K.-J. and Rose-John, S. (1999) IL-6 type cytokine receptor complexes: hexamer or tetramer or both? *Biol. Chem.*, **380**, 803–13.

7 Rose-John, S. and Neurath, M. (2004) IL-6 trans-signaling: the heat is on. *Immunity*, **20**, 2–4.

8 Reiss, K., Ludwig, A. and Saftig, P. (2006) Breaking up the tie: disintegrin-like metalloproteinases as regulators of cell migration in inflammation and invasion. *Pharmacol. Ther.*, **111**, 985–1006.

9 Clackson, T. and Wells, J.A. (1995) A hot spot of binding energy in a hormone-receptor interface. *Science*, **267**, 383–6.

10 Wells, J.A. (1996) Binding in the growth hormone receptor complex. *Proc. Natl Acad. Sci. USA*, **93**, 1–6.

11 Livnah, O., Stura, E.A., Middleton, S.A., Johnson, D.L., Jolliffe, L.K. and Wilson, I.A. (1999) Crystallographic evidence for preformed dimers of erythropoietin receptor before ligand activation. *Science*, **283**, 987–90.

12 Remy, I., Wilson, I.A. and Michnick, S.W. (1999) Erythropoietin receptor activation by a ligand-induced conformation change. *Science*, **283**, 990–3.

13 Ehlers, M., Grötzinger, J., de Hon, F.D., Müllberg, J., Brakenhoff, J.P., Liu, J., Wollmer, A. and Rose-John, S. (1994) Identification of two novel regions of human IL-6 responsible for receptor binding and signal transduction. *J. Immunol.*, **153**, 1744–53.

14 Kallen, K.-J., Grötzinger, J., Lelièvre, E., Vollmer, P., Aasland, D., Renné, C., Müllberg, J., Meyer zum Büschenfelde, K.-H. *et al.* (1999) Receptor recognition sites of 23 cytokines are organized as exchangeable modules: transfer of the LIFR binding site from CNTF to IL-6. *J. Biol. Chem.*, **274**, 11859–67.

15 Savino, R., Ciapponi, L., Lahm, A., Demartis, A., Cabibbo, A., Toniatti, C., Delmastro, P., Altamura, S. *et al.* (1994) Rational design of a receptor super-antagonist of human interleukin-6. *EMBO J.*, **13**, 5863–70.

16 Boulanger, M.J., Chow, D.-C., Brevnova, E.E. and Garcia, K.C. (2003) Hexameric structure and assembly of the interleukin-6/IL-6α receptor/gp130 complex. *Science*, **300**, 2101–4.

17 Chow, D.-C., He, X.-L., Snow, A.L., Rose-John, S. and Garcia, K.C. (2001) Structure of an extracellular gp130-cytokine receptor signalling complex. *Science*, **291**, 2150–5.

18 Kurth, I., Horsten, U., Pflanz, S., Dahmen, H., Kuster, A., Grotzinger, J., Heinrich, P.C. and Muller-Newen, G. (1999) Activation of the signal transducer glycoprotein 130 by both IL-6 and IL-11 requires two distinct binding epitopes. *J. Immunol.*, **162**, 1480–7.

19 Hammacher, A., Richardson, R.T., Layton, J.E., Smith, D.K., Angus, L.J., Hilton, D.J., Nicola, N.A., Wijdenes, J. *et al.* (1998) The immunoglobulin-like module of gp130 is required for signaling by interleukin-6, but not by leukemia inhibitory factor. *J. Biol. Chem.*, **273**, 22701–7.

20 Pflanz, S., Kurth, I., Grotzinger, J., Heinrich, P.C. and Muller-Newen, G. (2000) Two different epitopes of the

signal transducer gp130 sequentially cooperate on IL-6-induced receptor activation. *J. Immunol.*, **165**, 7042–9.

21 Auguste, P., Guillet, C., Fourcin, M., Olivier, C., Veziers, J., Pouplard Barthelaix, A. and Gascan, H. (1997) Signaling of type II oncostatin M receptor. *J. Biol. Chem.*, **272**, 15760–4.

22 Olivier, C., Auguste, P., Chabbert, M., Lelievre, E., Chevalier, S. and Gascan, H. (2000) Identification of a gp130 cytokine receptor critical site involved in oncostatin M response. *J. Biol. Chem.*, **275**, 5648–56.

23 Timmermann, A., Pflanz, S., Grötzinger, J., Küster, A., Kurth, I., Pitard, V., Heinrich, P.C. and Müller-Newen, G. (2000) Different epitopes are required for gp130 activation by interleukin-6, oncostatin M and leukemia inhibitory factor. *FEBS Lett.*, **468**, 120–4.

24 Hammacher, A., Wijdenes, J., Hilton, D.J., Nicola, N.A., Simpson, R.J. and Layton, J.E. (2000) Ligand-specific utilization of the extracellular membrane-proximal region of the gp130-related signalling receptors. *Biochem. J.*, **345**, 25–32.

25 Kurth, I., Horsten, U., Pflanz, S., Timmermann, A., Kuster, A., Dahmen, H., Tacken, I., Heinrich, P.C. *et al.* (2000) Importance of the membrane-proximal extracellular domains for activation of the signal transducer glycoprotein 130. *J. Immunol.*, **164**, 273–82.

26 Stuhlmann-Laeisz, C., Lang, S., Chalaris, A., Paliga, K., Sudarman, E., Eichler, J., Klingmüller, U., Samuel, M. *et al.* (2006) Forced dimerization of gp130 leads to constitutive STAT3 activation, cytokine independent growth and blockade of differentiation of embryonic stem cells. *Mol. Biol. Cell*, **17**, 2986–95.

27 Brakenhoff, J.P., Hart, M. and Aarden, L.A. (1989) Analysis of human IL-6 mutants expressed in *Escherichia coli*. Biologic activities are not affected by deletion of amino acids 1-28. *J. Immunol.*, **143**, 1175–82.

28 Krüttgen, A., Rose-John, S., Dufhues, G., Bender, S., Lütticken, C., Freyer, P. and Heinrich, P.C. (1990) The three carboxy-terminal amino acids of human interleukin-6 are essential for its biological activity. *FEBS Lett.*, **273**, 95–8.

29 Krüttgen, A., Rose-John, S., Moller, C., Wroblowski, B., Wollmer, A., Müllberg, J., Hirano, T., Kishimoto, T. *et al.* (1990) Structure-function analysis of human interleukin-6. Evidence for the involvement of the carboxy-terminus in function. *FEBS Lett.*, **262**, 323–6.

30 Coulie, P.G., Stevens, M. and Van Snick, J. (1989) High- and low-affinity receptors for murine interleukin 6. Distinct distribution on B and T cells. *Eur. J. Immunol.*, **19**, 2107–14.

31 van Dam, M., Müllberg, J., Schooltink, H., Stoyan, T., Brakenhoff, J.P., Graeve, L., Heinrich, P.C. and Rose-John, S. (1993) Structure-function analysis of interleukin-6 utilizing human/murine chimeric molecules. Involvement of two separate domains in receptor binding. *J. Biol. Chem.*, **268**, 15285–90.

32 Ehlers, M., Grötzinger, J., Fischer, M., Bos, H.K., Brakenhoff, J.P.J. and Rose-John, S. (1996) Identification of single amino acid residues of human Interleukin-6 involved in receptor binding and signal initiation. *J. Interferon Cytokine Res.*, **16**, 569–76.

33 Brakenhoff, J.P., Hart, M., De Groot, E.R., Di Padova, F. and Aarden, L.A. (1990) Structure-function analysis of human IL-6. Epitope mapping of neutralizing monoclonal antibodies with amino- and carboxyl-terminal deletion mutants. *J. Immunol.*, **145**, 561–8.

34 Kishimoto, T. (2005) IL-6: from laboratory to bedside. *Clin. Rev. Allergy Immunol.*, **28**, 177–86.

35 Brakenhoff, J.P., de Hon, F.D., Fontaine, V., ten Boekel, E., Schooltink, H., Rose-John, S., Heinrich, P.C., Content, J. *et al.* (1994) Development of a human interleukin-6 receptor antagonist. *J. Biol. Chem.*, **269**, 86–93.

36 de Hon, F.D., Ehlers, M., Rose-John, S., Ebeling, S.B., Bos, H.K., Aarden, L.A. and Brakenhoff, J.P. (1994) Development of an interleukin (IL) 6 receptor antagonist that inhibits IL-6-dependent growth of human myeloma cells. *J. Exp. Med.*, **180**, 2395–400.

37 Paonessa, G., Graziani, R., De Serio, A., Savino, R., Ciapponi, L., Lahm, A., Salvati, A.L., Toniatti, C. *et al.* (1995) Two distinct and independent sites on IL-6 trigger gp 130 dimer formation and signalling. *EMBO J.*, **14**, 1942–51.

38 McDonald, N.Q., Panayotatos, N. and Hendrickson, W.A. (1995) Crystal structure of dimeric human ciliary neurotrophic factor determined by MAD phasing. *EMBO J.*, **14**, 2689–99.

39 Kallen, K.-J., Grötzinger, J. and Rose-John, S. (2000) New perspectives in the design of cytokines and growth factors. *Trends Biotechnol.*, **18**, 455–61.

40 Müllberg, J., Geib, T., Jostock, T., Hoischen, S.H., Vollmer, P., Voltz, N., Heinz, D., Galle, P.R. *et al.* (2000) IL-6-receptor independent stimulation of human gp130 by viral IL-6. *J. Immunol.*, **164**, 4672–7.

41 Rose-John, S. and Heinrich, P.C. (1994) Soluble receptors for cytokines and growth factors: generation and biological function. *Biochem. J.*, **300**, 281–90.

42 Peters, M., Müller, A. and Rose-John, S. (1998) Interleukin-6 and soluble interleukin-6 receptor: direct Stimulation of gp130 and hematopoiesis. *Blood*, **92**, 3495–504.

43 Fischer, M., Goldschmitt, J., Peschel, C., Brakenhoff, J.P., Kallen, K.J., Wollmer, A., Grotzinger, J., Rose-John, S. *et al.* (1997) A bioactive designer cytokine for human hematopoietic progenitor cell expansion. *Nat. Biotechnol.*, **15**, 145.

44 Grötzinger, J., Kurapkat, G., Wollmer, A., Kalai, M. and Rose-John, S. (1997) The family of the IL-6-type cytokines: specificity and promiscuity of the receptor complexes proteins: structure, function, and genetics. *Proteins*, **27**, 96–109.

45 Rose-John, S., Schooltink, H., Lenz, D., Hipp, E., Dufhues, G., Schmitz, H., Schiel, X., Hirano, T. *et al.* (1990) Studies on the structure and regulation of the human hepatic interleukin-6 receptor. *Eur. J. Biochem.*, **190**, 79–83.

46 Audet, J., Miller, C.L., Rose-John, S., Piret, J.M. and Eaves, C.J. (2001) Distinct role of gp130 activation in promoting self-renewal divisions by mitogenically stimulated murine hematopoietic cells. *Proc. Natl Acad. Sci. USA*, **98**, 1757–62.

47 März, P., Herget, T., Lang, E., Otten, U. and Rose-John, S. (1997) Activation of gp130 by IL-6/soluble IL-6 receptor induces neuronal differentiation. *Eur. J. Neurosci.*, **9**, 2765–73.

48 März, P., Cheng, J.-C., Gadient, R.A., Patterson, P., Stoyan, T., Otten, U. and Rose-John, S. (1998) Sympathetic neurons can produce and respond to interleukin-6. *Proc. Natl Acad. Sci. USA*, **95**, 3251–6.

49 Klouche, M., Bhakdi, S., Hemmes, M. and Rose-John, S. (1999) Novel path of activation of primary human smooth muscle cells: upregulation of gp130 creates an autocrine activation loop by IL-6 and its soluble receptor. *J. Immunol.*, **163**, 4583–9.

50 Chalaris, A., Rabe, B., Paliga, K., Lange, H., Laskay, T., Fielding, C.A., Jones, S.A., Rose-John, S. *et al.* (2007) Apoptosis is a natural stimulus of IL6R shedding and contributes to the pro-inflammatory trans-signaling function of neutrophils. *Blood*, **110**, 1748–55.

51 Viswanathan, S., Benatar, T., Rose-John, S., Lauffenburger, D.A. and Zandstra, P.W. (2002) Ligand/receptor signaling threshold (LIST) model accounts for gp130-mediated embryonic stem cell self-renewal responses to LIF and HIL-6. *Stem Cells*, **20**, 119–38.

52 Humphrey, R.K., Beattie, G.M., Lopez, A.D., Bucay, N., King, C.C., Firpo, M., Rose-John, S. and Hayek, A. (2004) Maintenance of pluripotency in human embryonic stem cells is Stat3 independent. *Stem Cells*, **22**, 522–30.

53 Peters, M., Blinn, G., Solem, F., Fischer, M., Meyer zum Büschenfelde, K.-H. and Rose-John, S. (1998) In vivo and in vitro activity of the gp130 stimulating designer cytokine hyper-IL-6. *J. Immunol.*, **161**, 3575–81.

54 März, P., Özbek, S., Fischer, M., Voltz, N., Otten, U. and Rose-John, S. (2002) Differential response of neuronal cells to a fusion protein of ciliary neurotrophic factor and soluble CNTF-receptor (Hyper-CNTF) and leukemia inhibitory factor (LIF). *Eur. J. Biochem.*, **269**, 3023–31.

55 Sun, Y., März, P., Otten, U., Ge, J. and Rose-John, S. (2002) The Effect of gp130 stimulation on glutamate-induced excitotoxicity in primary hippocampal neurons. *Biochem. Biophys. Res. Commun.*, **295**, 532–9.

56 Pflanz, S., Tacken, I., Grotzinger, J., Jacques, Y., Minvielle, S., Dahmen, H., Heinrich, P.C. and Muller-Newen, G. (1999) A fusion protein of interleukin-11 and soluble interleukin-11 receptor acts as a superagonist on cells expressing gp130. *FEBS Lett.*, **450**, 117–22.

57 Wirtz, S., Tubbe, I., Galle, P.R., Schild, H.J., Birkenbach, M., Blumberg, R.S. and Neurath, M.F. (2006) Protection from lethal, septic peritonitis by neutralizing the biological function of interleukin 27. *J. Exp. Med.*, **203**, 1875–81.

58 Renné, C., Kallen, K.-J., Müllberg, J., Jostock, T., Grötzinger, J. and Rose-John, S. (1998) A new type of cytokine receptor antagonist directly targeting gp130. *J. Biol. Chem.*, **273**, 27213–19.

59 Jostock, T., Müllberg, J., Özbek, S., Atreya, R., Blinn, G., Voltz, N., Fischer, M., Neurath, M.F. *et al.* (2001) Soluble gp130 is the natural inhibitor of soluble IL-6R transsignaling responses. *Eur. J. Biochem.*, **268**, 160–7.

60 Atreya, R., Mudter, J., Finotto, S., Müllberg, J., Jostock, T., Wirtz, S., Schütz, M., Bartsch, B. *et al.* (2000) Blockade of IL-6 transsignaling abrogates established experimental colitis in mice by suppression of the antiapoptotic resistance of lamina propria T cells. *Nat. Med.*, **6**, 583–8.

61 Mitsuyama, K., Matsumoto, S., Rose-John, S., Suzuki, A., Hara, T., Tomiyasu, N., Handa, K., Tsuruta, O. *et al.* (2006) STAT3 activation via interleukin-6 trans-signaling contributes to ileitis in SAMP1/Yit mice. *Gut*, **55**, 1263–9.

62 Nowell, M.A., Richards, P.J., Horiuchi, S., Yamamoto, N., Rose-John, S., Topley, N., Williams, A.S. and Jones, S.A. (2003) Soluble IL-6 receptor governs IL-6 activity in experimental arthritis: blockade of arthritis severity by soluble glycoprotein 130. *J. Immunol.*, **171**, 3202–9.

63 Richards, P.J., Nowell, M.A., Horiuchi, S., McLoughlin, R.M., Fielding, C.A., Grau, S., Yamamoto, N., Ehrmann, M. *et al.* (2006) Functional characterization of a soluble gp130 isoform and its therapeutic capacity in an experimental model of inflammatory arthritis. *Arthritis Rheum.*, **54**, 1662–72.

64 Hurst, S.M., Wilkinson, T.S., McLoughlin, R.M., Jones, S., Horiuchi, S., Yamamoto, N., Rose-John, S., Fuller, G.M. *et al.* (2001) IL-6 and its soluble receptor orchestrate a temporal switch in the pattern of leukocyte recruitment. *Immunity*, **14**, 705–14.

65 Becker, C., Fantini, M.C., Schramm, C., Lehr, H.A., Wirtz, S., Nikolaev, A., Burg, J., Strand, S. *et al.* (2004) TGF-beta suppresses tumor progression in colon cancer by inhibition of IL-6 trans-signaling. *Immunity*, **21**, 491–501.

66 Becker, C., Fantini, M.C., Wirtz, S., Nikolaev, A., Lehr, H.A., Galle, P.R., Rose-John, S. and Neurath, M.F. (2005) IL-6 signaling promotes tumor growth in colorectal cancer. *Cell Cycle*, **4**, 217–20.

67 Rabe, B., Chalaris, A., May, U., Waetzig, G.H., Seegert, D., Williams, A.S., Jones, S.A., Rose-John, S. *et al.* (2008) Transgenic blockade of interleukin 6 transsignaling abrogates inflammation. *Blood*, **111**, 1021–8.

68 Rose-John, S., Waetzig, G.H., Scheller, J., Grotzinger, J. and Seegert, D. (2007) The IL-6/sIL-6R complex as a novel target for therapeutic approaches. *Expert. Opin. Ther. Targets*, **11**, 613–24.

69 Wang, T.W., Zhu, H., Ma, X.Y., Zhang, T., Ma, Y.S. and Wei, D.Z. (2006) Mutant library construction in directed molecular evolution: casting a wider net. *Mol. Biotechnol.*, **34**, 55–68.

70 Hoogenboom, H.R. (2005) Selecting and screening recombinant antibody libraries. *Nat. Biotechnol.*, **23**, 1105–16.

71 Conrad, U. and Scheller, J. (2005) Considerations on antibody-phage display methodology. *Comb. Chem. High Throughput Screen.*, **8**, 117–26.

72 Cwirla, S.E., Balasubramanian, P., Duffin, D.J., Wagstrom, C.R., Gates, C.M., Singer, S.C., Davis, A.M., Tansik, R.L. *et al.* (1997) Peptide agonist of the thrombopoietin receptor as potent as the natural cytokine. *Science*, **276**, 1696–9.

73 Frederickson, S., Renshaw, M.W., Lin, B., Smith, L.M., Calveley, P., Springhorn, J.P., Johnson, K., Wang, Y. *et al.* (2006) A rationally designed agonist antibody fragment that functionally mimics thrombopoietin. *Proc. Natl Acad. Sci. USA*, **103**, 14307–12.

74 Livnah, O., Stura, E.A., Johnson, D.L., Middleton, S.A., Mulcahy, L.S., Wrighton, N.C., Dower, W.J., Jolliffe, L.K. *et al.* (1996) Functional mimicry of a protein hormone by a peptide agonist: the EPO receptor complex at 2.8 Å. *Science*, **273**, 464–71.

75 Smith, G.P. (1985) Filamentous fusion phage: novel expression vectors that display cloned antigens on the virion surface. *Science*, **228**, 1315–17.

76 Hoess, R.H. (2001) Protein design and phage display. *Chem. Rev.*, **101**, 3205–18.

77 Smith, G.P. and Petrenko, V.A. (1997) Phage display. *Chem. Rev.*, **97**, 391–410.

78 Smothers, J.F., Henikoff, S. and Carter, P. (2002) Phage display. Affinity selection from biological libraries. *Science*, **298**, 621–2.

79 Thompson, J., Pope, T., Tung, J.S., Chan, C., Hollis, G., Mark, G. and Johnson, K.S. (1996) Affinity maturation of a high-affinity human monoclonal antibody against the third hypervariable loop of human immunodeficiency virus: use of phage display to improve affinity and broaden strain reactivity. *J. Mol. Biol.*, **256**, 77–88.

80 Daugherty, P.S., Chen, G., Iverson, B.L. and Georgiou, G. (2000) Quantitative analysis of the effect of the mutation frequency on the affinity maturation of single chain Fv antibodies. *Proc. Natl Acad. Sci. USA*, **97**, 2029–34.

81 Boder, E.T., Midelfort, K.S. and Wittrup, K.D. (2000) Directed evolution of antibody fragments with monovalent femtomolar antigen-binding affinity. *Proc. Natl Acad. Sci. USA*, **97**, 10701–5.

82 van den Beucken, T., Pieters, H., Steukers, M., van der Vaart, M., Ladner, R.C., Hoogenboom, H.R. and Hufton, S.E. (2003) Affinity maturation of Fab antibody fragments by fluorescent-activated cell sorting of yeast-displayed libraries. *FEBS Lett.*, **546**, 288–94.

83 Hanes, J., Schaffitzel, C., Knappik, A. and Pluckthun, A. (2000) Picomolar affinity antibodies from a fully synthetic naive library selected and evolved by ribosome display. *Nat. Biotechnol.*, **18**, 1287–92.

84 Mazor, Y., Blarcom, T.V., Mabry, R., Iverson, B.L. and Georgiou, G. (2007) Isolation of engineered, full-length antibodies from libraries expressed in *Escherichia coli*. *Nat. Biotechnol.*, **25**, 363–565.

85 Kurz, M., Gu, K. and Lohse, P.A. (2000) Psoralen photo-crosslinked mRNA-puromycin conjugates: a novel template for the rapid and facile preparation of mRNA-protein fusions. *Nucleic Acids Res.*, **28**, 83.

86 Getmanova, E.V., Chen, Y., Bloom, L., Gokemeijer, J., Shamah, S., Warikoo, V., Wang, J., Ling, V.S. and L. (2006) Antagonists to human and mouse vascular endothelial growth factor receptor 2 generated by directed protein evolution in vitro. *Chem. Biol.*, **13**, 549–56.

87 Green, N.M. (1975) Avidin. *Adv. Protein Chem.*, **29**, 85–133.

88 Foote, J. and Eisen, H.N. (1995) Kinetic and affinity limits on antibodies produced during immune responses. *Proc. Natl Acad. Sci. USA*, **92**, 1254–6.

89 Batista, F.D. and Neuberger, M.S. (1998) Affinity dependence of the B cell response to antigen: a threshold, a ceiling, and the importance of off-rate. *Immunity*, **8**, 751–9.

90 Dittrich, E., Haft, C.R., Muys, L., Heinrich, P.C. and Graeve, L. (1996) A di-leucine motif and an upstream serine in the interleukin-6 (IL-6) signal transducer gp130 mediate ligand-induced endocytosis and down-regulation of the IL-6 receptor. *J. Biol. Chem.*, **271**, 5487–94.

91 Zohlnhöfer, D., Graeve, L., Rose-John, S., Schooltink, H., Dittrich, E. and Heinrich, P.C. (1992) The hepatic interleukin-6 receptor. Down-regulation of the interleukin-6 binding subunit (gp80) by its ligand. *FEBS Lett.*, **306**, 219–22.

92 Queen, C., Schneider, W.P., Selick, H.E., Payne, P.W., Landolfi, N.F., Duncan, J.F., Avdalovic, N.M., Levitt, M. *et al.*

(1989) A humanized antibody that binds to the interleukin 2 receptor. *Proc. Natl Acad. Sci. USA*, **86**, 10029–33.

93 Bain, B., Brazil, M. (2003) Adalimumab. *Nat. Rev. Drug Discov.*, **2**, 693–4.

94 Fredericks, Z.L., Forte, C., Capuano, I.V., Zhou, H., Vanden Bos, T. and Carter, P. (2004) Identification of potent human anti-IL-1RI antagonist antibodies. *Protein Eng. Des. Sel.*, **17**, 95–106.

95 Vitaliti, A., Wittmer, M., Steiner, R., Wyder, L., Neri, D. and Klemenz, R. (2000) Inhibition of tumor angiogenesis by a single-chain antibody directed against vascular endothelial growth factor. *Cancer Res.*, **60**, 4311–14.

96 Gejima, R., Tanaka, K., Nakashima, T., Hashiguchi, S., Ito, Y., Yoshizaki, K. and Sugimura, K. (2002) Human single-chain Fv (scFv) antibody specific to human IL-6 with the inhibitory activity on IL-6-signaling. *Hum. Antibodies*, **11**, 121–9.

97 Wrighton, N.C., Farrell, F.X., Chang, R., Kashyap, A.K., Barbone, F.P., Mulcahy, L.S., Johnson, D.L., Barrett, R.W. *et al.* (1996) Small peptides as potent mimetics of the protein hormone erythropoietin. *Science*, **273**, 458–64.

98 Nakamura, T., Takasugi, H., Aizawa, T., Yoshida, M., Mizuguchi, M., Mori, Y., Shinoda, H., Hayakawa, Y. *et al.* (2005) Peptide mimics of epidermal growth factor (EGF) with antagonistic activity. *J. Biotechnol.*, **116**, 211–19.

99 Chirinos-Rojas, C.L., Steward, M.W. and Partidos, C.D. (1998) A peptidomimetic antagonist of TNF-alpha-mediated cytotoxicity identified from a phage-displayed random peptide library. *J. Immunol.*, **161**, 5621–6.

100 Akeson, A.L., Woods, C.W., Hsieh, L.C., Bohnke, R.A., Ackermann, B.L., Chan, K.Y., Robinson, J.L., Yanofsky, S.D. *et al.* (1996) AF12198, a novel low molecular weight antagonist, selectively binds the human type I interleukin (IL)-1 receptor and blocks in vivo responses to IL-1. *J. Biol. Chem.*, **271**, 30517–23.

101 England, B.P., Balasubramanian, P., Uings, I., Bethell, S., Chen, M.J., Schatz, P.J., Yin, Q., Chen, Y.F. *et al.* (2000) A potent dimeric peptide antagonist of interleukin-5 that binds two interleukin-5 receptor alpha chains. *Proc. Natl Acad. Sci. USA*, **97**, 6862–7.

102 Su, J.L., Lai, K.P., Chen, C.A., Yang, C.Y., Chen, P.S., Chang, C.C., Chou, C.H., Hu, C.L. *et al.* (2005) A novel peptide specifically binding to interleukin-6 receptor (gp80) inhibits angiogenesis and tumor growth. *Cancer Res.*, **65**, 4827–35.

103 Sato, A. and Sone, S. (2003) A peptide mimetic of human interferon (IFN)-beta. *Biochem. J.*, **371**, 603–8.

104 Toniatti, C., Cabibbo, A., Sporena, E., Salvati, A.L., Cerretani, M., Serafini, S., Lahm, A., Cortese, R. *et al.* (1996) Engineering human interleukin-6 to obtain variants with strongly enhanced bioactivity. *EMBO J.*, **15**, 2726–37.

105 Sporeno, E., Savino, R., Ciapponi, L., Paonessa, G., Cabibbo, A., Lahm, A., Pulkki, K., Sun, R.X. *et al.* (1996) Human interleukin-6 receptor super-antagonists with high potency and wide spectrum on multiple myeloma cells. *Blood*, **87**, 4510–19.

106 Hudson, K.R., Vernallis, A.B. and Heath, J.K. (1996) Characterization of the receptor binding sites of human leukemia inhibitory factor and creation of antagonists. *J. Biol. Chem.*, **271**, 11971–8.

107 Fairlie, W.D., Uboldi, A.D., McCoubrie, J.E., Wang, C.C., Lee, E.F., Yao, S., De Souza, D.P., Mifsud, S. *et al.* (2004) Affinity maturation of leukemia inhibitory factor and conversion to potent antagonists of signaling. *J. Biol. Chem.*, **279**, 2125–34.

108 Adam, N., Rabe, B., Suthaus, J., Grötzinger, J., Rose-John, S. and Scheller, J. (2009) Understanding receptor independent gp130 activation of viral interleukin-6. *J. Virol.*, in press.

109 Tenhumberg, S., Waetzig, G.H., Chalaris, A., Rabe, B., Seegert, D., Scheller, J., Rose-John, S. and Grötzinger, S. (2008) Structure guided optimization of the IL-6 transsignalling antagonist sgp 130Fc. *J. Biol. Chem.*, **283**, 27200–07.

3

Peptides Derived from Exon v6 of the CD44 Extracellular Domain Prevent Activation of Receptor Tyrosine Kinases and Subsequently Angiogenesis and Metastatic Spread of Tumor Cells

Helmut Ponta and Véronique Orian-Rousseau

3.1
Introduction

In humans, receptor tyrosine kinases (RTKs) form a group of 58 proteins charac-terised by a cytoplasmic tyrosine kinase domain, a transmembrane domain and an extracellular ligand-binding domain. Their classification in 20 different families is mainly due to the divergence in the ectodomain structure [1]. The RTKs promote cell signaling upon binding to specific ligands and regulate cell growth, differentia-tion, adhesion, migration and apoptosis [2]. Because of their involvement in these critical steps they are prone to trigger tumor formation or other hyperproliferative diseases such as psoriasis. In fact, for more then 30 RTKs a participation in nearly all cancer types has been demonstrated.

In normal cells, the activity of the RTKs and the cellular signaling they mediate are precisely coordinated and tightly regulated whereas cancer cells have escaped this control. It is astonishing how many different mechanisms can account for the deregulation of RTKs. They can be overexpressed [3, 4], subjected to autocrine stimulation in tumor cells that produce their own ligand [5, 6], they can cooperate with "signal amplifiers" [7], they can be mutated so that they become constitutively active and ligand independent [8–13] or they can be impaired in their turn over, for example, in the internalization process [14].

That RTKs are decisive factors in cell transformation and often also in tumor progression and metastasis makes them promising targets for tumor therapy. Two strategies have been successfully pursued so far. Immunological inhibitors have been developed to block ligand binding and receptor activation and pharmocologi-cal inhibitors have been identified that block the kinase activity of the RTKs. In the case of both strategies, drugs have already been tested in clinical trials and have been approved in the clinics. For instance Herceptin (Trastuzumab) is a monoclonal antibody directed against HER2, a member of the epidermal growth factor (EGF) receptor family, and was the first genomics-based therapeutic agent for tumor treatment [15]. Cetuximab, a monoclonal antibody directed against EGF-R, is currently in use in the treatment of colorectal cancer [16] although it

Peptides as Drugs. Discovery and Development. Edited by Bernd Groner
Copyright © 2009 WILEY-VCH Verlag GmbH & Co. KGaA, Weinheim
ISBN: 978-3-527-32205-3

also has the potential to interfere with the growth of other cancers [17]. The first inhibitors of the intrinsic tyrosine kinase activity of RTKs were genistein and herbimycin A isolated from fungal extracts. On the basis of these two drugs, ATP analogues of the quinazoline and pyrido-pyrimidine family that compete with ATP for binding to the ATP binding domain of the RTKs, mainly of the EGFR family, were developed [18, 19]. The most advanced drug is gleevec, a 2-phenylaminopyrimidine pharmacophore, that exhibits specificity for the non-receptor tyrosine kinase Abl, but affects as well the RTKs PDGF-R and Kit [20, 21].

Despite the fact that all these drugs are highly effective in animal models, their success in human cancer patients is still not optimal and leaves plenty of space for the development of additional strategies. Such strategies include the RNAi technology, the development of decoy receptors or the use of peptides or peptidomimetica that interfere with ligand binding or signal transduction.

3.2
CD44 Proteins and Their Involvement in RTK Activation

The finding that in most instances, RTKs require a coreceptor for their function has opened new avenues in cancer research. The first and for a long time the only example of such a coreceptor were the heparan sulfate modified surface proteins as coreceptors for members of the fibroblast growth factor receptors (FGF-Rs [22]). Recently, several other surface proteins such as cadherins, N-CAM, integrins or members of the CD44 family have been identified as coreceptors for a variety of RTKs [23]. We have intensively studied the coreceptor function of CD44v6 for the RTK c-Met and its Ron.

Members of the CD44 transmembrane protein family were originally detected as markers on immune cells [24] and several functions were assigned to these proteins often described under different names (for a review, see [25]). The identification of the genomic structure of CD44 revealed that the gene is composed of 20 exons. The first and last five exons are expressed in nearly all isoforms (if only these exons are expressed they give rise to the smallest but ubiquitously expressed CD44s isoform) and the central 10 "variant" exons v1-v10 can be integrated in many combinations due to alternative splicing [26, 27].

CD44 proteins play essential roles in a variety of physiological processes (for reviews see [25, 28]) including tissue development, limb development, neuronal axon guidance, hematopoiesis and in numerous immune responses. Furthermore, they have decisive functions in pathological processes such as cancer, inflammation and autoimmune diseases. Particularly interesting are the functions of CD44 proteins in the immune system. CD44s was described as a lymphocyte homing receptor that seems to play a role in lymphocyte emigration from the blood stream at the site of high endothelial venules [29, 30]. CD44 variant isoforms are transiently expressed upon lymphocyte activation and are instrumental in mediating B and T cell dependent immune responses [31]. In accordance to this observation, transgenic animals expressing specific variant isoforms of CD44 on thymocytes and peripheral T cells respond faster to activating stimuli [32]. An involvement of CD44 in hematopoiesis has been demonstrated by the use of CD44-specific antibodies [33, 34]. In long-term bone marrow cultures, antibodies directed against various epitopes of CD44 molecules either inhibited or enhanced hematopoiesis. The formation of cobblestone areas, an early stage of hemato-poiesis, was inhibited by panCD44 antibodies whereas CD44 variant specific anti-bodies interfered with myelopoeisis and lymphopoeisis [33–35].

Interest in CD44 increased with the discovery of its function as a receptor for a major component of the extracellular matrix, hyaluronan (HA [36]) and the finding that several variant isoforms of CD44 are able to confer the metastatic propensity to tumor cells [37]. Among these CD44 variant proteins, the ones containing exon v6 sequences seem to be particularly prone to mediate metastasis since the meta-static spreading of tumor cells could be blocked by CD44v6 specific antibodies and transfection of CD44v4-v7 or CD44v6,v7, induced metastatic spread in otherwise non-metastatic tumor cells [37, 38].

Since CD44v6 was shown to be associated with metastasis, worldwide many laboratories investigated the expression of CD44 in human tumor cells and showed that, for many different kinds of tumors, the expression of CD44, particularly of variant isoforms, is correlated with bad prognosis (reviewed by [39]). However, the mode of action of these CD44 variant proteins was for a long time a matter of debate. The suggestion that the binding to HA might be impaired by insertion of variant exons [40] turned out to be untrue. This function of CD44 is not the critical parameter in tumor growth. Several CD44 variant proteins, including the ones detected in metastatic tumor cells, have an even higher binding affinity to HA than CD44s [41, 42] and the abrogation of HA binding to metastatic tumor cells by expression of a hyaluronidase did not interfere with the metastatic process [43].

The identification of a heparan sulphate modification on CD44 variants contain-ing exon v3 [44] placed some of the variants into focus. These heparan sulfate proteoglycans (HSPG) are able to bind heparin-binding growth factors and thus could act as coreceptors for the authentic receptors [45]. Such a coreceptor function for FGF-Rs was identified for CD44 variants in limb development [46]. There, a CD44v3 variant is expressed on the apical ectodermal ridge and presents FGFs expressed by the same cells to the FGF receptors on the underlying mesenchymal cells thereby triggering their proliferation. The CD44 variant expressed on the ectodermal cells contains all variant exons and consequently antibodies directed against exon v3 as well as exon v6 could block proliferation of the mesenchymal cells [46].

3.3
CD44v6 Acts as a Coreceptor for c-Met and Ron

Although very interesting and promising with regard to the mode of action of some CD44 variant proteins, the function of CD44 as coreceptor for FGF-R concerned exclusively the CD44v3 isoforms that are modified by heparan sulfate and not the CD44v6 containing isoforms involved in tumor progression. Therefore, this mechanism could not explain the role of the CD44 variants in tumors. We wondered, however, whether such CD44v6 variants might also function as coreceptors for other RTKs using a different mode of action than in the case of HSPGs. The receptors that we have chosen for these tests were the c-Met receptor and its relative Ron.

c-Met, Ron and their respective ligands scatter factor or hepatocyte growth factor (here abbreviated as HGF) and macrophage stimulating protein (MSP) are of particular interest since they not only promote cell growth and apoptosis but also trigger a unique process called "branching morphogenesis" which combines cell dissociation and invasion through extracellular matrices [47–49]. Thus, these RTKs are involved in development, regeneration and organ remodelling. Under pathological conditions, for example, in transformed tumor cells, they mediate "invasive growth" into surrounding tissues giving rise to tumor cell dissemination and eventually to the formation of metastases.

In a variety of experiments, it was undoubtedly demonstrated that CD44 isoforms containing exon v6 sequences are instrumental for c-Met activation in several transformed cells and also in primary cells such as keratinocytes [50]. Antibodies against CD44v6 blocked the activation of the c-Met receptor, siRNA against CD44v6 abrogated c-Met activation, expression of the ectodomain of CD44v6 had a similar effect probably competing out HGF and c-Met, HGF and CD44v6 were all found in one complex. Finally, the transfection of CD44v6 in cells that express the c-Met receptor but did not respond to HGF treatment, rendered these cells HGF responsive [50, 51].

Not only was the ectodomain of CD44v6 required for the response of cells to HGF but the cytoplasmic tail of CD44v6 was also necessary. A mutant truncated in the cytoplasmic tail allowed activation of the c-Met receptor upon HGF treatment but did not induce signal transduction [52]. Furthermore, expression of CD44 cytoplasmic tails in c-Met responsive cells blocked signal transduction mediated by c-Met. Close analysis revealed that the cytoplasmic tail of CD44v6 binds ERM proteins (Ezrin, Radixin, Moesin) that in turn trap the cytoskeleton to CD44v6 and thus to the membrane. This recruitment of the cytoskeleton to the membrane, in the vicinity of the activated c-Met receptor, is a prerequisite for the activation of Ras by a guanidine exchange factor and for downstream signaling [52]. A scheme of all these functions is presented in Figure 3.1.

3.4
Three Amino Acids in CD44 Exon v6 Are Crucial for the CD44v6 Coreceptor Function, and Small Peptides Can Interfere with This Function

A CD44 isoform containing exclusively an exon from the variable region, exon v6, was sufficient to enable activation of the c-Met receptor (and its relative Ron as well [50]). The v6 exon comprises 42 amino acids or 126 base pairs. Linker scan

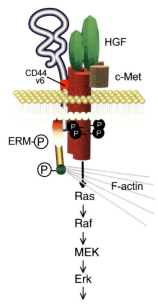

Figure 3.1 Scheme indicating the coreceptor function of CD44v6 for c-Met. For an explanation see text.

mutation analysis of rat CD44v6 revealed that when three of these amino acids in the center of exon v6 (EWQ) were replaced by alanines, the coreceptor function of CD44v6 for c-Met was lost [51]. This mutant was, however, not impaired in HA binding. Mutation of any of the other amino acids in the v6 exon had no impact on the function of the CD44 protein as a coreceptor. Interestingly, even mutation of only one or of two of the amino acids within the critical triplet did not destroy the coreceptor function (Figure 3.2).

Taken together, these results suggest that small peptides comprising these three critical amino acids might interfere with the coreceptor function of CD44v6 for c-Met. This was indeed the case. A 14 mer and even a 5 mer harboring the EWQ sequence completely blocked c-Met activation. Sequences outside EWQ had no impact on this inhibition, but the EWQ sequence alone as a 3mer, was inactive [51]. Mutation of the central tryptophan did not change the inhibitory property of the peptide, but when two of the three amino acids were changed, the inhibition of the coreceptor function was lost (Figure 3.3).

Interestingly, the homologous human and mouse sequences differ from the rat EWQ sequence. The human sequence is RWH whereas the mouse sequence corresponds to GWQ. Peptides containing these sequences act in a species-specific manner. The rat peptides interfered with c-Met activation only in rat cells, and accordingly the mouse and human peptides inhibited c-Met activation only in mouse and human cells respectively [51] (and Figure 3.3).

The fact that these peptides act in a species-specific manner was very surprising. Indeed, competition experiments in which the expression of the CD44v6

(a)

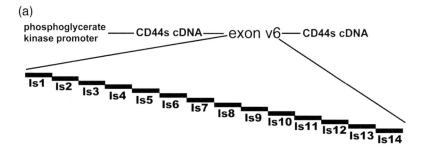

Is1	Is2	Is3	Is4	Is5
TGG GCA GAT	CCT AAT AGC	ACA ACA GAA	GAA GCA GCT	ACC CAG AAG
Trp Ala Asp	Pro Asn Ser	Thr Thr Glu	Glu Ala Ala	Thr Gln Lys

Is6	Is7	Is8	Is9	Is10
GAG AAG TGG	TTT GAG AAT	GAA TGG CAG	GGG AAG AAC	CCA CCC ACC
Glu Lys Trp	Phe Glu Asn	Glu Trp Gln	Gly Lys Asn	Pro Pro Thr

Is11	Is12	Is13	Is14	
CCA AGT GAA	GAC TCC CAT	GTG ACA GAA	GGG ACA ACT	G
Pro Ser Glu	Asp Ser His	Val Thr Glu	Gly Thr Thr	

(b)

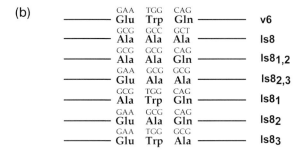

	GAA	TGG	CAG	
———	Glu	Trp	Gln	——— v6
	GCG	GCC	GCT	
———	Ala	Ala	Ala	——— Is8
	GCG	GCG	CAG	
———	Ala	Ala	Gln	——— Is8₁,₂
	GAA	GCG	GCG	
———	Glu	Ala	Ala	——— Is8₂,₃
	GCG	TGG	CAG	
———	Ala	Trp	Gln	——— Is8₁
	GAA	GCG	CAG	
———	Glu	Ala	Gln	——— Is8₂
	GAA	TGG	GCG	
———	Glu	Trp	Ala	——— Is8₃

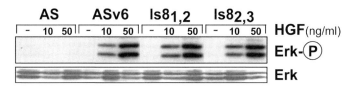

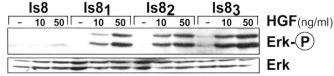

Figure 3.2 (a) Schematic representation of the linker scan mutants of CD44 exon v6 used to transfect the rat pancreas carcinoma cells Bsp73AS [51] (abbreviated to AS in panel b). The exon v6 was mutated in steps of 3 amino acids that were replaced by alanines. The mutated sequences contained a Not I site used to screen the mutants. Triplets already coding for alanines were changed to glycines. (b) Transfection of Bsp73AS cells with CD44v6 or with linker scan mutants rendered these cells responsive to HGF treatment, except in the case of Is8 (see also [51]). Only CD44v6 and Is8 transfectants are shown here. The activation of Erk (Erk-P) was used as a read-out for c-Met activation. Mutation of either one or two amino acids in the Is8 sequence (see scheme) did not interfere with the coreceptor function of CD44v6 for c-Met.

(a)

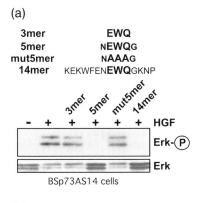

3mer	EWQ
5mer	NEWQG
mut5mer	NAAAG
14mer	KEKWFEN**EWQ**GKNP

BSp73AS14 cells

(b)

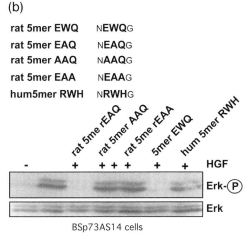

rat 5mer EWQ	NEWQG
rat 5mer EAQ	NEAQG
rat 5mer AAQ	NAAQG
rat 5mer EAA	NEAAG
hum5mer RWH	NRWHG

BSp73AS14 cells

Figure 3.3 (a) Peptides containing the sequence (EWQ) decisive for the coreceptor function of CD44v6 that was mutated in the ls8 mutant inhibit HGF responsive cells. A 3mer corresponding to the EWQ sequence has no effect whereas a 5mer or a 14mer are able to efficiently block HGF activation of Erk. A mutant peptide harboring 3 alanines is used as a control. The Bsp73AS14 cells have already been described [50]. (b) The effect of single amino acid exchanges in the 5mer peptide is shown.

ectodomain interferes with c-Met activation showed no such species specificity e. g. the rat ectodomain blocked the activation of c-Met in human cells [50] (and Figure 3.4). A solution to this seemingly contradictive finding came from the following experiment. The inhibition of c-Met activation by expression of the rat CD44v6 ectodomain in human cells was released by addition of the rat peptides (Figure 3.4). Thus the target of the rat peptides must be the rat CD44v6 ectodomain as the rat peptides cannot address human c-Met. We suspect that the CD44v6 molecules must adopt a specific folding so that they can act as coreceptors for c-Met and that the peptides interfere with this conformation (see scheme in Figure 3.4).

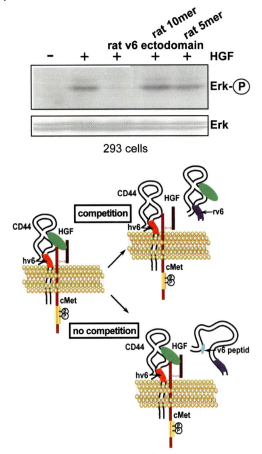

Figure 3.4 In the human 293 cells, the response to HGF treatment can be blocked by expression of the rat CD44v6 ectodomain. This inhibition can be released by a simultaneous treatment with rat CD44v6 specific peptides.

3.5
The Ectodomain of CD44v6 Binds to HGF

These results raise the question of the contribution of the ectodomain of CD44v6 to c-Met activation. Possibilities are that CD44v6 itself binds the ligand HGF and presents it to its authentic receptor or that CD44v6 stabilises the binding of the ligand to c-Met. To test these possibilities, binding of HGF to cells that either express only the c-Met receptor or only CD44v6 or both together was examined. Whereas cells that express both CD44v6 and c-Met show binding to HGF in FACS analysis, no binding was detected in cells expressing only c-Met (and in which the c-Met receptor could not be activated by HGF, for example, the Bsp73AS cells used in Figure 3.2 for transfection). In contrast, cells that express CD44v6 but not the c-Met receptor were able to bind HGF (Figure 3.5). Thus, one of the functions of the CD44v6 ectodomain appears to be the binding and the presention of the ligand HGF to the c-Met receptor. In agreement with this assumption, expression of the ectodomain of CD44v6 in the supernatant of CD44v6 expressing cells competed with binding of HGF to the cells (Figure 3.5). This binding is strictly dependent on the correct folding of the ectodomain since the peptides that abrogate c-Met activation inhibit also the HGF binding to cells expressing only CD44v6 (Figure 3.5).

The Ron receptor, a close relative of c-Met that is activated by its ligand MSP, also needs CD44v6 as a coreceptor. Its activation can be blocked by the same peptides that abrogate c-Met activation (these are of course the human CD44v6 peptides since Ron is a human receptor [51]). The mode of action of these peptides that interfere with the tertiary structure of CD44v6 can explain this at the first sight surprising finding.

3.6
Peptides Corresponding to Exon v6 of CD44 Inhibit Metastatic Spread of Tumor Cells

Originally, the role of CD44 isoforms in the metastatic process was shown on rat pancreatic tumor cells predominantly expressing CD44v4-v7 and CD44v6,v7. One of the key experiments was that transfection of expression vectors for either the CD44v4-v7 or the CD44v6,v7 variant proteins in non-metastatic rat pancreatic tumor cells rendered them metastatic [37, 38]. Interestingly, the recipient non-metastatic tumor cells express the c-Met receptor, but the receptor cannot be activated by HGF. In the CD44v4-v7 and CD44v6,v7 transfected cells, however, the c-Met receptor was fully reponsive to HGF [50]. If the coreceptor function of CD44v6 for c-Met would suffice for metastasis formation then the transfection of a CD44 variant containing only the exon v6 should also promote metastatic spread. Subcutaneous injection of such CD44v6 transfected tumor cells led in all cases to the formation of lung and lymph node metastases (in auxiliary lymph nodes on the side of injection; Table 3.1). Injection of the recipient ("non-metastatic") tumor cells into syngeneic rats only led to the development of primary tumors. Thus, similarly to CD44v4-v7 and CD44v6,v7 [37, 38], CD44v6 is sufficient to confer metastatic propensity to the non-metastatic tumor cells consistent with the assumption that the coreceptor function of CD44v6 for c-Met might be the decisive step for metastatic spread.

To further address this question, we tested whether the CD44v6 peptides that interfere with the activation of the c-Met receptor would also repress the metastatic spread of the rat pancreatic tumor cells. In a spontaneous metastasis assay, v6 or control peptides were injected at the site of tumor cell every second day. Injection

T47D cells
(-Met, +CD44v6)

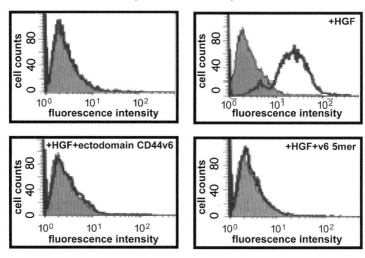

transfected T47D cells
(+Met, +CD44v6)

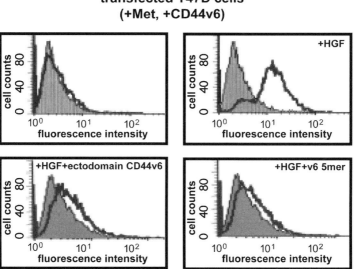

Figure 3.5 Binding of biotinylated HGF to human mammary carcinoma cells (T47D) that express CD44v6 and c-Met as indicated. Binding was measured in a fluorescence activated cell sorter using FITC-conjugated streptavidin for the detection of biotin.

Table 3.1 CD44v6-transfected Bsp73AS cells were injected subcutaneously into syngeneic BDX rats. Peptides or antibodies were injected three times per week directly into the tumor. Moribund animals were killed and further analyzed. The relative lymph node increase was calculated by comparing the weight of the axillary lymph node at the site of tumor injection with the one from the opposite site.

Treatment	Tumor volume (mm³)	Relative lymph nodeincrease	No. of lung metastases
PBS-treated			
Female 1	8380	1.30	43
Female 2	8432	1.45	15
Male 1	6800	1.00	>50
Male 2	11600	1.00	11
Treatment with ctrl peptide			
Female 3	1071	1.76	34
Female 4	3588	1.97	13
Male 3	6400	2.50	29
Male 4	34020	2.04	>50
Treatment with v6 mAbs			
Female 5	2145	1	0
Female 6	126	1	0
Male 5	7956	1	0
Male 6	9828	1	1
Treatment with v6 peptide			
Female 7	3800	1	1
Female 8	3348	1	0
Male 7	32938	1	0
Male 8	1368	1	0

PBS = phosphate-buffered saline.

of unrelated peptides had no influence on the formation of lymph node or lung metastases whereas the injection of the v6 peptides however, completely abrogated metastases formation (Table 3.1) similar to the injection of CD44 v6 specific antibodies. The growth of the primary tumor was not affected by the v6 peptides (Table 3.1).

3.7
The Significance of the Collaboration between CD44v6 and c-Met *In Vivo*

Given the importance of CD44 in many physiological processes and in the regulation of cellular fate, and given its decisive role as a coreceptor for c-Met, it was surprising that CD44 knockout mice were viable [53, 54]. A plausible explanation can be that functions of CD44 proteins are substituted by other proteins in the

CD44 knockout mice. Several lines of evidence speak for this interpretation. The main argument is derived from the finding that specific down-regulation of CD44 expression in the skin of mice resulted in a severe phenotype. The suppression of CD44 in skin keratinocytes was achieved by expression of CD44 antisense sequences under the control of the keratin-5 promoter [55] active at E10.5. In these animals severe skin defects were observed ranging from blistering, delayed wound healing and hair re-growth, to accumulation of hyaluronan and impaired tumor promotion [55, 56]. This discrepancy between the CD44 knockout mice that have no skin phenotype, and the severe skin phenotype in the "conditional" knockout mice is in agreement with a substitution of CD44 functions. Substitution of CD44 functions can apparently no longer occur at the time at which the K5 promoter gets activated and CD44 is shut off in keratinocytes. In agreement with such a "point of no further substitution" are minor defects observed in the total CD44 knockout mice. All these defects occur in processes that are established late in embryogenesis or in the adult organism, for example, in inflammatory processes or tissue regression [57–60].

The function of CD44 as a coreceptor for c-Met must also be taken over by other proteins in the CD44 knockout mice. Indeed, the mild phenotype observed in the case of the CD44 knockout differs from the c-Met knockout mice that die between embryonic days E12.5 to E16 from a placental defect [61]. In a first approach to demonstrate a substitution of CD44 and an interconnection between CD44 and c-Met *in vivo*, we crossed cd44 knockout mice with c-met heterozygote mice. The rationale for the cross is as follows: met heterozygote mice in a cd44$^{+/+}$ (or cd44$^{+/-}$) background develop normally. We hypothesize that a substituting coreceptor of c-Met in a cd44$^{-/-}$ mouse may not work as efficiently as CD44v6 and that met might therefore be haplo-insufficient in the context of the cd44$^{-/-}$ mice. This is exactly what we observed: the yield of alive mice with the genotype cd44$^{-/-}$;met$^{+/-}$ was dramatically reduced. Only 30% of animals with this genotype survived, 70% died from a breathing defect within a few hours after birth [62]. Their lungs were not inflated most likely as a result of an impaired synaptic transmission in the brain stem respiratory rhythm-generating network and of alterations in the phrenic nerve that innervates the diaphragm [62]. In conclusion, these crosses indicate i) that a substitution for the CD44 coreceptor function has occurred ii) that the substitute molecule exerts a function that allows normal embryonic development only in a met$^{+/+}$ background and iii) that CD44 and c-Met cooperate in wild type mice. These results also suggest that the coreceptor function of CD44 for c-Met is essential for synaptogenesis and the development of axon/nerve fibers in the peripheral and central nervous system.

3.8
The CD44v6 Peptides Interfere with Angiogenesis

In order to address the specificity of the coreceptor function of CD44v6, several other RTKs were examined for their response to treatment with CD44 specific antibodies. Whereas the PDGF receptor was not affected by this treatment, the activation of the NGF receptor, trk, was strongly inhibited [50]. In the case of the EGF-R family of RTKs it turned out that several CD44 isoforms are involved. EGF receptors are dimers composed of four different single chains, ErbB1-4 [63]. The various combinations are addressed by several ligands. Furthermore, the same combination can be activated by different ligands. Blocking experiments with CD44v6 specific antibodies revealed that in some cases CD44v6 containing iso-forms were necessary, for example, for the activation of EGF-R by EGF. On the contrary, activation by TGFα that addresses the same EGF receptor as EGF, cannot be blocked by CD44v6 antibodies (our unpublished results). This suggests that the ligand determines the specificity of the coreceptor. Activation by HB-EGF requires CD44 isoforms modified by heparan sulfate. In this case CD44v3 appears to be required for the processing of pro HB-EGF. CD44v3 binds and activates the metal-loprotease MMP7 that then can process proHB-EGF leading to the activation of the receptor [60].

Also the activation of the vascular endothelial growth factor receptor (VEGF-R2) can be blocked by CD44v6 antibodies on endothelial cells (EC; our unpublished results). Since it has been shown that VEGF can bind to HSPGs [64] it might be that the CD44 isoform on endothelial cells also contains exon v3, which can be modified by heparan sulfate and exon v6 sequences. Interestingly the exon v6 specific peptides that interfere with c-Met activation also block the activation of the VEGF receptor suggesting that the CD44 variant isoform might bind and present VEGF to its authentic receptor, similar to the case of HGF/c-Met.

There is ample evidence that CD44 isoforms play decisive roles in angiogenesis. bFGF and VEGF upregulate CD44 on endothelial cells in vivo and targeting of CD44 by specific antibodies leads to EC death [65]. EC proliferation and capillary formation in fibrin matrix is repressed by CD44 specific antibodies [66]. The adhe-sion of ECs to hyaluronan and their poliferation were dependent on CD44 [67]. CD44, together with bFGF are involved in tubule formation of ECs in collagen gels [68, 69] and the development of endothelial tubular network was impaired in CD44 knockout mice [70]. Finally CD44v3 was detected in EC cell lines and their chemotaxis was blocked by exon v3 specific antibodies [71]. We tested the response of CD44v6 peptides on migration of endothelial cells in wound healing assays, sprouting of endothelial cells from spheroids and tubule formation of endothelial cells on collagen. In all these assays, the exon v6 peptides interfered with the angiogenic propensity of the endothelial cells that were stimulated with VEGF (our unpublished results). Furthermore, although the VEGF-R2 receptor is the most prominent RTK involved in angiogenesis, c-Met (and EGF-R) also seems to play a role in this process [72]. Consequently the CD44v6 peptides also blocked the angiogenic response of ECs when they were stimulated with HGF alone or with both, VEGF and HGF together (our unpublished results).

Thus, the CD44v6 peptides not only inhibit effectively metastatic spread of pancreas carcinoma cells but also block angiogenesis, most likely by interfering with the coreceptor function of CD44v6 for c-Met and VEGF-R2 on endothelial cells.

3.9
Outlook

Since the discovery of the hybridoma technology by Köhler and Milstein [73] strategies to fight cancer focused on the development of monoclonal antibodies (mAbs) against tumor epitopes. Several mAbs that target cell surface receptors are now in clinical trials underscoring the success of this approach. Some of these antibodies that are not modified bind and inhibit tumor growth by interfering with proliferation induced by these receptors, for example, IMC-C225 cetuximab, an anti EGFR mAb [74]. Some are conjugated to toxins, for example, Mylotarg, a humanisied anti-CD33 mAb linked to calicheamicin [75]. Many of the antibodies are conjugated to radionuclides and serve as targeting agents to carry the radioactive load to the cancer cells.

Also CD44v6 mAbs have gone through clinical trials [76–78]. Labeled antibodies were used in a phase I therapy study on patients with head and neck squamous carcinoma [79–81] and a toxin conjugated CD44v6 mAb was applied in a phase I dose escalation study [82]. Since two of the seven patients treated with the toxin-conjugated mAbs showed severe skin toxicity the clinical study was discontinued [82].

A major limitation of mAbs as targets for cancer is their relatively large size with a molecular weight of 160 000. This size makes it difficult to reach the interior of a larger tumor mass where the supply with blood is inadequate. Reduction of their size by developing single chain antibodies with a molecular weight of 25 000 addresses this problem but does not overcome it. Another problem of therapies using mAbs is their non specific uptake into the reticuloendothelial system such as liver, spleen and bone marrow where they lead to dose-limiting toxicities particular in the case of radiolabeled or toxin conjugated mAbs [83, 84]. Cell surface binding peptides can overcome these drawbacks. They are considerably smaller than mAbs and in general do not bind to the reticuloendothelial system. Furthermore, they are easily synthesized chemically and therefore much cheaper than mAbs. Their degradation by the proteolytic systems can be prevented by chemical modifications such as incorporation of D-amino acids or cyclisation.

One of the first peptides identified by means of phage display library screens for selective binders to tumors, were peptides that bind to integrins such as RGD peptides (for review see [85, 86]). RGD is the recognition site of fibronectin for integrin $\alpha v\beta 3$. Cyclic RGD peptides and modification of the peptides are tested as antitumorigenic, antimetastatic and antiangiogenic agents [87–89].

Using a variety of combinational library methods, several peptides have been identified within the last years that interact with surface proteins on cancer cells or recognize proteins on the surface of endothelial cells and are thus promising candidates for interference with tumor growth and metastatic spread (for a review see [90]). Among these peptides are some that interfere with the activity of RTKs. An anti VEGF-R1 (flt1) hexapeptide interferes with the binding of VEGFs to VEGF-R1 and thereby blocks tumor growth and metastasis [91]. A peptide inhibiting VEGF binding to neuropilin-1, a coreceptor for VEGF-R, retards breast cancer angiogenesis and growth [92]. Among several laminin α5 synthetic peptides one peptide seems to bind to CD44 exon v3 modified by heparan sulfate and thereby interferes with binding and activation of a colon carcinoma cell by FGF2 [93]. This peptide apparently interferes with the coreceptor function of CD44v3 for FGF-R1. A peptide that prevents dimerisation of ErbB2 was recently designed using in silico docking studies and computational methods [94]. This rationally designed small antagonist peptide inhibited proliferation of human breast cancer cells.

A c-Met specific peptide was developed that prevents activation of the c-Met receptor upon binding to the C-terminal cytoplasmic tail. This peptide is highly selective as it does not inhibit EGF, PDGF or VEGF receptors [95]. To mediate its entry inside the cells the peptide has to be coupled to the Antennapedia internalization domain.

Our peptides developed on the basis of the coreceptor function of CD44v6 interfere with the activation of a variety of RTKs most of which are determinants of pathological developments and can be seen as a tool with broad specificity to fight cancer and other angiogenesis dependent diseases.

References

1 Robinson, D.R., Wu, Y.M. and Lin, S.F. (2000) The protein tyrosine kinase family of the human genome. *Oncogene*, **19**, 5548–57.

2 Hubbard, S.R. and Till, J.H. (2000) Protein tyrosine kinase structure and function. *Annu. Rev. Biochem.*, **69**, 373–98.

3 Libermann, T.A., Nusbaum, H.R., Razon, N., Kris, R., Lax, I., Soreq, H., Whittle, N., Waterfield, M.D., Ullrich, A. and Schlessinger, J. (1985) Amplification, enhanced expression and possible rearrangement of EGF receptor gene in primary human brain tumours of glial origin. *Nature*, **313**, 144–7.

4 Ullrich, A., Coussens, L., Hayflick, J.S., Dull, T.J., Gray, A., Tam, A.W., Lee, J., Yarden, Y., Libermann, T.A., Schlessinger, J. *et al.* (1984) Human epidermal growth factor receptor cDNA sequence and aberrant expression of the amplified gene in A431 epidermoid carcinoma cells. *Nature*, **309**, 418–25.

5 Derynck, R., Goeddel, D.V., Ullrich, A., Gutterman, J.U., Williams, R.D., Bringman, T.S. and Berger, W.H. (1987) Synthesis of messenger RNAs for transforming growth factors alpha and beta and the epidermal growth factor receptor by human tumors. *Cancer Res.*, **47**, 707–12.

6 Kaleko, M., Rutter, W.J. and Miller, A.D. (1990) Overexpression of the human insulinlike growth factor I receptor promotes ligand-dependent neoplastic transformation. *Mol. Cell Biol.*, **10**, 464–73.

7 Trusolino, L., Bertotti, A. and Comoglio, P.M. (2001) A signaling adapter function for alpha6beta4 integrin in the control of HGF-dependent invasive growth. *Cell*, **107**, 643–54.

8 Chappuis-Flament, S., Pasini, A., De Vita, G., Segouffin-Cariou, C., Fusco, A., Attie, T., Lenoir, G.M., Santoro, M. and Billaud, M. (1998) Dual effect on the RET receptor of MEN 2 mutations affecting specific extracytoplasmic cysteines. *Oncogene*, **17**, 2851–61.

9 Chesi, M., Nardini, E., Brents, L.A., Schrock, E., Ried, T., Kuehl, W.M. and Bergsagel, P.L. (1997) Frequent translocation t(4;14)(p16.3;q32.3) in multiple myeloma is associated with increased expression and activating mutations of fibroblast growth factor receptor 3. *Nat. Genet.*, **16**, 260–4.

10 Jeffers, M., Fiscella, M., Webb, C.P., Anver, M., Koochekpour, S. and Vande Woude, G.F. (1998) The mutationally activated Met receptor mediates motility and metastasis. *Proc. Natl. Acad. Sci. U. S. A.*, **95**, 14417–22.

11 Kannan, K. and Givol, D. (2000) FGF receptor mutations: dimerization syndromes, cell growth suppression, and animal models. *IUBMB Life*, **49**, 197–205.

12 Nishikawa, R., Ji, X.D., Harmon, R.C., Lazar, C.S., Gill, G.N., Cavenee, W.K. and Huang, H.J. (1994) A mutant epidermal growth factor receptor common in human glioma confers enhanced tumorigenicity. *Proc. Natl. Acad. Sci. U. S. A.*, **91**, 7727–31.

13 Schmidt, L., Duh, F.M., Chen, F., Kishida, T., Glenn, G., Choyke, P., Scherer, S.W., Zhuang, Z., Lubensky, I., Dean, M., Allikmets, R., Chidambaram, A., Bergerheim, U.R., Feltis, J.T., Casadevall, C., Zamarron, A., Bernues, M., Richard, S., Lips, C.J., Walther, M.M., Tsui, L.C., Geil, L., Orcutt, M.L., Stackhouse, T., Zbar, B. *et al.* (1997) Germline and somatic mutations in the tyrosine kinase domain of the MET proto-oncogene in papillary renal carcinomas. *Nat. Genet.*, **16**, 68–73.

14 Dikic, I. and Giordano, S. (2003) Negative receptor signalling. *Curr. Opin. Cell Biol.*, **15**, 128–35.

15 Bange, J., Zwick, E. and Ullrich, A. (2001) Molecular targets for breast cancer therapy and prevention. *Nat. Med.*, **7**, 548–52.

16 Snyder, L.C., Astsaturov, I. and Weiner, L.M. (2005) Overview of monoclonal antibodies and small molecules targeting the epidermal growth factor receptor pathway in colorectal cancer. *Clin. Colorectal. Cancer*, **5**, S71–80.Suppl 2

17 Bruns, C.J., Solorzano, C.C., Harbison, M.T., Ozawa, S., Tsan, R., Fan, D., Abbruzzese, J., Traxler, P., Buchdunger, E., Radinsky, R. and Fidler, I.J. (2000) Blockade of the epidermal growth factor receptor signaling by a novel tyrosine kinase inhibitor leads to apoptosis of endothelial cells and therapy of human pancreatic carcinoma. *Cancer Res.*, **60**, 2926–35.

18 Ciardiello, F. (2000) Epidermal growth factor receptor tyrosine kinase inhibitors as anticancer agents. *Drugs*, **60** (Suppl. 1), 25–32; discussion 41–2.

19 Hidalgo, M., Siu, L.L., Nemunaitis, J., Rizzo, J., Hammond, L.A., Takimoto, C., Eckhardt, S.G., Tolcher, A., Britten, C.D., Denis, L., Ferrante, K., Von Hoff, D.D., Silberman, S. and Rowinsky, E.K. (2001) Phase I and pharmacologic study of OSI-774, an epidermal growth factor receptor tyrosine kinase inhibitor, in patients with advanced solid malignancies. *J. Clin. Oncol.*, **19**, 3267–79.

20 Druker, B.J., Sawyers, C.L., Kantarjian, H., Resta, D.J., Reese, S.F., Ford, J.M., Capdeville, R. and Talpaz, M. (2001) Activity of a specific inhibitor of the BCR-ABL tyrosine kinase in the blast crisis of chronic myeloid leukemia and acute lymphoblastic leukemia with the Philadelphia chromosome. *N. Engl. J. Med.*, **344**, 1038–42.

21 Druker, B.J., Talpaz, M., Resta, D.J., Peng, B., Buchdunger, E., Ford, J.M., Lydon, N.B., Kantarjian, H., Capdeville, R., Ohno-Jones, S. and Sawyers, C.L. (2001) Efficacy and safety of a specific inhibitor of the BCR-ABL tyrosine kinase in chronic myeloid leukemia. *N. Engl. J. Med.*, **344**, 1031–7.

22 Yayon, A., Klagsbrun, M., Esko, J.D., Leder, P. and Ornitz, D.M. (1991) Cell surface, heparin-like molecules are required for binding of basic fibroblast growth factor to its high affinity receptor. *Cell*, **64**, 841–8.

23 Christofori, G. (2003) Changing neighbours, changing behaviour: cell adhesion molecule-mediated signalling during tumour progression. *EMBO J.*, **22**, 2318–23.

24 Dalchau, R., Kirkley, J. and Fabre, J.W. (1980) Monoclonal antibody to a human brain-granulocyte-T lymphocyte antigen probably homologous to the W 3/13 antigen of the rat. *Eur. J. Immunol.*, **10**, 745–9.

25 Naor, D., Sionov, R.V. and Ish-Shalom, D. (1997) CD44: structure, function and association with the malignant process, in *Advances in Cancer Research*, Vol. 71 (eds G.F. Vande Woude and G. Klein),

Harcourt Brace and Company, Academic Press, San Diego, pp. 243–318.

26 Screaton, G.R., Bell, M.V., Jackson, D.G., Cornelis, F.B., Gerth, U. and Bell, J.I. (1992) Genomic structure of DNA encoding the lymphocyte homing receptor CD44 reveals at least 12 alternatively spliced exons. *Proc. Natl. Acad. Sci. U. S. A.*, **89**, 12160–4.

27 Tölg, C., Hofmann, M., Herrlich, P. and Ponta, H. (1993) Splicing choice from ten variant exons establishes CD44 variability. *Nucleic Acids Res.*, **21**, 1225–9.

28 Ponta, H., Sherman, L. and Herrlich, P.A. (2003) CD44: from adhesion molecules to signalling regulators. *Nat. Rev. Mol. Cell Biol.*, **4**, 33–45.

29 Jalkanen, S.T., Bargatze, R.F., Herron, L.R. and Butcher, E.C. (1986) A lymphoid cell surface glycoprotein involved in endothelial cell recognition and lymphocyte homing in man. *Eur. J. Immunol.*, **16**, 1195–202.

30 Trowbridge, I.S., Lesley, J., Schulte, R., Hyman, R. and Trotter, J. (1982) Biochemical characterization and cellular distribution of a polymorphic, murine cell-surface glycoprotein expressed on lymphoid tissues. *Immunogenetics*, **15**, 299–312.

31 Arch, R., Wirth, K., Hofmann, M., Ponta, H., Matzku, S., Herrlich, P. and Zöller, M. (1992) Participation in normal immune responses of a splice variant of CD44 that encodes a metastasis-inducing domain. *Science*, **257**, 682–5.

32 Moll, J., Schmidt, A., van der Putten, H., Plug, R., Ponta, H., Herrlich, P. and Zoller, M. (1996) Accelerated immune response in transgenic mice expressing rat CD44v4-v7 on T cells. *J. Immunol.*, **156**, 2085–94.

33 Khaldoyanidi, S., Karakhanova, S., Sleeman, J., Herrlich, P. and Ponta, H. (2002) CD44 variant-specific antibodies trigger hemopoiesis by selective release of cytokines from bone marrow macrophages. *Blood*, **99**, 3955–61.

34 Miyake, K., Medina, K.L., Hayashi, S., Ono, S., Hamaoka, T. and Kincade, P.W. (1990) Monoclonal antibodies to Pgp-1/ CD44 block lympho-hemopoiesis in long- term bone marrow cultures. *J. Exp. Med.*, **171**, 477–88.

35 Moll, J., Khaldoyanidi, S., Sleeman, J.P., Achtnich, M., Preuss, I., Ponta, H. and Herrlich, P. (1998) Two different functions for CD44 proteins in human myelopoiesis. *J. Clin. Invest.*, **102**, 1024–34.

36 Aruffo, A., Stamenkovic, I., Melnick, M., Underhill, C.B. and Seed, B. (1990) CD44 is the principal cell surface receptor for hyaluronate. *Cell*, **61**, 1303–13.

37 Günthert, U., Hofmann, M., Rudy, W., Reber, S., Zöller, M., Haußmann, I., Matzku, S., Wenzel, A., Ponta, H. and Herrlich, P. (1991) A new variant of glycoprotein CD44 confers metastatic potential to rat carcinoma cells. *Cell*, **65**, 13–24.

38 Rudy, W., Hofmann, M., Schwartz-Albiez, R., Zoller, M., Heider, K.H., Ponta, H. and Herrlich, P. (1993) The two major CD44 proteins expressed on a metastatic rat tumor cell line are derived from different splice variants: each one individually suffices to confer metastatic behavior. *Cancer Res.*, **53**, 1262–8.

39 Naor, D., Nedvetzki, S., Golan, I., Melnik, L. and Faitelson, Y. (2002) CD44 in cancer. *Crit. Rev. Clin. Lab. Sci.*, **39**, 527–79.

40 Stamenkovic, I., Aruffo, A., Amiot, M. and Seed, B. (1991) The hematopoietic and epithelial forms of CD44 are distinct polypeptides with different adhesion potentials for hyaluronate-bearing cells. *EMBO J.*, **10**, 343–8.

41 Sleeman, J., Kondo, K., Moll, J., Ponta, H. and Herrlich, P. (1997) Variant exons v6 and v7 together expand the repertoire of glycosaminoglycans bound by CD44. *J. Biol. Chem.*, **272**, 31837–44.

42 Sleeman, J., Rudy, W., Hofmann, M., Moll, J., Herrlich, P. and Ponta, H. (1996) Regulated clustering of variant CD44 proteins increases their hyaluronate binding capacity. *J. Cell Biol.*, **135**, 1139–50.

43 Sleeman, J.P., Arming, S., Moll, J.F., Hekele, A., Rudy, W., Sherman, L.S., Kreil, G., Ponta, H. and Herrlich, P. (1996) Hyaluronate-independent metastatic behavior of CD44 variant-

expressing pancreatic carcinoma cells. *Cancer Res.*, **56**, 3134–41.

44 Jackson, D.G., Bell, J.I., Dickinson, R., Timans, J., Shields, J. and Whittle, N. (1995) Proteoglycan forms of the lymphocyte homing receptor CD44 are alternatively spliced variants containing the v3 exon. *J. Cell Biol.*, **128**, 673–85.

45 Bennett, K.L., Jackson, D.G., Simon, J.C., Tanczos, E., Peach, R., Modrell, B., Stamenkovic, I., Plowman, G. and Aruffo, A. (1995) CD44 isoforms containing exon v3 are responsible for the presentation of heparin-binding growth factor. *J. Cell Biol.*, **128**, 687–98.

46 Sherman, L., Wainwright, D., Ponta, H. and Herrlich, P. (1998) A splice variant of CD44 expressed in the apical ectodermal ridge presents fibroblast growth factors to limb mesenchyme and is required for limb outgrowth. *Genes Dev.*, **12**, 1058–71.

47 Montesano, R., Schaller, G. and Orci, L. (1991) Induction of epithelial tubular morphogenesis in vitro by fibroblast-derived soluble factors. *Cell*, **66**, 697–711.

48 Nakamura, T., Teramoto, H. and Ichihara, A. (1986) Purification and characterization of a growth factor from rat platelets for mature parenchymal hepatocytes in primary cultures. *Proc. Natl. Acad. Sci. U. S. A.*, **83**, 6489–93.

49 Stoker, M., Gherardi, E., Perryman, M. and Gray, J. (1987) Scatter factor is a fibroblast-derived modulator of epithelial cell mobility. *Nature*, **327**, 239–42.

50 Orian-Rousseau, V., Chen, L., Sleeman, J.P., Herrlich, P. and Ponta, H. (2002) CD44 is required for two consecutive steps in HGF/c-Met signaling. *Genes Dev.*, **16**, 3074–86.

51 Matzke, A., Herrlich, P., Ponta, H. and Orian-Rousseau, V. (2005) A 5-amino-acid peptide blocks Met and Ron dependent cell migration. *Cancer Res.*, **65**, 6105–10.

52 Orian-Rousseau, V., Morrison, H., Matzke, A., Kastilan, T., Pace, G., Herrlich, P. and Ponta, H. (2007) Hepatocyte Growth Factor-induced Ras Activation Requires ERM Proteins Linked to Both CD44v6 and F-Actin. *Mol. Biol. Cell*, **18**, 76–83.

53 Protin, U., Schweighoffer, T., Jochum, W. and Hilberg, F. (1999) CD44-deficient

mice develop normally with changes in subpopulations and recirculation of lymphocyte subsets. *J. Immunol.*, **163**, 4917–23.

54 Schmits, R., Filmus, J., Gerwin, N., Senaldi, G., Kiefer, F., Kundig, T., Wakeham, A., Shahinian, A., Catzavelos, C., Rak, J., Furlonger, C., Zakarian, A., Simard, J.J., Ohashi, P.S., Paige, C.J., Gutierrez-Ramos, J.C. and Mak, T.W. (1997) CD44 regulates hematopoietic progenitor distribution, granuloma formation, and tumorigenicity. *Blood*, **90**, 2217–33.

55 Kaya, G., Rodriguez, I., Jorcano, J.L., Vassalli, P. and Stamenkovic, I. (1997) Selective suppression of CD44 in keratinocytes of mice bearing an antisense CD44 transgene driven by a tissue-specific promoter disrupts hyaluronate metabolism in the skin and impairs keratinocyte proliferation. *Genes Dev.*, **11**, 996–1007.

56 Kaya, G., Rodriguez, I., Jorcano, J.L., Vassalli, P. and Stamenkovic, I. (1999) Cutaneous delayed-type hypersensitivity response is inhibited in transgenic mice with keratinocyte-specific CD44 expression defect. *J. Invest. Dermatol.*, **113**, 137–8.

57 Chen, D., McKallip, R.J., Zeytun, A., Do, Y., Lombard, C., Robertson, J.L., Mak, T.W., Nagarkatti, P.S. and Nagarkatti, M. (2001) CD44-deficient mice exhibit enhanced hepatitis after concanavalin A injection: evidence for involvement of CD44 in activation-induced cell death. *J. Immunol.*, **166**, 5889–97.

58 Cuff, C.A., Kothapalli, D., Azonobi, I., Chun, S., Zhang, Y., Belkin, R., Yeh, C., Secreto, A., Assoian, R.K., Rader, D.J. and Pure, E. (2001) The adhesion receptor CD44 promotes atherosclerosis by mediating inflammatory cell recruitment and vascular cell activation. *J. Clin. Invest.*, **108**, 1031–40.

59 Stoop, R., Kotani, H., McNeish, J.D., Otterness, I.G. and Mikecz, K. (2001) Increased resistance to collagen-induced arthritis in CD44-deficient DBA/1 mice. *Arthritis Rheum.*, **44**, 2922–31.

60 Yu, W.H., Woessner, J.F. Jr., McNeish, J.D. and Stamenkovic, I. (2002) CD44

anchors the assembly of matrilysin/ MMP-7 with heparin-binding epidermal growth factor precursor and ErbB4 and regulates female reproductive organ remodeling. *Genes Dev.*, **16**, 307–23.

61 Bladt, F., Riethmacher, D., Isenmann, S., Aguzzi, A. and Birchmeier, C. (1995) Essential role for the c-met receptor in the migration of myogenic precursor cells into the limb bud. *Nature*, **376**, 768–71.

62 Matzke, A., Sargsyan, V., Holtmann, B., Aramuni, G., Asan, E., Sendtner, M., Pace, G., Howells, N., Zhang, W., Ponta, H. and Orian-Rousseau, V. (2007) Haploinsufficiency of c-Met in cd44−/− mice identifies a collaboration of CD44 and c-Met in vivo. *Mol. Cell Biol.*, **27**, 8797–806.

63 Yarden, Y. (2001) The EGFR family and its ligands in human cancer. signalling mechanisms and therapeutic opportunities. *Eur. J. Cancer*, **37** (Suppl. 4), S3–8.

64 Jones, L.L., Liu, Z., Shen, J., Werner, A., Kreutzberg, G.W. and Raivich, G. (2000) Regulation of the cell adhesion molecule CD44 after nerve transection and direct trauma to the mouse brain. *J. Comp. Neurol.*, **426**, 468–92.

65 Griffioen, A.W., Coenen, M.J., Damen, C.A., Hellwig, S.M., van Weering, D.H., Vooys, W., Blijham, G.H. and Groenewegen, G. (1997) CD44 is involved in tumor angiogenesis; an activation antigen on human endothelial cells. *Blood*, **90**, 1150–9.

66 Trochon, V., Mabilat, C., Bertrand, P., Legrand, Y., Smadja-Joffe, F., Soria, C., Delpech, B. and Lu, H. (1996) Evidence of involvement of CD44 in endothelial cell proliferation, migration and angiogenesis in vitro. *Int. J. Cancer*, **66**, 664–8.

67 Savani, R.C., Cao, G., Pooler, P.M., Zaman, A., Zhou, Z. and DeLisser, H.M. (2001) Differential involvement of the hyaluronan (HA) receptors CD44 and receptor for HA-mediated motility in endothelial cell function and angiogenesis. *J. Biol. Chem.*, **276**, 36770–8.

68 Rahmanian, M. and Heldin, P. (2002) Testicular hyaluronidase induces tubular

structures of endothelial cells grown in three-dimensional collagen gel through a CD44-mediated mechanism. *Int. J. Cancer*, **97**, 601–7.

69 Rahmanian, M., Pertoft, H., Kanda, S., Christofferson, R., Claesson-Welsh, L. and Heldin, P. (1997) Hyaluronan oligosaccharides induce tube formation of a brain endothelial cell line in vitro. *Exp. Cell Res.*, **237**, 223–30.

70 Cao, G., Savani, R.C., Fehrenbach, M., Lyons, C., Zhang, L., Coukos, G. and Delisser, H.M. (2006) Involvement of endothelial CD44 during in vivo angiogenesis. *Am. J. Pathol.*, **169**, 325–36.

71 Forster-Horvath, C., Meszaros, L., Raso, E., Dome, B., Ladanyi, A., Morini, M., Albini, A. and Timar, J. (2004) Expression of CD44v3 protein in human endothelial cells in vitro and in tumoral microvessels in vivo. *Microvasc. Res.*, **68**, 110–18.

72 Suhardja, A. and Hoffman, H. (2003) Role of growth factors and their receptors in proliferation of microvascular endothelial cells. *Microsc. Res. Tech.*, **60**, 70–5.

73 Kohler, G. and Milstein, C. (1975) Continuous cultures of fused cells secreting antibody of predefined specificity. *Nature*, **256**, 495–7.

74 Kim, E.S., Khuri, F.R. and Herbst, R.S. (2001) Epidermal growth factor receptor biology (IMC-C225). *Curr. Opin. Oncol.*, **13**, 506–13.

75 Sievers, E.L. and Linenberger, M. (2001) Mylotarg: antibody-targeted chemotherapy comes of age. *Curr. Opin. Oncol.*, **13**, 522–7.

76 Schrijvers, A.H., Quak, J.J., Uyterlinde, A.M., van Walsum, M., Meijer, C.J., Snow, G.B. and van Dongen, G.A. (1993) MAb U36, a novel monoclonal antibody successful in immunotargeting of squamous cell carcinoma of the head and neck. *Cancer Res.*, **53**, 4383–90.

77 Stroomer, J.W., Roos, J.C., Sproll, M., Quak, J.J., Heider, K.H., Wilhelm, B.J., Castelijns, J.A., Meyer, R., Kwakkelstein, M.O., Snow, G.B., Adolf, G.R. and van Dongen, G.A. (2000) Safety and biodistribution of 99mTechnetium-labeled anti-CD44v6 monoclonal antibody BIWA

1 in head and neck cancer patients. *Clin. Cancer Res.*, **6**, 3046–55.

78 Van Hal, N.L., Van Dongen, G.A., Rood-Knippels, E.M., Van Der Valk, P., Snow, G.B. and Brakenhoff, R.H. (1996) Monoclonal antibody U36, a suitable candidate for clinical immunotherapy of squamous-cell carcinoma, recognizes a CD44 isoform. *Int. J. Cancer*, **68**, 520–7.

79 Borjesson, P.K., Postema, E.J., Roos, J.C., Colnot, D.R., Marres, H.A., van Schie, M.H., Stehle, G., de Bree, R., Snow, G.B., Oyen, W.J. and van Dongen, G.A. (2003) Phase I therapy study with (186) Re-labeled humanized monoclonal antibody BIWA 4 (bivatuzumab) in patients with head and neck squamous cell carcinoma. *Clin. Cancer Res.*, **9**, 3961S–72S.

80 Heider, K.H., Kuthan, H., Stehle, G. and Munzert, G. (2004) CD44v6: a target for antibody-based cancer therapy. *Cancer Immunol. Immunother.*, **53**, 567–79.

81 Postema, E.J., Borjesson, P.K., Buijs, W.C., Roos, J.C., Marres, H.A., Boerman, O.C., de Bree, R., Lang, M., Munzert, G., van Dongen, G.A. and Oyen, W.J. (2003) Dosimetric analysis of radioimmunotherapy with 186Re-labeled bivatuzumab in patients with head and neck cancer. *J. Nucl. Med.*, **44**, 1690–9.

82 Tijink, B.M., Buter, J., de Bree, R., Giaccone, G., Lang, M.S., Staab, A., Leemans, C.R. and van Dongen, G.A. (2006) A phase I dose escalation study with anti-CD44v6 bivatuzumab mertansine in patients with incurable squamous cell carcinoma of the head and neck or esophagus. *Clin. Cancer Res.*, **12**, 6064–72.

83 Neumeister, P., Eibl, M., Zinke-Cerwenka, W., Scarpatetti, M., Sill, H. and Linkesch, W. (2001) Hepatic veno-occlusive disease in two patients with relapsed acute myeloid leukemia treated with anti-CD33 calicheamicin (CMA-676) immunoconjugate. *Ann. Hematol.*, **80**, 119–20.

84 Thomas, G.E., Esteban, J.M., Raubitschek, A. and Wong, J.Y. (1995) gamma-Interferon administration after 90yttrium radiolabeled antibody therapy: survival

and hematopoietic toxicity studies. *Int. J. Radiat. Oncol. Biol. Phys.*, **31**, 529–34.

85 Arap, W., Pasqualini, R. and Ruoslahti, E. (1998) Cancer treatment by targeted drug delivery to tumor vasculature in a mouse model. *Science*, **279**, 377–80.

86 Koivunen, E., Restel, B.H., Rajotte, D., Lahdenranta, J., Hagedorn, M., Arap, W. and Pasqualini, R. (1999) Integrin-binding peptides derived from phage display libraries. *Methods Mol. Biol.*, **129**, 3–17.

87 Buerkle, M.A., Pahernik, S.A., Sutter, A., Jonczyk, A., Messmer, K. and Dellian, M. (2002) Inhibition of the alpha-nu integrins with a cyclic RGD peptide impairs angiogenesis, growth and metastasis of solid tumours in vivo. *Br. J. Cancer*, **86**, 788–95.

88 Fujii, H., Nishikawa, N., Komazawa, H., Orikasa, A., Ono, M., Itoh, I., Murata, J., Azuma, I. and Saiki, I. (1996) Inhibition of tumor invasion and metastasis by peptidic mimetics of Arg-Gly Asp (RGD) derived from the cell recognition site of fibronectin. *Oncol. Res.*, **8**, 333–42.

89 Haier, J., Goldmann, U., Hotz, B., Runkel, N. and Keilholz, U. (2002) Inhibition of tumor progression and neoangiogenesis using cyclic RGD-peptides in a chemically induced colon carcinoma in rats. *Clin. Exp. Metastasis*, **19**, 665–72.

90 Aina, O.H., Sroka, T.C., Chen, M.L. and Lam, K.S. (2002) Therapeutic cancer targeting peptides. *Biopolymers*, **66**, 184–99.

91 Bae, D.G., Kim, T.D., Li, G., Yoon, W.H. and Chae, C.B. (2005) Anti-flt1 peptide, a vascular endothelial growth factor receptor 1-specific hexapeptide, inhibits tumor growth and metastasis. *Clin. Cancer Res.*, **11**, 2651–61.

92 Starzec, A., Vassy, R., Martin, A., Lecouvey, M., Di Benedetto, M., Crepin, M. and Perret, G.Y. (2006) Antiangiogenic and antitumor activities of peptide inhibiting the vascular endothelial growth factor binding to neuropilin-1. *Life Sci.*, **79**, 2370–81.

93 Hibino, S., Shibuya, M., Hoffman, M.P., Engbring, J.A., Hossain, R., Mochizuki, M., Kudoh, S., Nomizu, M. and Kleinman, H.K. (2005) Laminin alpha5

chain metastasis- and angiogenesis-inhibiting peptide blocks fibroblast growth factor 2 activity by binding to the heparan sulfate chains of CD44. *Cancer Res.*, **65**, 10494–501.

94 Nakajima, H., Mizuta, N., Sakaguchi, K., Fujiwara, I., Yoshimori, A., Takahashi, S., Takasawa, R. and Tanuma, S. (2008) Development of HER2-antagonistic peptides as novel anti-breast cancer drugs by in silico methods. *Breast Cancer*, **15**, 65–72.

95 Bardelli, A., Longati, P., Williams, T.A., Benvenuti, S. and Comoglio, P.M. (1999) A peptide representing the carboxyl-terminal tail of the met receptor inhibits kinase activity and invasive growth. *J. Biol. Chem.*, **274**, 29274–81.

4
Peptide Aptamers Targeting the Viral E6 Oncoprotein Induce Apoptosis in HPV-positive Cancer Cells

Felix Hoppe-Seyler, Susanne Dymalla, Markus A. Moosmeier, and Karin Hoppe-Seyler

4.1
Human Papillomaviruses and Oncogenesis

Human papillomaviruses (HPVs) are small, nonenveloped viruses with a circular DNA genome of approximately 8 kb in length [1]. Based on the degree of their sequence homology in the viral L1 gene, more than 200 types of HPVs have been identified, which can be further divided into subtypes [2]. All HPVs exhibit a similar genomic organization. As exemplified for HPV type 18 (HPV18) in Figure 4.1, the viral genome can be separated into: (i) a region coding for early proteins (E1, E2, E4–E7) which play a role in viral replication and transcription; (ii) a region coding for the two viral late proteins (L1, L2) which compose the viral capsid; and (iii) a transcriptional control region, alternatively called the long control region (LCR) or upstream regulatory region (URR), containing cis-elements required for viral replication and transcription, including the common promoter for the E6 and E7 genes at the 3'-terminus.

HPVs are strictly epitheliotropic, and can cause benign lesions of the skin (e.g., common warts) and mucous membranes (condylomas). In addition, HPVs have attracted much attention in cancer medicine, since the discovery was made that certain HPV types – the so-called "oncogenic" or "high-risk" HPVs – are closely associated with the development of cancer in humans [1]. HPV-associated cancers include carcinomas of the oropharynx, such as oral, tonsillar, and laryngeal cancers, and carcinomas of the anogenital region, such as anal, vulvar, penile, and cervical cancer [1].

Other HPV types, most notably the so-called *Epidermodysplasia verruciformis* (*EV*)-types (e.g., HPV5 and HPV8) are associated with the development of squamous cell carcinomas of the skin in *EV* patients [3, 4]. This rare disease is characterized by an increased susceptibility towards cutaneous HPV infections. Approximately one-third of *EV* patients develop squamous cell carcinomas of the skin later in life, predominantly at sun-exposed areas [3].

Specific cutaneous HPV types, particularly *EV* types, are also found in a high percentage of squamous carcinomas of the skin in transplant recipients receiving

Peptides as Drugs. Discovery and Development. Edited by Bernd Groner
Copyright © 2009 WILEY-VCH Verlag GmbH & Co. KGaA, Weinheim
ISBN: 978-3-527-32205-3

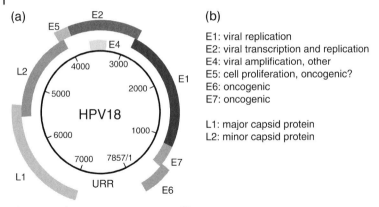

Figure 4.1 The genomic composition of human
papillomaviruses, exemplified for HPV18. (a) The circular viral
genome can be subdivided into early (E) and late (L) regions,
separated by the transcriptional control region.
URR = Upstream Regulatory Region; (b) Functional activities
of the HPV proteins.

immunosuppression. These patients have an approximately 50–100-fold increased
risk for skin cancer development, and this represents a major problem for transplantation medicine. In addition, specific cutaneous HPV types are also found in
a substantial portion of nonmelanoma skin cancers among the immunocompetent
population [4–6]. Yet, in these latter forms of nonmelanoma skin cancer, the
pathogenic role of HPVs in cancer development is still unclear and remains the
subject of controversy. Unlike the situation for cervical cancer, the detectable copy
number of HPV genomes is much lower than one per cell [7], indicating that the
majority of the tumor cells does not contain HPV DNA. Under these circum-
stances, a causative role for HPVs could be explained by a "hit-and-run" mechanism, in which cutaneous HPVs induce the cancer but are no longer required for
maintenance of the transformed phenotype. Alternatively, HPVs can be readily
detected in the normal skin of healthy individuals, so that the presence of cutaneous HPVs in these cancers could be unrelated to tumor formation and rather
represent an epiphenomenon.

4.1.1
Cervical Cancer

Thus far, the best-studied HPV-associated cancer is cervical cancer. With an
annual incidence of approximately 500 000 new cases, and an annual mortality of
over 250 000, cervical cancer represents the second most common malignancy in
females worldwide [8]. Epidemiological studies have indicated that the worldwide
burden of HPV-associated cancers will increase by over 40% until the year 2020,
mainly due to the population dynamics in developing countries, where the disease
is particularly prominent [8].

Virtually all cervical cancers contain the DNA of specific HPV types; the most prevalent are HPV16 and HPV18, which are found in approximately 55% and 16% of all cases, respectively [9]. In cervical cancers, every tumor cell contains HPV DNA. There is common consensus that oncogenic HPVs are not simply innocent bystanders in this disease, but rather are causative agents which interfere with cellular regulatory pathways. Accordingly, both HPV16 and HPV18 have been officially classified as human carcinogens by the World Health Organization [10]. Yet, whereas infection with oncogenic HPVs is considered an essential component for virtually all cervical cancer cases, it is not sufficient for cancer development. This can be deduced from the observations that: (i) only a small proportion of females infected with an oncogenic HPV type eventually develop cervical cancer; (ii) cervical cancers are monoclonal, indicating that they originate from only a single HPV-positive cell in the infected epithelium; and (iii) there is typically a long latency between the primary infection and the development of cancer, usually in the range of several decades. Thus, additional genetic events are required, besides the activity of an oncogenic HPV type, in order to develop cervical cancer.

The high prevalence and causative role of HPV16 and HPV18 in cervical cancer has been considered for the design of recently developed prophylactic vaccines. These are available as bivalent vaccines, protecting against HPV16 and HPV18, or tetravalent vaccines, protecting against HPV16 and HPV18, and also against HPV6 and HPV11 which cause approximately 90% of external genital warts [11]. Although these vaccines hold great promise for a future prevention of HPV-associated cancers, there remain many hurdles to be overcome before their widespread application. One major problem when introducing the vaccine is currently its high price (ca. US$375 in the United States). This issue is particularly relevant for poor countries, where the majority of cervical cancers occurs. It has been estimated that every 5-year delay in bringing the vaccine to developing countries will result in the cancer-related death of 1.5–2 million women [12]. Moreover, it is important to note that there are at least two generations of females that are already infected, and therefore will not benefit from a prophylactic vaccine. In view of these facts, and the medical impact of the disease, novel treatment strategies against cervical cancer are still urgently required.

4.1.2
The E6 and E7 Genes

In HPV-associated cancers, the viral genomes are often integrated into the host cell chromosomes – an event which is associated with loss of portions of the viral DNA. However, two viral genes, designated E6 and E7, are regularly retained and expressed in all tumor cells of HPV-positive cervical cancers [13]. This, at an early stage of HPV research, suggested that the E6 and E7 genes might play a key role for viral transformation and, indeed, subsequent analyses have found that both genes possess transforming potential in a variety of experimental systems [1]. Furthermore, early experiments blocking viral E6/E7 expression by antisense constructs resulted in an inhibition of growth, and also indicated that both genes played a crucial role in the maintenance of the malignant phenotype of HPV-positive cancer cells [14].

During the past few years, a large body of information has been collected concerning the molecular pathways targeted by the HPV E6 and E7 proteins during the transformation process. Both viral oncoproteins are relatively small, with E6 having a length of approximately 150 amino acids and E7 approximately 100 amino acids, depending on the individual HPV type. Both, E6 and E7 undergo a large number of protein–protein interactions, many of which are believed to be crucial for their transforming activity. For example, the E7 protein has been identified as a proliferative stimulus in HPV-positive cancer cells by binding to and inactivating cellular pocket proteins, such as the retinoblastoma tumor suppressor protein, pRb, and the related p107 and p130 proteins [15]. In addition, E7 can interact and interfere with cyclin-dependent kinase inhibitors, such as p21 or p27 [15]. Moreover, E7 can act as a mitotic mutator, leading to chromosomal missegregation and aneuploidy [16].

E6, on the other hand, has been shown to possess anti-apoptotic potential [17]. As one important underlying mechanism, this could be attributed to the finding that E6 can counteract the activity of the pro-apoptotic p53 tumor suppressor protein. In this scenario, E6 induces the proteolytic degradation of p53 by forming a trimeric complex with p53 and the cellular ubiquitin-protein ligase E6AP (E6-associated protein) [18, 19]. As a result, the p53 response is disturbed in HPV-positive cancer cells, although it is not completely inactivated and can be restored upon E6 inhibition [20, 21]. As a consequence of the distorted p53 activity, critical p53-dependent growth and apoptosis regulatory pathways are no longer efficiently induced. For example, proper induction of the pro-apoptotic p53/PUMA/Bax cascade is prevented in HPV-positive cancer cells and contributes to their survival [22]. In view of the interaction with p53, it is furthermore noteworthy that the E6 protein of oncogenic HPV types has also been reported to interact with the transcriptional coactivator p300. This can interfere with the transcriptional activation of downstream targets by p53 [23].

In addition, there is evidence that E6 can modulate other apoptosis regulators. For example, E6 has the potential to interfere with CD95 or FADD, two important activators of the extrinsic apoptosis pathway, to induce the degradation of Bak, an activator of the intrinsic apoptosis pathway, and to activate c-IAP2, an anti-apoptotic factor common to both pathways [24–27]. Other potential pathways targeted by E6 during the transformation process include activation of telomerase in keratinocytes [28] and the interaction with several so-called PDZ proteins, such as hDlg and hScrib, human homologues of *Drosophila melanogaster* tumor suppressor proteins [29, 30], or different MAGI proteins [31]. Binding to PDZ proteins is mediated by a short amino acid motif located at the extreme C-terminus, which is only found in high-risk E6 proteins and leads to the degradation of PDZ proteins, many of which have anti-proliferative capacities.

Whereas, both E6 and E7 possess some transforming potential on their own, this activity is increased when both genes are coexpressed [32, 33], as it is the case in HPV-positive cancer cells. This indicates that both oncogenes cooperate during HPV-associated carcinogenesis. A possible model for this functional cooperativity

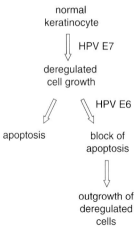

Figure 4.2 Hypothetical model for the functional cooperativity of the HPV E6 and E7 oncoproteins during cellular transformation. E7 deregulates cell growth, for example by interfering with the activity of pocket proteins and cyclin-dependent kinase inhibitors (see text). Normal cells react to the deregulated growth stimulus by inducing apoptosis. The concomitant expression of E6, however, blocks apoptosis and allows the survival of deregulated cells.

is depicted in Figure 4.2. In this scenario, E7 primarily acts as an abnormal proliferative stimulus, for example by interfering with pRb-mediated cell cycle control. Normal cells would react to such abnormal growth stimuli, as exerted by activated cellular or viral oncogenes, by inducing apoptosis [34]. As a cellular surveillance mechanism, this would ultimately eliminate cells exhibiting a disturbed proliferation control. However, the concomitant expression of the anti-apoptotic E6 protein can counteract this apoptotic response, for example by blocking p53 function, eventually allowing the outgrowth of deregulated cells. According to this model, the targeted inhibition of E6 should restore apoptotic sensitivity of HPV-positive cancer cells and result in their elimination.

4.2
Peptide Aptamers Targeting the HPV E6 Oncoprotein

Peptide aptamers are proteinaceous agents, classically consisting of a randomized peptide moiety which is presented in the context of a supporting scaffold protein. They are isolated from randomized expression libraries by virtue of their ability to bind to a given target protein, using the yeast two-hybrid technology [35, 36]. By binding to distinct surface domains of their target, peptide aptamers have the potential to interfere with the normal protein–protein contacts of their target protein, and to block its intracellular activity with high specificity and efficiency. A list of peptide aptamers which can induce distinct cellular phenotypes is provided in Table 4.1. Inhibitory peptide aptamers have been generated against a

Table 4.1 Bioactive peptide aptamers.

Targets	Reported effects	Reference(s)
Cell cycle		
Human Cdk2	Inhibit substrate phosphorylation, cell cycle block	[35, 37]
D. m. Cdks	Eye deformations *in vivo* (typical for cell cycle defects)	[38]
E2F	Cell cycle block	[39]
D. m. Cyclin J	Mitotic defects	[40]
Signal transduction/apoptosis		
mt and wt Ras	Inhibit Ras-mediated activation of downstream targets	[41]
Trio	Inhibit activation of RhoA	[42]
EGFR	Block EGFR phosphorylation, antiproliferative	[43]
Stat3	Growth arrest, apoptosis	[44]
Smad proteins	Block TGFβ signaling pathway	[45, 46]
BCL-6	Prevent differentiation of proliferating B cells	[47]
FLASH	Block extrinsic apoptosis pathway	[48]
CK2	Pro-apoptotic	[49]
ErbB2	Interference with AKT signaling	[50]
Calcineurin	Antiproliferative	[51]
AMPK	Inhibition of AMPK kinase activity	[52]
Viral proteins		
HPV16 E6	Pro-apoptotic	[53]
HPV16 E7	Pro-apoptotic	[54]
HBV core	Block viral capsid formation and replication	[55]
TSWV N	Resistance of plants to tospoviruses	[56]
TGMV	Block viral replication	[57]
DHBV core	Block viral capsid formation and replication	[58]
RSV Nr-13	Pro-apoptotic	[59]
HIV-1 integrin	Integrase inhibition	[60]
HCV NS3	Inhibit HCV replication	[61]
Others		
PrP	Block cellular prion formation	[62]

D. m. = Drosophila melanogaster.

variety of different target proteins. These include cell cycle regulators, proteins involved in signal transduction, or structural viral proteins.

The present authors' group has developed a GAL4-based peptide aptamer screening system which consists basically of three components: (i) a *bait*, corresponding to a given target protein, expressed as a fusion protein with the yeast GAL4 DNA binding domain; (ii) a *prey*, corresponding to a peptide expression library of randomized 20mer peptides, anchored with both ends in the context of the *Escherichia coli* Thioredoxin A (TrxA) scaffold protein and linked to the GAL4 transcriptional activation domain; and (iii) a *yeast strain*, containing three different selectable marker genes [53]. The presentation of the peptide moiety in the context of a supporting protein scaffold is associated with a number of theoretical advantages, which include a higher binding affinity to the target and improved stability, when compared with flexible peptides with free ends [63, 64]. Thus, peptide aptamers resemble antibodies, in which a variable antigen-binding domain is presented in the context of a rigid protein backbone. It should, however, be noted that a scaffold appears not to be absolutely required to identify peptides which can strongly bind to and efficiently interfere with the activity of a target protein (K. Hoppe-Seyler *et al.*, unpublished results). The use of different marker genes under the control of different promoters in the yeast reporter strain helps to reduce the number of false positives. These could be, for example, due to peptide aptamers which stabilize a certain marker gene product, or to peptide aptamers which may indirectly or directly stimulate the promoter activity of a marker gene promoter, independent of an interaction with the target protein.

The fact that the screening for peptide aptamers is performed intracellularly in yeast cells, provides some advantages above commonly used *in vitro* screening assays for interacting peptides, such as the phage display technology. For example, the peptide aptamer screening technique preselects for molecules which are stable inside eukaryotic cells. Moreover, it selects for molecules which are properly folded to bind to their target in the intracellular milieu. In contrast, peptides or intrabodies isolated by using *in vitro* binding techniques may be unstable or differently folded, once they are intracellularly expressed [65]. In addition, intracellular peptide aptamer screens occur in a rich environment where the presence of competing proteins can enhance specificity.

In a search for potential E6 inhibitors, a series of peptide aptamers was identified which specifically bind to the HPV16 E6 oncoprotein [53]. Among these, at least two peptide aptamers induced apoptosis in HPV-positive cancer cells, upon intracellular expression. This effect was specific to HPV-positive cells and associated with an increase of intracellular p53 protein levels. These results were in line with the idea that an inhibition of E6 activity would reconstitute endogenous p53 protein levels in HPV-positive cancer cells. They furthermore indicate that the targeted interference with E6 activity should represent a most promising therapeutic strategy in HPV-positive cancer cells.

This conclusion was subsequently supported by a series of studies in which E6 function in HPV-positive cancer cells was blocked by other experimental approaches. These included RNA interference, antisense constructs or intracellular antibodies. All strategies resulted in profound anti-oncogenic activities in HPV-positive cancer cells, showing that E6 inhibition either induced apoptosis [66–68], growth arrest [69, 70], or both [71]. These phenotypic differences may be due to varying efficiencies of the employed inhibitory agents, or to differences in the analyzed cell systems. It is also necessary to account for possible secondary effects on E7 expression, since the maintenance of E7 activity may be a necessary pro-apoptotic stimulus in HPV-positive cancer cells, following E6 inhibition (see Figure 4.1). Notably, as a noncellular protein, E6 is not expressed in normal, healthy cells. Specific E6-inhibitors could therefore allow the selective targeting of HPV-positive cells, without affecting virus-negative healthy cells. This contrasts the effects of conventional chemo- or radiotherapeutic agents which usually also harm normal tissue. Clearly, the induction of apoptosis, rather than growth inhibition, should be the preferred therapeutic effect of E6-inhibitors. This would result in the elimination of the tumor cells and, in contrast to transient growth inhibition, may not require the continuous application of a therapeutic agent.

4.3
E6-Targeting Peptide Aptamers: Therapeutic Perspectives

In principle, one could envision following several strategies, to develop peptide aptamers into a therapeutic perspective:

- The peptide aptamers should be helpful tools for evaluating a given protein as a potential therapeutic target.

- The peptide aptamers may themselves be developed into protein drugs.

- The interaction of a peptide aptamer with its target protein may form a basis for identifying small molecules of therapeutic value which could serve as functional mimics of bioactive peptide aptamers.

4.3.1
Therapeutic Target Protein Evaluation by Peptide Aptamers

Peptide aptamers have not only been proven to serve as helpful tools for basic research in order to explore the function of a protein in a particular disease, but they may also serve as valuable tools for the validation of novel therapeutic targets. Specifically, antagonizing a certain protein function with a ligand, and thereby correcting the pathogenic phenotype of a cell, identifies this protein as a potential therapeutic target. Notably, due to the nature of the screening method, knowledge of the structure of the target protein is not a prerequisite for the identification of inhibitory peptide aptamers.

It is important to note that peptide aptamers can contact distinct surface regions on their target protein. For example, the results of some early studies showed that a peptide aptamer binding to Cdk2 interfered only with histone H1 phosphorylation, but not with the phosphorylation of pRb, which is another substrate for Cdk2 [72]. This distinct substrate specificity is most likely due to at least partially, nonoverlapping binding sites for histone H1 and pRb on Cdk2. The bioactive peptide aptamer most likely blocks the sites on Cdk2 which are needed for the interaction with histone H1, but not those interacting with pRb [72]. More recent studies, employing systematic site-directed mutagenesis, showed that peptide aptamers can recognize many different distinct domains on their target proteins, ranging from flat surfaces to molecular pocket structures [73]. It is likely that inhibitory peptide aptamers antagonize protein functions by preferentially binding to active site structures. In this way, they should serve as helpful tools for defining functionally relevant surface domains on the target protein in structure–function analyses.

Due to their ability to bind to distinct surface regions, peptide aptamers should provide an important advantage for the validation of therapeutic targets when compared to commonly used strategies, such as blocking gene expression by RNAi. The latter technology prevents expression of the complete protein, and so is likely to interfere with all interactions of the target protein in its physiological cellular network. So, by inhibiting only distinct protein–protein interactions, peptide aptamer-induced perturbations of the molecular network surrounding the target protein would be expected to be more subtle and more closely resemble the effects of a therapeutic agent specifically targeting the same domain [73].

Applying these considerations to the effects observed for E6 binding peptide aptamers, it can be concluded that: (i) continuous E6 function is required for the survival of HPV-positive cancer cells, thereby providing a molecular explanation for the apparent selection pressure of HPV-positive cancer cells to maintain E6 expression; (ii) E6 is a promising therapeutic target for intervention strategies, since E6-binding molecules can induce apoptosis, selectively in HPV-positive cancer cells; and (iii) E6 targeting peptide aptamers which block the anti-apoptotic activity of E6 may define a surface region on E6 which is crucial to mediate its anti-apoptotic function. This region could serve as an interesting docking domain to be targeted by pharmacological inhibitors.

Knowledge concerning the structure of a target–with or without a bioactive peptide aptamer bound to it–may provide a deeper understanding of the structure–function relationship. It also could reveal potential binding pockets, and serve as a basis for optimizing aptamer activity. Structural investigations of E6 have long been hindered by difficulties in purifying the protein in a stable folded form. However, recent advances in purifying the monomeric C-terminal part of HPV16 E6 have led to a nuclear magnetic resonance (NMR)-based, three-dimensional (3-D) model of E6 [74]. These data could be helpful for further exploring the binding of peptide aptamers to E6, and for defining the critical amino acid residues and contact points. Structural information regarding E6 and E6-blocking peptide aptamers should be informative about the potential of E6 to serve as a valid therapeutic target, and provide additional insight into the intrinsic therapeutic potential of aptamers. In addition, structural data may serve as a basis for *in silico* screening methods for small-molecule aptamer mimics.

4.3.2
The Intrinsic Therapeutic Potential of Peptide Aptamers

As specific and efficient intracellular inhibitors of their target, peptide aptamers themselves may be developed into protein drugs. Very much like protein therapy in general, this endeavor must still overcome several technical hurdles, including potential immunogenicity, metabolic instability, and efficient delivery. Thus, the exploitation of peptide aptamers as potential therapeutics will require the optimization of both biopharmaceutic (solubility, permeability, stability, immunogenicity) and pharmacokinetic (volume of distribution, clearance rate, target binding behavior, serum half-life) parameters.

Nonmodified peptides are usually rapidly cleared from the bloodstream, commonly due either to enzymatic degradation by serum proteases or to rapid renal clearance. As there is no general strategy for stabilizing peptide aptamers at hand, potential approaches could be based on conventional methods. For example, attempts to prolong the short-half lives of peptide aptamers could be based on intrinsic modifications of the peptide or by linking peptide aptamers to stabilizing conjugates.

Until recently, however, technical difficulties in the purification and biochemical *in vitro* analysis of many peptide aptamers were encountered which were due to some unfavorable properties of the *E. coli* Thioredoxin A (TrxA) scaffold. This protein was originally chosen as a scaffold for peptide aptamers due to its relatively small size (ca. 12 kDa), its stability and solubility, and the fact that its 3-D structure is well known [35, 64]. Moreover, the platform protein itself should be functionally inert. In the case of TrxA, peptides are introduced into a constrained loop within the active center of the molecule, thereby destroying its enzymatic activity. Unfortunately, many TrxA-based peptide aptamers exhibit the tendency to form insoluble aggregates. Paradoxically, under certain instances, this may even be beneficial for their inhibitory function upon intracellular expression, for example by coaggregating the bound target protein and sequestering it into aggresomes [58]. On the other hand, however, in many cases these solubility problems have precluded detailed biochemical analyses *in vitro* and also complicated protein transduction studies. Recently, a modified human TrxA (hTrxA) molecule was developed from which five internal cysteines had been removed [75]. Several hTrxA-based peptide aptamers were found to be efficiently produced in bacteria and could be purified with high yield. Moreover, replacing the bacterial TrxA with hTrxA in peptide aptamers specifically binding to Stat3 did not affect the target binding [75]. Thus, it is hoped that the hTrxA scaffold will facilitate the *in vitro* analyses and modifications of those bioactive peptide aptamers which have already proved their intracellular efficacy.

Possible intrinsic peptide aptamer alterations to enhance stability could make use of amino acid modifications. It is noteworthy here that proteases are less active on modified L-amino acids [76] and on chemical or stereochemical modifications of single or multiple amino acids [77]. Chemical optimization has already been demonstrated as an attractive approach for DNA and RNA aptamers. For example, the introduction of non-natural oligonucleotides or a mirror image approach utilizing isomeric L-oligonucleotides were associated with increased serum stabilities [78–80]. Yet, whereas modified oligonucleotides can be easily implemented *de novo* into the *in vitro* selection process, potential positive effects of D-amino acids on bioactive peptide aptamers will need to be investigated subsequent to the initial screening process. These time-consuming and expensive evaluations of synthetic peptide aptamer variants could potentially be overcome by recent advances in generating peptides on microchips [81, 82]. This will allow the large-scale *in vitro* screening of the properties of peptide aptamers consisting of non-natural amino acids.

Alternative approaches to alter the stability of peptide aptamers by intrinsic modifications include the possibility to enhance peptide folds by intramolecular stabilization. This renders peptides less prone to protease degradation. For example, alpha-helical peptides, which have been stabilized by linking suitable amino acids by an all-hydrocarbon bridge, were shown to be active in cell culture. Such stapled peptides were conformationally constrained and displayed enhanced serum half-life and permeability [83, 84]. Other modifications may include the disulfide bridging of cysteine residues and cyclization [85, 86]. In order to implement all of these modifications for optimizing peptide aptamers, detailed structural data for the peptide aptamer and its target would be advantageous.

The conjugation of bioactive peptides represents another common approach to alter stability, and includes linkage to polyethylene glycol (PEG) or dendrimer formations [87, 88]. For example, PEGylation of the clinically approved RNA aptamer drug pegaptanib caused an increase in the serum half-life to 10 days [89].

For all of these potential modifications, it will be important to consider that optimizing peptide aptamer stability may alter other biopharmaceutic or pharmacokinetic parameters, or affect the peptide aptamer's biological activity. For example, PEGylation has been linked to the improved solubility, lower renal clearance and decreased immunogenicity of peptides. On the other hand, the influence of substituting L-amino acids by D-enantiomers on immunogenicity has been the subject of much controversy [77]. Constraining peptide conformations by intra-molecular stapling or bridging is being investigated as a strategy to improve binding to its target [83].

Another major problem for the therapeutic delivery of peptides and proteins is the fact that these molecules, due to their biophysical properties, usually do not penetrate through the intact cell membrane. However, this technical hurdle may be overcome by their fusion to so-called protein transduction domains (PTDs), which are small peptides that can transport linked molecules through the plasma membrane [90]. Particularly intriguing for HPV-associated lesions, which typically affect the skin and mucosa, are reports indicating an efficient uptake of PTD-linked molecules into intact human [91], porcine [92], or mouse [93] skin, following topical application. Furthermore, as a human protein, hTrxA may be less immunogenic in humans than its bacterial counterpart [75], and this may represent a possible benefit for therapeutic application.

4.3.3
Identification of Functional Peptide Mimics by Displacement Screening

The interaction between a peptide aptamer and its target protein can also serve as a basis for the establishment of high-throughput screening assays that could lead to the identification of therapeutically useful small-molecular-weight compounds. As discussed above, it is conceivable that a bioactive peptide aptamer, which induces a therapeutically desirable cellular phenotype, binds to a pathogenetically important domain on its target protein. For example, a peptide or peptide aptamer which binds to the HPV E6 oncoprotein and induces apoptosis in HPV-positive cancer cells, is likely to do this by binding to a surface domain which is important for the anti-apoptotic function of E6. Based on these considerations, small molecules which bind to the same or to an overlapping region on E6 could act as functional peptide aptamer mimics and also induce apoptosis in HPV-positive cancer cells.

Large-scale screening assays could assist in the identification of molecules which bind to the therapeutically relevant surface domain of the target protein, as defined by an inhibitory peptide aptamer. This could be achieved by selecting competitive inhibitors of peptide aptamer binding – that is, molecules which can displace the peptide aptamer from its target protein. Small-molecular-weight compounds with a similar binding behavior may exert the same inhibitory activities as a peptide aptamer, but allow circumvention of several of the pharmacological problems still associated with protein drugs. For example, molecules contained in the compound library can be preselected for their drug-likeness, structural and shape diversity, novelty, and compliance with medicinal chemistry requirements. Possible high-throughput assays to screen for functional peptide aptamer mimics include conventional *in vitro* competition binding assays based on fluorescence polarization (FP), Förster resonance energy transfer (FRET), or the AlphaScreen (amplified luminescent proximity homogeneous assay, PerkinElmer) system. The feasibility of a competition binding high-throughput screening has been already demonstrated utilizing RNA and DNA aptamers [94].

Although this approach seems practicable, screening for aptamer mimics has not yet been routinely integrated into the drug discovery process. This is most likely due to the fact that the targeting of protein–protein interactions is widely considered to be difficult and less attractive for drug discovery, primarily due to the lack of well-defined binding pockets [95]. However, there is today a growing list of compounds which interfere with cancer-relevant protein–protein interactions [96]. In addition, there is a current lack of structural data on peptide aptamers or on peptide aptamer–protein complexes, and the principles and patterns of target recognition are poorly understood. Hence, the identification of small-molecule compounds which can selectively act as peptide aptamer mimics on a certain target protein could assist in exploring the 'druggability' of a target and in pursuing of structural investigations into aptamer–target interactions.

4.4
Perspectives

Tumor viruses are associated with approximately 15–20% of human malignancies, making them the second most common, defined risk factor for cancer development; exceeded only by tobacco smoking [97]. Besides HPVs, recognized tumor viruses include hepatitis B virus (HBV) and hepatitis C virus (HCV), which are linked to hepatoma development, the Epstein–Barr virus (EBV), which is linked to lymphomas and nasopharyngeal cancer, HTLV-1, linked to adult T-cell leukemia, or Kaposi's sarcoma-associated herpes virus (KSHV), linked to Kaposi sarcoma and primary effusion lymphoma [98]. In addition, other viruses are currently being intensively investigated for a role in human cancer development, such as human endogenous retroviruses (HERVs) [99] or torque teno viruses (TTVs) [100].

Research on oncogenic HPVs has the advantage that the viral oncogenes are clearly defined and extensively studied. The viral E6 and E7 genes are crucial both for the transformation process and for the maintenance of the transformed phenotype of HPV-positive cancer cells. Notably, they target and inactivate tumor suppressor pathways which are affected in many cancers by genetic modifications, such as by DNA mutations or epigenetic silencing. The best-studied examples are the inactivation of p53- or pRb-regulated pathways by the HPV E6 and E7 onco-proteins, respectively. Both pathways are also inactivated in the majority of all human cancers. Clearly, however, there are additional tumor-relevant pathways targeted by E6 and E7 which, thus far, have not been studied in detail. For example, transcriptome analyses have revealed changes in the expression of many cellular genes, following the inhibition of viral E6/E7 expression in HPV-positive cancer cells [101–104]. These included genes affected in other cancers that are not associ-ated with viral infections. Thus, the HPV E6 and E7 proteins should prove to be extremely useful experimental tools, not only to effect an understanding of HPV-associated tumorigenesis, but also for the study of molecular carcinogenesis in general.

The prominent role played by the viral E6 and E7 oncoproteins in maintaining the transformed phenotype of HPV-positive cancer cells has important advantages for therapeutic considerations. By targeting viral oncoproteins for functional inhibition, it should – in theory – be possible to develop highly specific therapeutic strategies which affect only virus-positive cells. E6-targeting peptide aptamers may therefore represent a basis for the design of novel, virus-specific therapeutic agents with which to treat HPV-positive lesions.

In many cases, HPV-associated mucosal lesions are readily accessible, and the topical application of therapeutic agents should be feasible. However, if one general property of PTDs were to be an efficient permeation into the skin [91–93], it is possible that PTD-linked peptide aptamers targeting E6 could be developed for the topical treatment of HPV-associated preneoplastic and neoplastic lesions. This issue could be tested preclinically by using a mouse model of HPV-induced cervical cancer in which the tumorigenic phenotype is E6-dependent [105]. If suc-cessful, similar efforts could then be extended to identify agents with antiviral actions against other HPV types, for example those associated with skin cancer or with benign diseases, such as skin warts, anogenital warts, and recurrent laryngeal papilloma.

References

1 zur Hausen, H. (2002) *Nat. Rev. Cancer,* **2**, 342–50.

2 de Villiers, E.M., Fauquet, C., Broker, T.R., Bernard, H.U. and zur Hausen, H. (2004) *Virology*, **324**, 17–27.

3 Majewski, S., Jablonska, S. and Orth, G. (1997) *Clin. Dermatol.,* **15**, 321–34.

4 Pfister, H. (2003) *J. Natl Cancer Inst. Monogr.,* **31**, 52–6.

5 de Jong-Tieben, L.M., Berkhout, R.J., Smits, H.L., Bouwes Bavinck, J.N., Vermeer, B.J., van der Woude, F.J. and ter Schegget, J. (1995) *J. Invest. Dermatol.*, **105**, 367–71.

6 Shamanin, V., zur Hausen, H., Lavergne, D., Proby, C.M., Leigh, I.M., Neumann, C., Hamm, H., Goos, M., Haustein, U.F., Jung, E.G., Plewig, G., Wolff, H. and de Villiers, E.M. (1996) *J. Natl Cancer Inst.*, **88**, 802–11.

7 Weissenborn, S.J., Nindl, I., Purdie, K., Harwood, C., Proby, C., Breuer, J., Majewski, S., Pfister, H. and Wieland, U. (2005) *J. Invest. Dermatol.*, **125**, 93–7.

8 Parkin, D.M. and Bray, F. (2006) *Vaccine*, **24** (Suppl. 3), S11–25.

9 Schiffman, M., Castle, P.E., Jeronimo, J., Rodriguez, A.C. and Wacholder, S. (2007) *Lancet*, **370**, 890–907.

10 International Agency for Research on Cancer (IARC) (1995) *IARC Monographs on the Evaluation of Carcinogenic Risks to Humans*, Vol. **64**, IARC, Lyon.

11 Lowy, D.R. and Schiller, J.T. (2006) *J. Clin. Invest.*, **116**, 1167–73.

12 Agosti, J.M. and Goldie, S.J. (2007) *N. Engl. J. Med.*, **356**, 1908–10.

13 Schwarz, E., Freese, U.K., Gissmann, L., Mayer, W., Roggenbuck, B., Stremlau, A. and zur Hausen, H. (1985) *Nature*, **314**, 111–14.

14 von Knebel Doeberitz, M., Oltersdorf, T., Schwarz, E. and Gissmann, L. (1988) *Cancer Res.*, **48**, 3780–6.

15 Münger, K., Basile, J.R., Duensing, S., Eichten, A., Gonzalez, S.L., Grace, M. and Zacny, V.L. (2001) *Oncogene*, **20**, 7888–98.

16 Duensing, S., Lee, L.Y., Duensing, A., Basile, J., Piboonniyom, S., Gonzalez, S., Crum, C.P. and Münger, K. (2000) *Proc. Natl Acad. Sci. USA*, **97**, 10002–7.

17 Mantovani, F. and Banks, L. (2001) *Oncogene*, **20**, 7874–87.

18 Scheffner, M., Werness, B.A., Huibregtse, J.M., Levine, A.J. and Howley, P.M. (1990) *Cell*, **63**, 1129–36.

19 Huibregtse, J.M., Scheffner, M. and Howley, P.M. (1991) *EMBO J.*, **10**, 4129–35.

20 Butz, K., Shahabeddin, L., Geisen, C., Spitkovsky, D., Ullmann, A. and Hoppe-Seyler, F. (1995) *Oncogene*, **10**, 927–36.

21 Goodwin, E.C. and DiMaio, D. (2000) *Proc. Natl Acad. Sci. USA*, **97**, 12513–18.

22 Vogt, M., Butz, K., Dymalla, S., Semzow, J. and Hoppe-Seyler, F. (2006) *Oncogene*, **25**, 4009–15.

23 Zimmermann, H., Koh, C.H., Degenkolbe, R., O'Connor, M.J., Müller, A., Steger, G., Chen, J.J., Lui, Y., Androphy, E. and Bernard, H.U. (2000) *J. Gen. Virol.*, **81**, 2617–23.

24 Aguilar-Lemarroy, A., Gariglio, P., Whitaker, N.J., Gariglio, P., zur Hausen, H., Krammer, P.H. and Rösl, F. (2002) *Oncogene*, **21**, 165–75.

25 Filippova, M., Parkhurst, L. and Duerksen-Hughes, P.J. (2004) *J. Biol. Chem.*, **279**, 25729–44.

26 Yuan, H., Fu, F., Zhuo, J., Wang, W., Nishitani, J., An, D.S., Chen, I.S. and Liu, X. (2005) *Oncogene*, **24**, 5069–78.

27 Thomas, M. and Banks, L. (1998) *Oncogene*, **17**, 2943–54.

28 Klingelhutz, A.J., Foster, S.A. and McDougall, J.K. (1996) *Nature*, **380**, 79–82.

29 Gardiol, D., Kühne, C., Glaunsinger, B., Lee, S.S., Javier, R. and Banks, L. (1999) *Oncogene*, **18**, 5487–96.

30 Nakagawa, M. and Huibregtse, J.M. (2000) *Mol. Cell. Biol.*, **20**, 8244–53.

31 Thomas, M., Laura, R., Hepner, K., Guccione, E., Sawyers, C., Lasky, L. and Banks, L. (2002) *Oncogene*, **21**, 5088–96.

32 Hawley-Nelson, P., Vousden, K.H., Hubbert, N.L., Lowy, D.R. and Schiller, J.T. (1989) *EMBO J.*, **8**, 3905–10.

33 Münger, K., Phelps, W., Bubb, V., Howley, P.M. and Schlegel, R. (1989) *J. Virol.*, **63**, 4417–21.

34 Evan, G.I. and Vousden, K.H. (2001) *Nature*, **411**, 342–8.

35 Colas, P., Cohen, B., Jessen, T., Grishina, I., McCoy, J. and Brent, R. (1996) *Nature*, **380**, 548–50.

36 Hoppe-Seyler, F., Crnkovic-Mertens, I., Tomai, E. and Butz, K. (2004) *Curr. Mol. Med.*, **4**, 529–38.

37 Colas, P., Cohen, B., Ko Ferrigno, P., Silver, P.A. and Brent, R. (2000) *Proc. Natl Acad. Sci. USA*, **97**, 13720–5.

38 Kolonin, M.G. and Finley, R.L., Jr (1998) *Proc. Natl Acad. Sci. USA*, **95**, 14266–71.

39 Fabrizzio, E., Le Cam, L., Polanowska, J., Kaczorek, M., Lamb, N., Brent, R. and Sardet, C. (1999) *Oncogene*, **18**, 4357–63.

40 Kolonin, M.G. and Finley, R.L., Jr (2000) *Dev. Biol.*, **227**, 661–72.

41 Xu, C.W. and Luo, Z. (2002) *Oncogene*, **21**, 5753–7.

42 Schmidt, S., Diriong, S., Méry, J., Fabbrizio, E. and Debant, A. (2002) *FEBS Lett.*, **523**, 35–42.

43 Buerger, C., Nagel-Wolfrum, K., Kunz, C., Wittig, I., Butz, K., Hoppe-Seyler, F. and Groner, B. (2003) *J. Biol. Chem.*, **278**, 37610–21.

44 Nagel-Wolfrum, K., Buerger, C., Wittig, I., Butz, K., Hoppe-Seyler, F. and Groner, B. (2004) *Mol. Cancer Res.*, **2**, 170–82.

45 Cui, Q., Lim, S.K., Zhao, B. and Hoffmann, F.M. (2005) *Oncogene*, **24**, 3864–74.

46 Zhao, B.M. and Hoffmann, F.M. (2006) *Mol. Biol. Cell*, **17**, 3819–31.

47 Chattopadhyay, A., Tate, S.A., Beswick, R.W., Wagner, S.D. and Ko Ferrigno, P. (2006) *Oncogene*, **25**, 2223–33.

48 Kim, G.S., Park, Y.A., Choi, Y.S., Choi, Y.H., Choi, H.W., Jung, Y.K. and Jeong, S. (2006) *Biochem. Biophys. Res. Commun.*, **343**, 1165–70.

49 Martel, V., Filhol, O., Colas, P. and Cochet, C. (2006) *Oncogene*, **25**, 7343–53.

50 Kunz, C., Borghouts, C., Buerger, C. and Groner, B. (2006) *Mol. Cancer Res.*, **4**, 983–98.

51 de Chassey, B., Mikaelian, I., Mathieu, A.L., Bickle, M., Olivier, D., Nègre, D., Cosset, F.L., Rudkin, B.B. and Colas, P. (2007) *Mol. Cell. Proteomics*, **6**, 451–9.

52 Miller, R.A., Binkowski, B.F. and Belshaw, P.J. (2007) *J. Mol. Biol.*, **365**, 945–57.

53 Butz, K., Denk, C., Ullmann, A., Scheffner, M. and Hoppe-Seyler, F. (2000) *Proc. Natl Acad. Sci. USA*, **97**, 6693–7.

54 Nauenburg, S., Zwerschke, W. and Jansen-Dürr, P. (2001) *FASEB J.*, **15**, 592–4.

55 Butz, K., Denk, C., Fitscher, B., Crnkovic-Mertens, I., Ullmann, A., Schröder, C.H. and Hoppe-Seyler, F. (2001) *Oncogene*, **20**, 6579–86.

56 Rudolph, C., Schreier, P.H. and Uhrig, J.F. (2003) *Proc. Natl Acad. Sci. USA*, **100**, 4429–34.

57 Lopez-Ochoa, L., Ramirez-Prado, J. and Hanley-Bowdoin, L. (2006) *J. Virol.*, **80**, 5841–53.

58 Tomai, E., Butz, K., Lohrey, C., von Weizsäcker, F., Zentgraf, H. and Hoppe-Seyler, F. (2006) *J. Biol. Chem.*, **281**, 21345–52.

59 Nouvion, A.L., Thibaut, J., Lohez, O.D., Venet, S., Colas, P., Gillet, G. and Lalle, P. (2007) *Oncogene*, **26**, 701–10.

60 Armon-Omer, A., Levin, A., Hayouka, Z., Butz, K., Hoppe-Seyler, F., Loya, S., Hizi, A., Friedler, A. and Loyter, A. (2008) *J. Mol. Biol.*, **376**, 971–82.

61 Trahtenherts, A., Gal-Tanamy, M., Zemel, R., Bachmatov, L., Loewenstein, S., Tur-Kaspa, R. and Benhar, I. (2008) *Antiviral Res.*, **77**, 195–205.

62 Gilch, S., Kehler, C. and Schätzl, H.M. (2007) *Mol. Biol.*, **371**, 362–73.

63 Ladner, R.C. (1995) *Trends Biotechnol.*, **13**, 426–30.

64 Geyer, C.R. and Brent, R. (2000) *Methods Enzymol.*, **328**, 171–208.

65 Cattaneo, A. and Biocca, S. (1999) *Trends Biochem.*, **17**, 115–20.

66 Butz, K., Ristriani, T., Hengstermann, A., Denk, C., Scheffner, M. and Hoppe-Seyler, F. (2003) *Oncogene*, **22**, 5938–45.

67 Griffin, H., Elston, R., Jackson, D., Ansell, K., Coleman, M., Winter, G. and Doorbar, J. (2006) *J. Mol. Biol.*, **355**, 360–78.

68 Yamato, K., Fen, J., Kobuchi, H., Nasu, Y., Yamada, T., Nishihara, T., Ikeda, Y., Kizaki, M. and Yoshinouchi, M. (2006) *Cancer Gene Ther.*, **13**, 234–41.

69 Koivusalo, R., Mialon, A., Pitkänen, H., Westermarck, J. and Hietanen, S. (2006) *Cancer Res.*, **66**, 11817–24.

70 Courtête, J., Sibler, A.P., Zeder-Lutz, G., Dalkara, D., Oulad-Abdelghani, M., Zuber, G. and Weiss, E. (2007) *Mol. Cancer Ther.*, **6**, 1728–35.

71 DeFilippis, R.A., Goodwin, E.C., Wu, L. and DiMaio, D. (2003) *J. Virol.*, **77**, 1551–63.

72 Cohen, B.A., Colas, P. and Brent, R. (1998) Proc. Natl Acad. Sci. USA, 95, 14272–7.

73 Baines, I.C. and Colas, P. (2006) Drug Discov. Today, 11, 334–41.

74 Nomine, Y., Masson, M., Charbonnier, S., Zanier, K., Ristriani, T., Deryckere, F., Sibler, A.P., Desplancq, D., Atkinson, R.A., Weiss, E., Orfanoudakis, G., Kieffer, B. and Trave, G. (2006) Mol. Cell, 21, 665–78.

75 Borghouts, C., Kunz, C., Delis, N. and Groner, B. (2008) Mol. Cancer Res., 6, 267–81.

76 Fauchere, J.L. and Thurieau, C. (1992) Adv. Drug Res., 23, 127–59.

77 Fischer, P.M. (2003) Curr. Protein Pept. Sci., 4, 339–56.

78 Klussmann, S., Nolte, A., Bald, R., Erdmann, V.A. and Furste, J.P. (1996) Nat. Biotechnol., 14, 1112–15.

79 Pagratis, N.C., Bell, C., Chang, Y.F., Jennings, S., Fitzwater, T., Jellinek, D. and Dang, C. (1997) Nat. Biotechnol., 15, 68–73.

80 Somasunderam, A., Ferguson, M.R., Rojo, D.R., Thiviyanathan, V., Li, X., O'Brien, W.A. and Gorenstein, D.G. (2005) Biochemistry, 44, 10388–95.

81 Beyer, M., Nesterov, A., Block, I., Konig, K., Felgenhauer, T., Fernandez, S., Leibe, K., Torralba, G., Hausmann, M., Trunk, U., Lindenstruth, V., Bischoff, F.R., Stadler, V. and Breitling, F. (2007) Science, 318, 1888.

82 Evans, D., Johnson, S., Laurenson, S., Davies, A.G., Ko Ferrigno, P. and Walti, C. (2008) J. Biol., 7, 3.

83 Walensky, L.D., Kung, A.L., Escher, I., Malia, T.J., Barbuto, S., Wright, R.D., Wagner, G., Verdine, G.L. and Korsmeyer, S.J. (2004) Science, 305, 1466–70.

84 Bernal, F., Tyler, A.F., Korsmeyer, S.J., Walensky, L.D. and Verdine, G.L. (2007) J. Am. Chem. Soc., 129, 2456–7.

85 Barthe, P., Rochette, S., Vita, C. and Roumestand, C. (2000) Protein Sci., 9, 942–55.

86 Li, P. and Roller, P.P. (2002) Curr. Top. Med. Chem., 2, 325–41.

87 Cloninger, M.J. (2002) Curr. Opin. Chem. Biol., 6, 742–8.

88 Yang, H. and Lopina, S.T. (2006) J. Mater. Res. A, 76, 398–407.

89 Apte, R.S., Modi, M., Masonson, H., Patel, M., Whitfield, L. and Adamis, A.P. (2007) Ophthalmology, 114, 1702–12.

90 Snyder, E.L. and Dowdy, S.F. (2005) Expert Opin. Drug Deliv., 2, 43–51.

91 Rothbard, J.B., Garlington, S., Lin, Q., Kirschberg, T., Kreider, E., McGrane, P.L., Wender, P.A. and Khavari, P.A. (2000) Nat. Med., 6, 1253–7.

92 Lopes, L.B., Brophy, C.M., Furnish, E., Flynn, C.R., Sparks, O., Komalavilas, P., Joshi, L., Panitch, A. and Bentley, M.V. (2005) Pharm. Res., 22, 750–7.

93 Song, H.Y., Lee, J.A., Ju, S.M., Yoo, K.Y., Won, M.H., Kwon, H.J., Eum, W.S., Jang, S.H., Choi, S.Y. and Park, J. (2008) Biochem. Pharmacol., 75, 1348–57.

94 Green, L.S., Bell, C. and Janjic, N. (2001) Biotechniques, 30, 1094–100.

95 Arkin, M.R. and Wells, J.A. (2004) Nat. Rev. Drug Discov., 3, 301–17.

96 Arkin, M. (2005) Curr. Opin. Chem. Biol., 9, 317–24.

97 Parkin, D.M. (2006) Int. J. Cancer, 118, 3030–44.

98 McLaughlin-Drubin, M.E. and Munger, K. (2008) Biochim. Biophys. Acta, 1782, 127–50.

99 Löwer, R. (1999) Trends Microbiol., 7, 350–6.

100 de Villiers, E.M., Schmidt, R., Delius, H. and Krammer, H. (2002) J. Mol. Med., 80, 44–50.

101 Wells, S.I., Aronow, B.J., Wise, T.M., Williams, S.S., Couget, J.A. and Howley, P.M. (2003) Proc. Natl Acad. Sci. USA, 100, 7093–8.

102 Thierry, F., Benotmane, M.A., Demeret, C., Mori, M., Teissier, S. and Desaintes, C. (2004) Cancer Res., 64, 895–903.

103 Kelley, M.L., Keiger, K.E., Lee, C.J. and Huibregtse, J.M. (2005) J. Virol., 79, 3737–47.

104 Kuner, R., Vogt, M., Sültmann, H., Buness, A., Dymalla, S., Bulkescher, J., Fellmann, M., Butz, K., Poustka, A. and Hoppe-Seyler, F. (2007) J. Mol. Med., 85, 1253–62.

105 Shai, A., Brake, T., Somoza, C. and Lambert, P.F. (2007) Cancer Res., 67, 1626–35.

5
The Prevention of HIV Infection with Viral Entry Inhibitors

Lisa Egerer, Anne Hubert, Dorothee von Laer, and Ursula Dietrich

5.1
Introduction: The Potential of Peptides as Drugs in the Treatment of HIV Infection

The HIV-1 replication cycle offers multiple targets for therapeutic interventions based on the inhibition of viral protein functions or protein–protein and protein–RNA interactions (Figure 5.1). Due to their small size and their specific binding properties, peptides can be selected from random peptide libraries for any structured target. The peptide may then serve as a drug by itself or, alternatively, a structural analysis of the peptide bound to the target may represent a lead for the development of low-molecular-weight drugs with improved therapeutic properties.

Peptides generally do not enter cells; such entry can only be accomplished by the provision of carriers, the presence of a protein transduction domain, or a stabilized α-helical structure. From a therapeutic point of view it is therefore much easier to target extracellular structures on the viral or cellular surfaces. This can result in the inhibition of HIV-1 entry and, indeed, the first entry inhibitor to be licensed by the Food and Drug Administration (FDA) for the treatment of HIV-1 infection was a peptide (T20, *enfuvirtide*) derived from the HIV-1 transmembrane protein, gp41. The mode of action of this peptide was shown to be via the competitive interference of formation of the six-helix bundle structure, an essential step during viral and cellular membrane fusion in the HIV-1 entry process (see below).

Some naturally occurring peptides and polypeptides that are generated upon viral infections as components of the innate or adaptive immune system also interfere with HIV-1 infection at the level of entry. These include defensins, chemokines or antibodies. A few monoclonal antibodies monoclonal antibody (mAbs) or antibody fragments have been identified that target essential domains in the HIV-1 glycoproteins or cellular receptors involved in HIV-1 entry (for a review, see Ref. [1]).

These mAbs have been extensively studied *in vitro*, in animal models, as well as in clinical trials for therapeutic or prophylactic interventions. A broadly neutralizing activity of these mAbs has been demonstrated in these systems, and the

Peptides as Drugs. Discovery and Development. Edited by Bernd Groner
Copyright © 2009 WILEY-VCH Verlag GmbH & Co. KGaA, Weinheim
ISBN: 978-3-527-32205-3

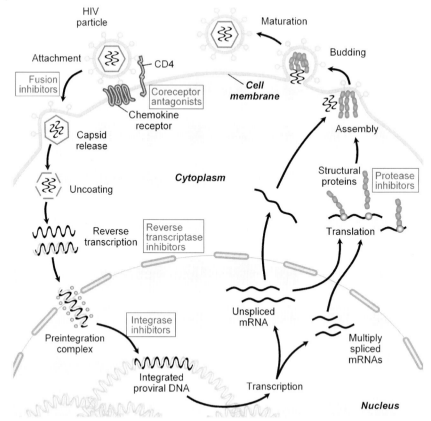

Figure 5.1 The HIV replication cycle. HIV particles attach to the target cell by binding to CD4 and a chemokine receptor. The viral and cellular membranes fuse and the capsid is released into the cytosol. Upon uncoating, the viral RNA genome is reverse-transcribed into cDNA by the viral enzyme Reverse Transcriptase. As part of the preintegration complex, the proviral cDNA is transported into the nucleus and integrated into the host cell genome by the viral Integrase. The integrated proviral cDNA is transcribed and translation occurs from full-length as well as from multiply spliced mRNAs. Full-length mRNA genomes and structural viral proteins assemble at the plasma membrane. Here, new virus particles are released from the cell by budding and may, following maturation, infect new target cells. As indicated in boxes, several steps of the viral life cycle can be inhibited by therapeutic intervention.

epitope structure recognized by some mAbs has been extensively studied. However it has not yet been possible to generate immunogens capable of inducing such antibodies upon immunization and, although immune sera were found to bind to their target, they had no neutralizing abilities [2]. An alternative method of inhibiting HIV-1 entry is based on peptide mimetics of cellular HIV receptor domains, such as the CD4 miniproteins or extracellular domains of the CCR5 coreceptor, that bind to the virus and thereby neutralize the infection.

Addressing intracellular targets with peptides is more difficult, mainly because delivery of peptides into the cells requires a great deal of assistance, since short hydrophilic peptides generally do not cross the plasma membranes in their own right. Rather, the peptides may be taken up by cells, if coupled to carrier systems such as liposomes or nanoparticles, or they can be fused to a protein transduction domain. Alternatively, they may be expressed within cells after transduction with viral vectors. Despite these difficulties, a number of peptide ligands have been identified which show promise as intracellular targets *in vitro*, including ligands for the complex RNA structure Ψ that is responsible for packaging full-length RNA genomes into nascent virus particles, or the Gag multimerization domain which is implicated in viral assembly [3–5].

Although these peptide ligands have been shown to inhibit HIV-1 *in vitro*, due to the above-mentioned difficulties and to their short half-lives *in vivo*, they will most likely serve in the derivation of peptidomimetics or low-molecular-weight drugs aimed at inhibiting HIV-1 at particular steps within its replication cycle. In this chapter, attention will be focused exclusively on those peptides which inhibit the entry of HIV-1 into target cells.

5.2
The HIV Entry Process

The entry of HIV into target cells is mediated by the viral envelope glycoproteins gp120 and gp41 (Figure 5.2). Gp120, is linked noncovalently to gp41, a class I transmembrane protein that anchors the gp120/gp41 heterodimer to the cell or viral surface. Three gp120/gp41 complexes associate to form trimeric spikes on the viral envelope. The actual cell entry is a multistep process that is initiated by the binding of gp120 to its primary receptor on the target cell, CD4 [6]. Such binding induces a conformational change in the viral envelope glycoprotein complex that causes the coreceptor binding domain on gp120 to be exposed. The HIV-1 variants differ in their coreceptor usage; most strains employ the chemokine receptors CCR5 or CXCR4, or both, and are correspondingly classified as CCR5-tropic (R5), CXCR4-tropic (X4) or dual-tropic (R5X4).

Binding to the coreceptor initiates a fusion of the viral and cellular membranes – the key step that finally allows internalization of the viral capsid containing the viral genome, and thus infection of the target cell. The critical domains in gp41 are the N-terminal hydrophobic fusion peptide, followed by two heptad repeats (HR1 and HR2), as well as a C-terminal membrane anchor. The HR1 of the three gp41 molecules within a gp120/gp41 complex form a coiled-coil structure, with fusion being initiated by insertion of the N- terminal fusion peptide of gp41 into the target cell membrane. Subsequently, the three HR2 domains fold back and pack into the grooves of the gp41 HR1 coiled-coil to form a trimer of hairpins. This six-helix bundle serves to bring the membranes into close proximity, enabling fusion pore formation and release of the viral capsid into the cytoplasm.

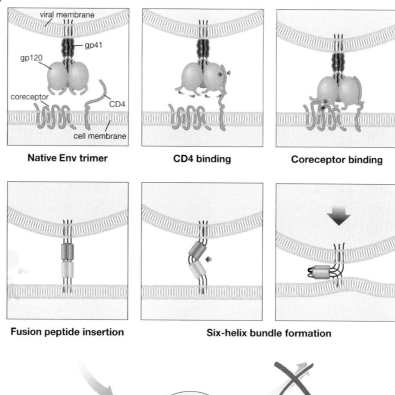

Native Env trimer   **CD4 binding**   **Coreceptor binding**

Fusion peptide insertion   **Six-helix bundle formation**

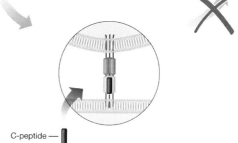

C-peptide —

Figure 5.2 The HIV entry process. HIV entry into target cells is mediated by the viral envelope glycoproteins gp120 and gp41 upon binding to the CD4 molecule, and a coreceptor on the target cell plasma membrane. Subsequent conformational changes in gp41 bring the viral and cellular membranes in close proximity and finally allow fusion pore formation. C peptides derived from the C-terminal HR2 of gp41 block membrane fusion by binding to the coiled-coil of HR1 helices and thus inhibit six-helix bundle formation (see circle).

5.3
Peptides that Inhibit Receptor or Coreceptor Binding

5.3.1
Physiological Antimicrobial Peptides

A number of physiological soluble factors such as cytokines, chemokines and anti-microbial peptides (AMPs) are known to be secreted from cells of the innate and adaptive immune system, and subsequently combat the invading pathogens (including HIV-1) in a concerted action. The epithelial barriers that surround higher organisms constitute the first line of defense, with the epithelial cells of the skin contributing to an innate pathogen resistance by producing AMPs with a broad spectrum of antimicrobial activities [7]. AMPs have been isolated from the skin of frogs, including peptides that are active against infections with enveloped viruses. Three frog-derived peptides, Caerin 1.1 (IC_{50}: $1.2\,\mu M$), Caerin 1.9 (IC_{50}: $7.8\,\mu M$), and Maculatin 1.1 (IC_{50}: $11.3\,\mu M$), were shown to be highly effective against HIV infection by disrupting the integrity of the virion membrane and preventing entry of the virus into target cells at concentrations that were not toxic to the cells [8]. These peptides also prevented the transfer of HIV from dendritic cells to T cells, thus making them promising candidates for HIV prophylaxis at mucosal sites.

In general, the AMPs are amphipathic α-helical peptides comprising 11 to 26 amino acids with clusters of positively charged and hydrophobic amino acids on opposite sides of the molecules. The positively charged amino acids bind to the negatively charged head groups of pathogen membranes. The two major AMP classes are cathelicidins and defensins, but only one human cathelicidin has yet been described that seems to play a role in the control of Herpes simplex virus (HSV) infections, thus underlining the importance of cathelicidins in the antiviral host defense of the skin [9].

5.3.1.1 Defensins
The defensins are cysteine-rich cationic peptides with a molecular weight of 3–5 kDa, and are produced either by epithelial cells or neutrophils. Depending on the location of the disulfide bonds, the defensins are classified as α-, β- or θ-defensins. Human defensins were first reported to show antiviral activities against HIV-1 in 1993 [10]. The α-defensins are mostly produced by neutrophils, and block several steps in the HIV-1 replication cycle. Earlier studies reported inhibition within infected cells either by interference with signal transduction and import of the preintegration complex into the nucleus, or via an indirect role involving the induction of chemokines [11]. More recently, however, α-defensins 1 and 2 have been shown to interfere with HIV-1 infection at the level of interaction of gp120 with the CD4 receptor [12]. Consequently, these α-defensins demonstrate activity against a broad spectrum of primary HIV-1 isolates, independently of their subtype or coreceptor specificity.

The mechanism of entry inhibition by α-defensins was elucidated in more detail, and shown to be dual in nature, with the peptides binding directly not only to the D1 domain of the CD4 implicated in gp120 binding, but also to the CD4-binding regions and CD4-induced epitopes on gp120. Due to their high local concentrations at mucosal sites, α-defensins may very likely contribute to the host antiviral immune defense *in vivo* at these sites. Interestingly, another human defensin – human β-defensin 3 – has also been shown to interfere with HIV-1 entry, but in this case as an antagonist of the coreceptor CXCR4, thereby opening new routes for drug design [13].

A different mode of action was described for *retrocyclin*, a synthetic macrocyclic θ-defensin, which binds to the HR2 ectodomain of gp41 and interferes with six-helix bundle formation [14]. Despite these clear antiviral roles of defensins, it should be mentioned here that, in a recent study, an enhancing activity of human defensins 5 and 6 was also demonstrated on HIV-1 infection in the context of *Gonococcus* coinfection, using a cervicovaginal tissue culture system. Notably, these findings underline the complexity of defensins as immune mediators in HIV-1 infection [15].

An additional physiological antiviral factor which has been shown to differ clearly from the defensins is the CD8 cell antiviral factor (CAF), as first identified by J. Levy [16]. Although the identity of CAF has not yet been fully elucidated, it appears to inhibit retroviral transcription within the cell, and so will not be discussed in detail at this point.

5.3.2
Chemokines

The finding that HIV-1 is dependent on chemokine receptors to enter cells was made during the mid-1990s. These receptors are required in addition to the well-studied CD4 receptor, and this observation was a major breakthrough in HIV research (for a review, see Ref. [17]). The identification of CCR5 and CXCR4 as essential coreceptors for HIV-1 entry was the missing link in understanding the antiviral activity of physiological peptides – the chemokines – that are secreted by different cells of the immune system during inflammation. Chemokines are small cysteine-rich polypeptides of 8–10 kDa, and are present in all vertebrates. These chemotaxis-inducing cytokines play an important role in immune defense and development, and consequently the chemokine system is often manipulated by invading pathogens. According to the position of the cysteines, chemokines are classified as C-, CC-, CXC- or CX3C, and exert their function by binding to G-protein-coupled receptors such as CCR5 or CXCR4. HIV-1 gp120 – and, in particular, the third variable region V3 – seems to structurally mimic the chemokines that interact with the corresponding chemokine receptors [18].

Based on the antiviral activity of the natural chemokine ligands of CCR5 (CCL5/RANTES, CCL3/MIP1α, CCL4/MIP1β) and CXCR4 (CXCL12/SDF-1), chemokine derivatives have been developed with the aim of interfering with HIV-1 entry at the crucial step of coreceptor binding. N-terminally modified RANTES analogues have been engineered, such as AOP-RANTES, NNY-RANTES or PSC-RANTES, and this has resulted in entry inhibitors with subnanomolar affinity and improved pharmacological profiles [19, 20]. The antiviral activity is mediated by receptor blockage as well as by receptor downmodulation [21]. Potent semisynthetic chemokine analogues are promising leads for the development of microbicidal compounds for topical applications in the prophylaxis of HIV transmission [22].

5.3.3
Synthetic Peptides and Peptidomimetics

Based on the sequences of gp120 or its receptors, a number of peptides have been derived with the aim of interfering specifically with this interaction – and consequently with HIV-1 entry into target cells – without affecting normal receptor functions in antigen presentation (CD4) or chemotaxis (CCR5, CXCR4).

One class comprises peptides or polypeptides derived from the CD4 receptor, or peptides mimicking CD4 domains essential for gp120 binding. The first protein, which was described during the mid-1990s, was a recombinant antibody-like fusion protein where the variable domains of the light and heavy chains of human IgG2 were substituted with the D1 and D2 immunoglobulin-like domains of CD4 [23]. This molecule was developed further for clinical application (PRO 542), and shown capable of potently neutralizing primary HIV-1 isolates *in vitro*. Moreover, it also showed promising antiviral activity *in vivo* [24, 25]. However, further clinical studies in HIV-1 infected children revealed nonlinear pharmacokinetics; that is, doubling the dose did not result in any improved antiviral effects, most likely due to Fc-mediated uptake and inactivation of the IgG-like molecules [26].

Another approach for developing CD4-related polypeptides was based on modeling and rational design using structural information [27]. These CD4 miniprotein mimetics (M33) contain some non-natural amino acids, and exhibit the functional characteristics of native CD4 in terms of gp120 binding and they are stable at low pH and resistant to protease degradation. Optimized CD4 mimetics (M47, M48) were selected from tailored peptide libraries synthesized through combinatorial chemistry [28]. The best constructs in terms of HIV-1 entry inhibition were variants of the M48 CD4 miniprotein mimetic, that had been designed specifically to target the Phe42 cavity on gp120 critical for binding to native CD4 (M48-UX). These compounds inhibited diverse HIV-1 subtype B isolates independently of their coreceptor usage in the low nanomolar range, although for subtype C strains the EC_{50} values were tenfold higher [28].

Nevertheless, the best constructs also inhibited replication-competent HIV-1 in cocultures of T cells with macrophages, and completely prevented viral infection when the cultures were treated from 2 h before until 24 h after infection at nontoxic concentrations. Currently, these CD4 miniproteins are being optimized further and represent a promising class of HIV microbicides.

Other studies have described the development of peptidomimetics targeting the CD4 receptor itself, with the aim of interfering with gp120 binding, but not with MHC Class II antigen presentation [29, 30]. The best constructs bound CD4 in the low micromolar range, although functional data on HIV inhibition or antigen presentation were not available [31]. A further approach was the development of a rationally designed synthetic mimetic of the discontinuous CD4 binding site on HIV-1 gp120. Based on structural information, the individual components of the discontinuous epitope of the HIV-1 neutralizing antibody b12 that binds to the CD4 binding site on gp120 were synthesized onto a molecular scaffold [32]. The best peptide competed with gp120 for binding to CD4 and mAb b12 in the low micromolar range [33].

Recently, an interesting class of metallocene peptide conjugate, generated by a combination of peptide and click chemistry, was described. These conjugates bind gp120 in a mode that interferes with both CD4 and coreceptor binding, probably by altering the conformation of gp120 upon binding [34, 35]. Furthermore, the best compound (HNG-156), as selected by surface plasmon resonance (SPR) interaction with gp120, inhibited HIV-1$_{Ba-L}$ in the low nanomolar range [34]. This improved mode of inhibition may be due to a slower off-rate from gp120.

In addition to targeting the inhibition of gp120 with CD4, other peptidic compounds have been developed with the aim of interfering with gp120 binding to coreceptors. The first compound to be described was Peptide T, a threonine-rich peptide which corresponded to amino acids 185–192 of the V2 region of HIV-1 gp120, and which was shown to inhibit the entry of CCR5-using HIV-1 by binding to the coreceptor [36]. A derivative of Peptide T, known as D-Ala-Peptide T-amide (DAPTA), resulted in a reduced viral load in HIV-positive patients and improvement in patients with cognitive impairment and a low CD4 count [37].

Following the identification of domains in the CCR5 coreceptor essential for gp120 binding by mutational analyses, domain swapping between susceptible and nonsusceptible receptors as well as phage display [38–41], synthetic peptides were derived from these functionally important domains that interfere with gp120 binding to CCR5. In particular, peptides derived from the N-terminus of CCR5, where tyrosines are sulfated as in the natural receptor, were shown to interact with CCR5-using gp120 and to inhibit these isolates *in vitro*, although only in the micromolar range [42–44]. Furthermore, these peptides could functionally reconstitute a CCR5 receptor lacking the N-terminal domain [45].

Recently, the binding of a tyrosine-sulfated peptide derived from the N-terminus of CCR5 to gp120 in complex with CD4 has been identified and studied using nuclear magnetic resonance (NMR) spectroscopy [46]. However, other extracellular loops (ECLs) of CCR5 also contribute to gp120 binding: for example, ECL2 interacts with the V3 loop of CCR5-using gp120 [47], while ECL1 has been shown to contain an amino acid motif essential for the infectivity of R5 strains [41]. Consequently, peptides derived from these ECLs are also able to inhibit HIV-1 strains [48]. Recently, the structure of a tyrosine-sulfated peptide corresponding to the N-terminus of CCR5 in complex with gp120/CD4 has been reported, providing new insights into this attractive target for HIV-1 entry inhibition [46].

CXCR4 is more difficult to target due to its role in essential physiological functions, such as the homing of T cells to sites of inflammation and bone marrow homeostasis. Interestingly, poly-arginine-rich peptides originally designed or selected to interfere with binding of the transcriptional activator Tat to the Tat-responsive region TAR in the viral RNA, were shown also to interfere with HIV-1 entry by binding to CXCR4 [49, 50]. A similar effect was found by others ([51]; also C. Königs and U. Dietrich, unpublished results). CXCR4 arginine-rich antagonistic peptides also comprise natural peptides derived from self-defense proteins such as polyhemusins, isolated from the horseshoe crab (T22, T140) [52]. These were the starting point for optimized highly potent and selective β-hairpin mimetic CXCR4 inhibitors with excellent anti-HIV activity and pharmacokinetic profiles [53]. The best compound, POL3026, was found to inhibit CXCR4-using HIV-1 as well as dual-tropic isolates, in the subnanomolar range [54].

5.4
Inhibitors of the Viral and Cellular Membrane Fusion Process

Currently available fusion inhibitors inhibit either the first step of membrane fusion or insertion of the viral fusion peptide into the target cell membrane, or they may prevent the subsequent six-helix bundle formation. Most fusion inhibitory peptides belong to the latter class, and inhibit six-helix bundle formation by binding to a prehairpin intermediate. These so-called N- and C-peptides are derived from the highly conserved amino acid sequences of the N- and C-heptad repeats (HR1 and HR2) of gp41, respectively.

Antiviral C peptides were first described by Wild *et al.* [55]. During the fusion process, antiviral C peptides interact with the coiled-coil formed by the N-terminal hydrophobic helices (HR1) of the prehairpin structure [56]. Thus, the binding sites for HR2 are blocked and the formation of the six-helix bundle and membrane fusion is prevented (Figure 5.2, see circle). C peptides have been shown to potently and broadly neutralize not only various primary and laboratory adapted HIV isolates, with IC_{50} values in the low nanomolar range [57–59], but also SIV strains [60–62].

Although several C peptides have been described, the most prominent family member is T20 (DP178, *enfuvirtide*; Fuzeon®), this being the first entry inhibitor to be approved for clinical treatment of HIV-1 infection by the US Food and Drug Administration (FDA) [63]. T20 is a synthetically produced soluble peptide of 36 amino acids, and represents a portion of the natural sequence of the gp41 HR2 of the HIV-1_{LAI} strain (corresponding to amino acids 638–673 of the HIV-1_{HxB2} Env protein) [55]. *In vitro* experiments with T20 revealed that the peptide inhibits the entry of both HIV-1 primary and laboratory isolates into their target cells, with IC_{50} values in the low nanomolar range [55]. In clinical Phase III trials, an optimal dose of 100 mg enfuvirtide (T20), twice daily, resulted in a clearly reduced viral load (two logs) and an increase in the patients' CD4 cell count [58, 64]. However, the peptide is not orally bioavailable and so must be injected subcutaneously; it also has a very short serum half-life of only 2–4 h [58]. For these reasons, and because a high peptide dose is required, the annual cost for therapy is approximately US$20 000 per patient. Unfortunately, yet another major problem with enfuvirtide treatment has been the rapid emergence of resistant virus variants [65].

Several novel C peptides are also active against viruses that are resistant to enfuvirtide. These C peptides are amino-terminally elongated and interact with a highly conserved hydrophobic groove at the C-terminus of the central HR1 coiled-coil structure. The interaction with this conserved pocket improves the inhibitory activity of peptides [66–68] and also delays the development of viral escape mutants [69, 70]. The hydrophobic amino acids W628, W631 and I635 (numbering according to the HIV-1$_{HxB2}$ Env protein) within the elongated C peptides are the major determinants for interaction with the conserved binding pocket [71], and can for instance be found in C34 [72], T-649 [73], or the second-generation C peptide T-1249, which is derived from HIV-1, HIV-2, and SIV sequences [74].

Using molecular design, C peptides with a greatly enhanced helical structure were engineered, resulting in a superior affinity to HR1. These peptides show significantly improved bundle stability, antiviral activity and pharmacokinetics [75, 76]. *Sifuvirtide*, for example, was designed by Y. He and coworkers after a series of alterations, starting from the gp41 sequence of the HIV-1 subtype E [77]. Compared to T20, sifuvirtide shows improved affinity to HR1 and thus a higher bundle stability. The peptide also demonstrates superior inhibitory activities against a wide variety of primary and laboratory-adapted HIV-1 isolates, including nonsubtype E viruses and also T20-resistant virus strains. The safety of sifuvirtide was proven in a clinical Phase Ia trial. In further clinical pharmacokinetics studies the half-life in humans was found to be 26 h, compared to 3.8 h for T20, making sifuvirtide a promising candidate for the treatment of HIV/AIDS patients in the future.

N peptides are HR1-derived sequences that, in contrast to C peptides, are weak inhibitors with IC$_{50}$ values in the micromolar range [78], although this is most likely due to their strong tendency to aggregate [79]. N peptides prevent membrane fusion either by binding to the HR2 domain of the prehairpin intermediate in analogy to C peptides [80], or by intercalation into the HR1 coiled-coil, thus disrupting this structure [81].

Another more potent fusion inhibitor is the 5-Helix protein [82], which resembles a six-helix bundle lacking one of the outer HR2 helices. The cavity created by the absence of one HR2 helix generates a binding site for the HR2 domain of gp41, thereby blocking six-helix bundle formation and the fusion process. 5-Helix has been shown to potently and broadly inhibit HIV-1 entry in the low nanomolar range [82].

Human blood contains a number of natural antiviral peptides, including the chemokines or defensins as described above, which can be purified from human hemofiltrates. By using this approach, another fusion inhibitory peptide – VIRIP (virus-inhibitory peptide) – was isolated recently for which a different mechanism of action has been described [83]. The active peptide sequence (LEAIPMSIPPEVK-FNKPFVF) was found to correspond to a fragment of human α1-antitrypsin, the most abundant circulating serine protease inhibitor. A synthetic peptide corresponding to this fragment inhibited HIV-1 in peripheral blood mononuclear cells (PBMCs) with an IC$_{50}$ of 4–20 μM, irrespective of viral subtype or coreceptor usage. VIRIP did not inhibit viruses belonging to the HIV-2/SIVmac group or non-HIV control viruses. VIRIP was then further optimized by structure–activity relation-ship (SAR) analysis, with the best compounds showing a 100-fold improved anti-viral activity.

Both, NMR and Biacore analysis confirmed a direct interaction of the VIRIP derivative VIR-165 with a peptide corresponding to amino acids 1 to 23 of the HIV-1 gp41 fusion peptide. Due to the broad antiviral activity of VIRIP, and the conserved nature of the fusion peptide of gp41, compounds targeting this particu-lar step during membrane fusion are promising candidates for the development of drugs interfering with HIV-1 entry.

5.5
Entry Inhibitory Peptides Selected by the Phage Display Technology

The phage display technology is highly suited to the rapid identification of peptide ligands for any structured targets (e.g., proteins or RNA), due to the linkage of phenotype and genotype (for a review, see Ref. [84]). An elegant variant of the selection procedure – mirror image phage display – uses synthetic D-amino acid targets for the biopanning procedure. The selected L-amino acid peptide ligands are transformed into their D-amino acid counterparts that should then bind the natural L-amino acid targets [85]. The advantage of D-amino acid peptides is their increased stability due to their resistance to protease degradation, which results in an increased serum half-life.

HIV-1 glycoproteins or their receptors have been used in a number of studies as targets in phage display experiments. Here, the intention was to select peptides that interfered with HIV-1 entry such that, when gp120 was used as the target, a peptide (12p1) was selected that interfered with binding to CD4 and the corecep-tors [86]. Mutational analysis then showed that 12p1 would bind to gp120 prior to CD4 binding at an adjacent site, thereby limiting the capacity of the viral glyco-protein to bind to CD4 and coreceptors [87]. Recently, peptide conjugates with potent antiviral activity against HIV-1$_{Ba-L}$ were derived from 12p1 by SAR analysis (see above and Ref. [35]).

Other peptides were selected that bind to the coreceptors CCR5 and CXCR4, respectively [88, 89], or that mimic the coreceptor domains important for gp120 binding [41, 90, 91]. These peptides could potentially interfere with gp120 binding to coreceptors, but the antiviral activity of the selected peptides, when analyzed, was in the high micromolar range.

By using the single-chain polypeptide N36(L8)C34 that mimics the gp41 six-helix bundle core structure as a target, HXXNPF consensus peptides were selected from phage-displayed peptide libraries. These peptides bind to the N-terminal heptad peptides of the fusion active gp41 core and inhibit syncytium formation [92, 93]. In other studies, the hydrophobic pocket of the gp41 N-trimer was used as a target for phage display screens.

A first generation of D-peptides was selected for this pocket using mirror image phage display, and the resultant molecules were shown to inhibit a laboratory-adapted HIV-1 strain in the high micromolar range [94]. A constrained decamer library was built based on the consensus sequence of the selected peptides ($CX_5EWXWLC$), and this resulted in the selection of an artificial 8mer with optimized binding properties for the pocket [95]. Subsequently, a constrained octamer library was generated (CX_4WXWLC) and the selected peptides were optimized further, using structural information. A trimeric version of the optimal peptide inhibited various HIV-1 strains in the picomolar range. This approach, which was based on a combination of mirror image phage display and structure-guided optimization, resulted in promising fusion inhibitors for therapeutic applications due to the favorable pharmacological properties of D-peptides.

5.6
Limitations of Peptides in the Treatment of HIV Infection

Although many peptides with high activities in tissue culture have been described, only a few peptidic drugs have been approved and subsequently marketed. A number of characteristics of peptides limit their broad clinical use. For example, peptides containing non-host amino acid sequences are potentially immunogenic, and although small peptides given without any adjuvant generally show minimal immunogenicity, a prolonged application can induce an immune response. Enfuvirtide, for example, does not contain any known dominant cytotoxic T lymphocyte (CTL) epitopes [96], but many HIV-1-infected patients have preexisting antibodies [97]. However, the presence of anti-enfuvirtide antibodies does not seem to impede therapeutic efficacy [98]. Although, after prolonged application patients develop local reactions at the injection site, systemic anaphylactic reactions are rare [99].

Peptides have unfavorable pharmacokinetics; typically, they are not absorbed after oral application but rather are degraded in the gastrointestinal tract by local proteases. Following parenteral administration, most peptides are eliminated rapidly by protease/peptidase degradation and renal clearance. Enfuvirtide, for example, has a serum half-life of 3–4 h, which leads to a need for the frequent administration of high-level peptide doses (in the case of enfuvirtide, 90 mg administered twice daily). This issue has been addressed by employing unusual or D- (rather than the natural L-) amino acids, which renders the peptides protease-resistant. Further improvements might be derived from the use of nonpeptidic backbones, peptidomimetics and/or formulations to improve stability, and also by the chemical modification of peptides to create protease-resistant and less toxic prodrug molecules. In fact, this approach has been used for the drug *colistimethate* (Colymycin®) [100, 101].

Another important issue here is the peptides' very high cost of manufacture, which has limited not only the testing and development of large numbers of drug candidates but also the range of targets to which the molecules can be applied. When using solid-phase chemical synthesis, the peptide production cost ranges from $100 to $600 per gram – which is an average daily dose for most systemic therapeutics. Clearly, all therapeutic strategies must take this factor into account, and there is a consequent growing need for less expensive peptide-production platforms.

Many attempts have been made to produce designer peptides by a variety of recombinant DNA methods, using bacteria and fungi as well as plant and animal production systems, although none of these expression systems has yet proved to be commercially feasible. A recent breakthrough in this regard was the use of a natural fungal peptide *plectasin* as a template, combined with a fungal expression system to produce an antimicrobial peptide at the scale and purity required for therapeutic administration [102]. One potential solution to costly peptide production and a short *in vivo* half-life would be to produce the therapeutic peptides *in vivo*, ideally directly at the site of virus replication (as discussed below).

5.7
Strategies to Prolong the *In Vivo* Half-Life of Antiviral Peptides

One major disadvantage of peptidic drugs is their short half-life *in vivo*, this being due to their proteolytic degradation coupled with a lack of oral bioavailability. One way to circumvent these problems would be the generation of D-peptides consisting of unnatural amino acids that would not be cleaved by proteases. As noted above, potent D-peptide fusion inhibitors have been generated based on mirror image phage display, although to date these have not advanced to clinical trials [95].

Another method of improving the stability and therapeutic potential of peptides would be their *multimerization*. This commonly occurs in many natural proteins, and offers potential advantages with respect to therapeutic applications. Multimerization can increase peptide stability, result in a higher binding strength due to multiple valencies in the molecule, improve pharmacokinetic properties, and also offer the possibility to combine several functional domains into one molecule.

With respect to HIV-1 entry inhibitors, the first multimeric molecule to enter clinical trials was PRO 542, a tetrameric CD4-IgG2 molecule containing D1 and D2 domains of the CD4 receptor (see above and Figure 5.3). The multimers were expressed in Chinese hamster ovary (CHO) cells and secreted into the culture supernatants as functional tetramers. Subsequently, the plasma half-life in rabbits was increased to more than one day for the tetramers, as compared to 15 min for the monomer [23]. The antiviral activity of the tetrameric antibody is most likely due to a crosslinking of the functional envelope spikes on the virions [103]. Although clinical application of the multimers showed no toxic side effects, the Fc-portion of the molecule resulted in a Fc-receptor-mediated uptake and consequently in clearance from the circulation, leading to nonlinear pharmacokinetics in a pediatric study [26].

In addition to the linkage to IgG-like molecules, other natural protein domains have been used to multimerize peptides. One such system was developed by the Cohen group in France, and is based on the human complement 4b binding protein (C4bp) ([104, 105]) (Figure 5.3). The human plasma protein C4bp has a

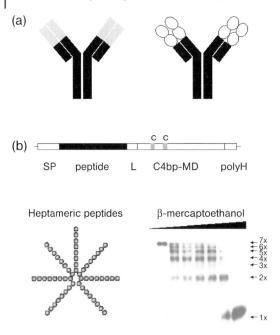

Figure 5.3 Principles of multimerization of therapeutic peptides. (a) Tetramerization of CD4 (D1 and D2 domains, white ellipses) by substitution of the variable domains (gray) of the light and heavy chains of an IgG molecule; (b) Heptamerization of a therapeutic peptide by fusion to the multimerizing domain of the human plasma protein C4bp (C4bp-MD). Heptameric peptides can be purified from cell culture supernatants under nonreducing conditions. The Western blot shows intermediate multimeric peptides depending on the concentration of β-mercaptoethanol. SP, signal peptide; L, linker; polyH, His-tag; C, cysteines mediating multimerization.

spider-like structure consisting of seven α-chains and one β-chain [106]. The α-chain contains at its C-terminus a domain of 60 amino acids that is responsible for multimerization induced by the formation of intermolecular cysteine bridges between the individual domains; otherwise, this domain is functionally inert. For multimerization, a nucleotide sequence encoding the peptide to be multimerized can be linked 5′ to the cDNA sequence of the C4bp multimerizing domain. Upon transfection of expression vectors into eukaryotic cells, the fusion proteins multimerize spontaneously in the endoplasmic reticulum and are secreted into the culture supernatant, if they also possess a signal peptide [104, 107]. Interestingly, the multimers are heptameric, like the natural C4bp molecule; moreover, the C4bp multimerizing domain is not immunogenic and is rather well suited for therapeutic applications.

The C4bp multimerizing system was first used to multimerize the soluble CD4 receptor [105]. Heptameric CD4 molecules were secreted into the culture supernatants of transfected 293T cells, after which the antiviral activity of heptameric CD4 molecules was seen to be threefold higher than that of monomeric sCD4 in HelaP4 cells infected with HIV-1$_{LAI}$. Organoids were then generated from transfected clones and surgically implanted into the peritoneal cavity of young mice. At 13 weeks after transplantation, the plasma levels of heptameric sCD4 were up to 2.5 µg ml^{-1}, but no sCD4 was detected for organoids secreting mono-meric sCD4, due to the shorter half-life. Thus, multimerization results in more stable peptides *in vivo*.

The group of U. Dietrich developed the C4bp multimerizing system to express soluble therapeutic peptides that are too small to be routed correctly through the cellular compartments for proper folding and post-translational modification. In order to establish the system, T20-related fusion inhibitory peptide C46 was expressed in a heptameric form in eukaryotic cells. This recombinant protein also comprised an N-terminal signal peptide, a linker joining the peptide with the C4bp multimerizing domain, and a His-tag for purification (see Figure 5.3) [108]. Multimeric C46 was purified from the culture supernatants and tested for antiviral activity *in vitro* in single-round infection assays using different HIV-1 pseudotypes.

In general, the multimers showed a slightly enhanced antiviral activity when compared to the monomers, although the enhancement was not proportional to the degree of multimerization. This effect was most likely due to the increased size of the molecule, which must fit between the viral and cellular membranes after receptor binding. However, the C46 multimers were much more stable *in vivo* in mice and showed improved pharmacological properties. It appears, there-fore, that multimerization may confer improved properties to peptide drugs, even when the drug potency *per se* is not considerably different.

In another study, fusion inhibitory peptides derived from HR2 were oligomer-ized by design through an increase in the helical structure of peptides related to T20 [75]. This led to self-oligomerization and high-affinity binding to HR1 pep-tides, with the best peptides being 3600-fold more active than enfuvirtide against viruses resistant to HR2 peptides in antiviral assays. Furthermore, resistance against these optimized peptides has not yet been observed *in vitro*. Interestingly, the engineered peptides also had extended half-lives of up to 35 h in cynomolgus monkeys. The superior antiviral properties of these oligomeric HR2 peptides, coupled with their enhanced pharmacokinetics, make them attractive candidates for further clinical development.

An innovative approach for increasing the antiviral activity of inhibitory peptides targeting viral entry was recently described, based on a combination of peptides targeting two different steps in the HIV-1 entry process in a single molecule [109]. This "molecular combination therapy" was carried out with a bifunctional fusion inhibitor (BFFI) which consisted of the variable domains of an antibody against CCR5 (Mab 004) and a peptide, which inhibits membrane fusion (T2635), fused to its C-terminus. In single-round infection assays, the BFFI was 86-fold more potent than the fusion inhibitory peptide alone, 30-fold more active than the antibody alone, and it also inhibited diverse HIV-1 isolates in the picomolar range. Thus, this molecule represents a prototypic bifunctional entry inhibitor and a promising can-didate for further development of synergistic HIV-1 entry inhibitors.

A further advance with respect to clinical applications of HIV-1 entry inhibitors (notably for microbicides) has been the engineering of commensal bacteria such as *Lactobacillus* to secrete HIV-1 fusion inhibitory peptides with potent antiviral activity [110]. The HR2-related peptides were expressed in the bacteria and secreted into the supernatant; HIV-1 isolates could then be neutralized up to 98% by using diluted culture supernatant (1:10). As commensal bacteria play an important role in not only intestinal but also vaginal fluids, the production of highly potent anti-HIV peptides *in situ* may be very well suited to preventing sexually transmitted HIV-1 infections.

5.8
Antiviral Peptides in Gene Therapy of HIV Infection

The major limitations to treatment with synthetic peptides have been outlined above, and include the cost of production, the short *in vivo* half-life, and the lack of oral bioavailability. Yet, each of these limitations could potentially be overcome by employing gene therapeutic procedures. It is conceivable that a cell could be altered genetically to contain a gene that would encode a therapeutic protein and so provide the patient with cells that could secretes a therapeutic protein/peptide. Several groups have shown that HIV-1 replication can be efficiently inhibited by the expression of antiviral genes in the target cells for HIV; this strategy has been termed "intracellular immunization" [111], and has two potential modes of action. First, if sufficient levels of gene-protected cells can be obtained, viral replication would be expected to decline due to a lack of available target cells. Second, the control of virus replication by the immune system would be expected to improve with an increasing number of T-helper cell clones specific for HIV antigens that are protected against viral infection. These gene-protected helper cells could support the immune control of viral replication, without the risk of infection facilitated by the activation of T cells against HIV antigens.

The basic problem of intracellular immunization strategies is that the total number of target cells for HIV-1 in the patient is very large, more than 10^{11}. The quantitative genetic modification of the entire target cell population – whether by T cell or stem cell targeting – is unlikely to be feasible in the foreseeable future. Thus, the application of cells containing an antiviral gene is not expected to lead to a substantial level of gene protection with a significant reduction of available nonmodified target cells, unless the genetically protected cells have a selective advantage over the nonmodified cells and accumulate with time [112]. Indeed, several antiviral genes have been developed that are expected to confer such a selective advantage, as they have been shown to effectively suppress viral replication and protect cells from the viral cytopathic effect in HIV-infected cell cultures.

Several types of antiviral proteins have been used in gene therapeutic approaches. Dominant-negative mutants of viral proteins inhibit the function of wild-type viral proteins; examples of these are the transdominant Rev and Tat mutants (see below [113, 114]). The expression of mutated cellular proteins, such as sCD4 or eIF-5A

(a)   (b)

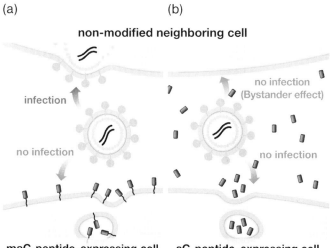

Figure 5.4 Mode of action of membrane-anchored and secretable entry inhibitors. (a) Cells that were genetically modified to express a membrane-anchored (ma) C-peptide on the plasma membrane are effectively protected from HIV entry. In HIV-infected mixed cultures, unmodified neighboring cells can be infected and rapidly disappear, while gene-protected cells have a selective advantage and accumulate over time; (b) Cells expressing secretable (s) entry inhibitory C peptides are expected to exert a "bystander effect", thus preventing viral infection of gene-modified as well as of nonmodified neighboring cells.

[115], can also interfere with essential functions of their wild-type cellular counterparts and interfere with functions essential in the viral life cycle – for example, CD4 receptor binding and the expression of unspliced viral genomic RNA. The ectopic expression of certain cytokines has been shown to inhibit HIV replication; examples include interferon α/β and interleukin-16 [116–119]. Finally, antibodies that bind and inactivate viral proteins can either be expressed within the cell as single-chain fragments (scFvs: anti-Rev, anti-IN, anti-RT) or secreted as a neutralizing antibody into the supernatant [120–122].

Although, currently, the fusion inhibitory C peptides described above belong to the most active antiviral biomolecules, peptides of less than 50 amino acids are not translated and secreted efficiently, and this poses new challenges for the development of gene therapeutic regimens aiming at the *in vivo* secretion of therapeutic peptides. The therapeutic peptide sequence must be linked to a scaffold for efficient expression. Recently, von Laer and coworkers succeeded in the expression of antiviral levels of C peptides by fusing the C peptide sequence to a scaffold that anchors it to the cell membrane (Figure 5.4a).

Membrane-anchored C peptides (maC peptides) effectively inhibit the entry of a broad range of HIV isolates [123, 124]. These peptides are derived from the C-terminal heptad repeat of the HIV gp41 envelope glycoprotein. A retroviral vector (M87o) was developed to express high levels of a 46-amino acid maC peptide

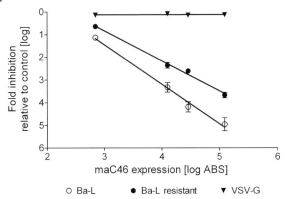

○ Ba-L   ● Ba-L resistant   ▼ VSV-G

Figure 5.5 Dose–response assay showing the correlation of maC46 expression on the cell surface with HIV-1 inhibition for wild-type and maC46-resistant HIV-1$_{Ba-L}$. PM-1 cell lines expressing different amounts of surface maC46 expression levels were determined by binding of the mAb 2F5, the corresponding antibody binding sites (ABS) per cell are depicted on the x-axis. The established cell lines were infected with a lentiviral vector encoding enhanced green fluorescent protein (eGFP), pseudotyped with the viral envelope glycoproteins cloned from wild-type Ba-L (Ba-L) or from the selected maC46-resistant Ba-L isolate (Ba-L_resistant). The G protein of the vesicular stomatitis virus (VSV-G) was used as a control. Fold inhibition relative to the level of infection on native PM-1 cells is given on the y-axis.

(maC46). In M87o, maC46 peptide is expressed as a fusion protein, with an N-terminal signal peptide to mediate translocation into the endoplasmic reticulum, followed by the C46 sequence, a flexible linker derived from human IgG2 and the membrane anchor from human CD34. The replication of several primary HIV isolates from different clades (B, D, E, O), and even of HIV-2, was effectively inhibited in transduced bulk cultures of T-helper cell lines and primary T cells [124].

The predicted mode of action at the level of virus entry of maC46 was confirmed by single-round infections with different replication-incompetent viral pseudotypes [125, 126]. A more than 10 000-fold inhibition of HIV-1 Env-mediated viral entry was seen in cells expressing maC46 [127]. This strong antiviral activity conferred a sufficient selective advantage to allow the rapid accumulation of maC46-expressing T cells in HIV-infected mixed cultures of gene-protected and unmodified cells [124].

Interestingly, maC46 was also found to be highly active against virus strains resistant to enfuvirtide (T20), when Hermann and coworkers selected an HIV-1 strain with reduced sensitivity to maC46. Here, after over 200 days of passaging on suboptimal and slowly increasing concentrations of maC46, a virus strain with a tenfold-reduced sensitivity to maC46 emerged (Figure 5.5). The virus had five mutations at highly conserved positions in the viral envelope, three in gp120, and one mutation each in the HR1 and HR2 of gp41. No mutations developed in the domain around the GIV motif in HR1, which generally is associated with resistance to C peptide fusion inhibitors. The GIV mutation is thought to reduce the binding affinity of enfuvirtide to the gp41 HR1 coiled-coil.

In contrast, the mutations that reduced sensitivity of HIV to maC46 were not found to reduce binding affinity to C46, but either to enhance the intramolecular binding affinity between gp41 HR1 and HR2 or accelerate the entry process. Thus, resistance to maC46 does not readily develop and requires multiple cooperating mutations at highly conserved positions of the viral envelope glycoproteins gp120 and gp41. This finding is extremely interesting, since the reason for this "resistance to resistance" for maC46 is most likely the large interaction surface between the viral envelope gp41 HR1 and the C46 peptide [128]. Interacting domains tend to be much smaller for low-molecular-weight compounds, and even for most mAbs.

A Phase I clinical trial was conducted to test the safety and potential antiviral activity of autologous T cells expressing maC46 (M87o) in 10 AIDS patients with severe immunodeficiency and HAART (highly active antiretroviral therapy) failure [129]. No major toxicities were observed, and neither cellular nor humoral immune responses to the transgene product maC46 were detected. While a significant rise in T-helper cell counts was seen, the viral load was unaffected. Although gene marking could be detected throughout the one-year follow-up, the levels were too low to account for the marked rise in CD4 counts.

The results of *in vitro* studies have shown clearly that the maC46 transgene product effectively protects cells from HIV infection, and thus indeed confers a selective advantage to the gene-modified cells in HIV-infected cell cultures [124, 130]. However, a clear accumulation of gene-modified cells over time was not seen in the treated patients. There are several possible explanations for this discrepancy [129]. First, the gene-modified cells may have downregulated expression of the transgene *in vivo*. The antiviral efficacy of maC46 correlates strongly with the level of maC46 expressed on the cell surface, as shown in Figure 5.5 (F.G. Hermann and D. von Laer, unpublished data) [124]. In addition, the gene-modified cells may have lost their repopulation potential during *ex vivo* expansion and thus may *per se* have a selective disadvantage.

Transferred autologous T cells only carry T-cell receptors (TCRs) with specificities already present within the reduced T-cell repertoire of the patient. They must compete with these cells to survive and to proliferate. In addition, the proportion of HIV-infected T cells is <1% [131–133], and thus the total turnover of T-helper cells is much lower in the patient than in HIV-infected T-cell cultures. Therefore, the selective pressure is relatively low in the HIV-infected patient, and most likely much lower than for the gene-corrected cells used successfully to genetically correct T-cell precursors and mature T cells in children with severe combined immune deficiency [134–139].

Finally, the architecture of the lymph nodes, which provide a major support for T-cell regeneration, is destroyed in these advanced patients with persistently high levels of virus replication. Thus, HIV-infected patients with a short history of high-level virus replication where the lymph node function is not yet severely impaired, but the replicating virus is already exerting a considerable selective advantage to the gene-protected cells, would be expected to profit most from "intracellular immunization" gene therapy strategies. However, mathematical models predict that the system is labile, and that the selective advantage conferred by an antiviral gene may be insufficient to allow an efficient accumulation of gene-modified cells *in vivo* [140].

The need to accumulate gene-protected cells could be circumvented by using an *in vivo*-secreted antiviral entry inhibitor (iSAVE). iSAVE (poly)peptides are expected to produce a "bystander effect" on neighboring nonmodified cells and to exert an overall antiviral effect even at low levels of gene marking (Figure 5.4b). Here, the modification of both T cells as well as hematopoietic progenitor cells appears to have great therapeutic potential, as gene-modified cells would be expected to home to lymphatic tissues, which are also the major sites of viral replication; this would in turn lead to high local concentrations of the secreted antiviral gene product [141]. However, the number of reports on secreted antiviral gene products in the field of gene therapy is still very limited; examples include neutralizing antibodies, soluble CD4 and interferon β [121, 141, 142]. In principle, these gene products hold considerable promise, as an overall antiviral effect could be achieved, even at relatively low levels of gene marking.

Until now, although no attempts to secrete antiviral C peptides from gene-modified cells have been reported, this approach holds great promise as C peptides are the most active antiviral protein or peptide described to date. The fact that high serum levels ($>1\,\mu g\,ml^{-1}$) are required for therapeutic efficacy (i.e., three orders of magnitude above effective *in vitro* concentrations), coupled with the low steady-state volume of distribution (5–7 l), indicate that enfuvirtide penetrates the lymphatic tissue – the predominant site of HIV replication and intended site of antiviral drug activity – very inefficiently. In addition, the rapid clearance of enfuvirtide, together with its unfavorable biodistribution, is expected to lead to fluctuations in local drug concentrations in the lymphatic tissues that may permit periodic local low-level virus replication, thus favoring the emergence of viral resistance.

Although viral resistance has been shown to emerge less readily against longer C peptides, such as C46 [70, 128], the production process unfortunately limits the size of the synthetic antiviral C peptides produced. For iSAVE C peptides, however, the size is not restricted and secretion into the lymphatic tissue is expected to lead to high and stable locally effective concentrations of peptide. Thus, iSAVE C peptides would be expected to prove relatively "resistant to resistance".

Short peptides are only inefficiently translated and exported through the secretory pathway. Physiological peptides, such as neuropeptides, are thus generally processed from larger secreted protein precursors (see Ref. [143]). It is proposed that future research investigations should focus on the development of strategies that will allow the high-level secretion of therapeutic peptides *in vivo*, as such technology would have a broad applicability beyond antiviral therapy.

References

1 Lin, G. and Nara, P.L. (2007) Designing immunogens to elicit broadly neutralizing antibodies to the HIV-1 envelope glycoprotein. *Curr. HIV Res.*, **5**, 514.

2 Ollman Saphire, E., Montero, M., Menendez, A., van Houten, M.B., Irving, N.E., Pantophlet, R., Zwick, M.B., Parren, P.W.H.I., Burton, D.R., Scott, J.K. and Wilson, I.A. (2007) Structure of a high-affinity "mimotope" peptide bound to HIV-1-neutralizing antibody b12 explains its inability to elicit gp120 cross-reactive antibodies. *J. Mol. Biol.*, **369**, 696.

3 Dietz, J., Koch, J., Kaur, A., Raja, C., Stein, S., Grez, M., Pustowka, A., Mensch, S., Ferner, J., Möller, L., Bannert, N., Tampe, R., Divita, G., Mely, Y., Schwalbe, H. and Dietrich, U. (2008) Inhibition of HIV-1 by a peptide ligand of the genomic RNA packaging signal Psi. *ChemMedChem*, **3**, 749.

4 Sticht, J., Humbert, M., Findlow, S., Bodem, J., Muller, M., Dietrich, U., Werner, J. and Krausslich, H.G. (2005) A peptide inhibitor of HIV-1 assembly in vitro. *Nat. Struct. Mol. Biol.*, **12**, 671.

5 Zhang, H., Zhao, Q., Bhattacharya, S., Waheed, A.A., Tong, X., Hong, A., Heck, S., Curreli, F., Goger, M., Cowburn, D., Freed, E.O. and Ebnath, A.K. (2008) A cell-penetrating helical peptide as a potential HIV-1 inhibitor. *J. Mol. Biol.*, **378**, 565.

6 Freed, E.O. and Martin, M.A. (2007) *Fields Virology*, Vol. **2** (eds D.M. Knipe, P.M. Howley, D.E. Griffin, R.A. Lamb, M.A. Martin, B. Roizman and S.E. Straus), Lippincott Williams & Wilkins, Philadelphia, pp. 2107–85.

7 Namjoshi, S., Caccetta, R. and Benson, H.A.E. (2007) Skin peptides: biological activity and therapeutic opportunities. *J. Pharm. Sci.*, **97**, 2524.

8 Van Compernolle, S.E., Taylor, R.J., Oswald-Richter, K., Jiang, J., Youree, B.E., Bowie, J.H., Tyler, M.J., Conlon, J.M., Wade, D., Aiken, C., Dermody, T., KewalRamani, V., Rollins-Smith, L. and Unutmaz, D. (2005) Antimicrobial peptides from amphibian skin potently inhibit human immunodeficiency virus infection and transfer of virus from dendritic cells to T cells. *J. Virol.*, **79**, 11598.

9 Howell, M.D., Wollenberg, A., Gallo, R.L., Flaig, M., Streib, J.E., Wong, C., Pavicic, T., Boguniewicz, M. and Leung, D.Y. (2006) Cathelicidin deficiency predisposes to eczema herpeticum. *J. Allergy Clin. Immunol.*, **117**, 836.

10 Nakashima, H., Yamamoto, N., Masuda, M. and Fujii, N. (1993) Defensins inhibit HIV replication in vitro. *AIDS*, **7**, 1129.

11 Chang, T.L., Vargas, J.J., Del Portillo, A. and Klotman, M.E. (2005) Dual role of alpha-defensin-1 in anti-HIV-1 innate immunity. *J. Clin. Invest.*, **115**, 765.

12 Furci, L., Sironi, F., Tolazzi, M., Vassena, L. and Lusso, P. (2007) α-defensins block the early steps of HIV-1 infection: interference with the binding of gp120 to CD4. *Blood*, **109**, 2928.

13 Feng, Z., Dubyak, G.R., Lederman, M.M. and Weinberg, A. (2006) Cutting edge: human beta defensin 3 – a novel antagonist of the HIV-1 coreceptor CXCR4. *J. Immunol.*, **177**, 782.

14 Gallo, S.A., Wang, W., Rawat, S.S., Jung, G., Waring, A.J., Cole, A.M., Lu, H., Yan, X., Daly, N.L., Craik, D.J., Jiang, S., Lehrer, R.I. and Blumenthal, R. (2006) Theta-defensins prevent HIV-1 Env-mediated fusion by binding gp41 and blocking 6-helix bundle formation. *J. Biol. Chem.*, **281**, 18787.

15 Klotman, M.E., Rapista, A., Teleshova, N., Micsenyi, A., Jarvis, G.A., Lu, W., Porter, E. and Chang, T.L. (2008) Neisseria gonorrhoeae-induced human defensins 5 and 6 increase HIV infectivity: role in enhanced transmission. *J. Immunol.*, **180**, 6176.

16 Levy, J.A. (2003) The search for the CD8+ cell anti-HIV factor (CAF). *Trends Immunol.*, **24**, 628.

17 Lusso, P. (2006) HIV and the chemokine system: 10 years later. *EMBO J.*, **25**, 447.

18 Sharon, M., Kessler, N., Levy, R., Zolla-Pazner, S., Görlach, M. and

Anglister, J. (2003) Alternative conformations of HIV-1 V3 loops mimic beta hairpins in chemokines, suggesting a mechanism for coreceptor selectivity. *Structure*, **11**, 225.

19 Hartley, O., Gaertner, H., Wilken, J., Thompson, D., Fish, R., Ramos, A., Pastore, C., Dufour, B., Cerini, F., Melotti, A., Heveker, N., Picard, L., Alizon, M., Mosier, D., Kent, S. and Offord, R. (2004) Medicinal chemistry applied to a synthetic protein: development of highly potent HIV entry inhibitors. *Proc. Natl Acad. Sci. USA*, **101**, 16460.

20 Miranda, L.P., Shao, H.Y., Williams, J., Chen, S.Y., Kong, T., Garcia, R., Chinn, Y., Fraud, N., O'Dwyer, B., Ye, J., Wilken, J., Low, D.E., Cagle, E.N., Carnevali, M., Lee, A., Song, D., Kung, A., Bradburne, J.A., Paliard, X. and Kochendoerfer, G.G. (2007) A chemical approach to the pharmaceutical optimization of an anti-HIV protein A chemical approach to the pharmaceutical optimization of an anti-HIV protein. *J. Am. Chem. Soc.*, **129**, 13153.

21 Pastore, C., Picchio, G.R., Galimi, F., Fish, R., Hartley, O., Offord, R.E. and Mosier, D.E. (2003) Two mechanisms for human immunodeficiency virus type 1 inhibition by N-terminal modifications of RANTES. *Antimicrob. Agents Chemother.*, **47**, 509.

22 Gaertner, H., Offord, R., Botti, P., Kuenzi, G. and Hartley, O. (2008) Semisynthetic analogues of PSC-RANTES, a potent anti-HIV protein. *Bioconjug. Chem.*, **19**, 480.

23 Allaway, G.P., Davis-Bruno, K.L., Beaudry, G.A., Garcia, E.B., Wong, E.L., Ryder, A.M., Hasel, K.W., Gauduin, M.C., Koup, R.A., McDougal, J.S. and Maddon, P.J. (1995) Expression and characterization of CD4-IgG2, a novel heterotetramer that neutralizes primary HIV type 1 isolates. *AIDS Res. Hum. Retroviruses*, **11**, 533.

24 Trkola, A., Pomales, A.B., Yuan, H., Korber, B., Maddon, P.J., Allaway, G.P., Katinger, H., Barbas, C.F., Burton, D.R., Ho, D.D. and Moore, J.P. (1995) Cross-clade neutralization of primary isolates of human immunodeficiency virus type 1 by human monoclonal antibodies and tetrameric CD4-IgG. *J. Virol.*, **69**, 6609.

25 Shearer, W.T., Israel, R.J., Starr, S., Fletcher, C.V., Wara, D., Rathore, M., Church, J., DeVille, J., Fenton, T., Graham, B., Samson, P., Staprans, S., McNamara, J., Moye, J., Maddon, P.J. and Olson, W.C. (2000) Recombinant CD4-IgG2 in human immunodeficiency virus type 1-infected children: phase 1/2 study. The Pediatric AIDS Clinical Trials Group Protocol 351 Study Team. *J. Infect. Dis.*, **182**, 1774.

26 Fletcher, C.V., DeVille, J.G., Samson, P.M., Moye, J.H.J., Church, J.A., Spiegel, H.M., Palumbo, P., Fenton, T., Smith, M.E., Graham, B., Kraimer, J.M., Shearer, W.T., Group, P.A.C.T. and Group, P.S. (2007) Nonlinear pharmacokinetics of high-dose recombinant fusion protein CD4-IgG2 (PRO 542) observed in HIV-1-infected children. *J. Allergy Clin. Immunol.*, **119**, 747.

27 Martin, L., Stricher, F., Misse, D., Sironi, F., Pugniere, M., Barthe, P., Prado-Gotor, R., Freulon, I., Magne, X., Roumestand, C., Menez, A., Lusso, P., Veas, F. and Vita, C. (2003) Rational design of a CD4 mimic that inhibits HIV-1 entry and exposes cryptic neutralization epitopes. *Nat. Biotech.*, **21**, 71.

28 Van Herrewege, Y., Morellato, L., Descours, A., Aerts, L., Michiels, J., Heyndrickx, L., Martin, L. and Vanham, G. (2008) CD4 mimetic miniproteins: potent anti-HIV compounds with promising activity as microbicides. *J. Antimicrob. Chemother.*, **61**, 818.

29 Neffe, A.T. and Meyer, B. (2004) A peptidomimetic HIV-entry inhibitor directed against the CD4 binding site of the viral glycoprotein gp120. *Angew. Chem. Int. Ed. Engl.*, **43**, 2937.

30 Neffe, A.T., Bilang, M. and Meyer, B. (2006) Synthesis and optimization of peptidomimetics as HIV entry inhibitors against the receptor protein CD4 using STD NMR and ligand docking. *Org. Biomol. Chem.*, **4**, 3259.

31 Neffe, A.T., Bilang, M., Grüneberg, I. and Meyer, B. (2007) Rational optimization of the binding affinity of CD4 targeting peptidomimetics with potential anti HIV activity. *J. Med. Chem.*, **50**, 3482.

32 Franke, R., Hirsch, T. and Eichler, J. (2006) A rationally designed synthetic mimic of the discontinuous CD4-binding site of HIV-1 gp120. *J. Recept. Signal Transduct. Res.*, **26**, 453.

33 Franke, R., Hirsch, T., Overwin, H. and Eichler, J. (2007) Synthetic mimetics of the CD4 binding site of HIV-1 gp120 for the design of immunogens. *Angew. Chem. Int. Ed. Engl.*, **46**, 1253.

34 Gopi, H., Cocklin, S., Pirrone, V., McFadden, K., Tuzer, F., Zentner, I., Ajith, S., Baxter, S., Jawanda, N., Krebs, F.C. and Chaiken, I.M. (2009) Introducing metallocene into a triazole peptide conjugate reduces its off-rate and enhances its affinity and antiviral potency for HIV-1 gp120. *J. Mol. Recognit.*, **22**, 169.

35 Gopi, H., Umashankara, M., Pirrone, V., LaLonde, J., Madani, N., Tuzer, F., Baxter, S., Zentner, I., Cocklin, S., Jawanda, N., Miller, S.R., Schön, A., Klein, J.C., Freire, E., Krebs, F.C., Smith, A.B., Sodroski, J. and Chaiken, I. (2008) Structural determinants for affinity enhancement of a dual antagonist peptide entry inhibitor of human immunodeficiency virus type-1. *J. Med. Chem.*, **51**, 2638.

36 Ruff, M.R., Polianova, M., Yang, Q.E., Leoung, G.S., Ruscetti, F.W. and Pert, C.B. (2003) Update on D-ala-peptide T-amide (DAPTA): a viral entry inhibitor that blocks CCR5 chemokine receptors. *Curr. HIV Res.*, **1**, 51.

37 Goodkin, K., Vitiello, B., Lyman, W.D., Asthana, D., Atkinson, J.H., Heseltine, P.N., Molina, R., Zheng, W., Khamis, I., Wilkie, F.L. and Shapshak, P. (2006) Cerebrospinal and peripheral human immunodeficiency virus type 1 load in a multisite, randomized, double-blind, placebo-controlled trial of D-Ala1-peptide T-amide for HIV-1-associated cognitive-motor impairment. *J. Neurovirol.*, **12**, 178.

38 Atchison, R.E., Gosling, J., Monteclaro, F.S., Franci, C., Digilio, L., Charo, I.F. and Goldsmith, M.A. (1996) Multiple extracellular elements of CCR5 and HIV-1 entry: dissociation from response to chemokines. *Science*, **274**, 1924.

39 Doranz, B.J., Lu, Z.H., Rucker, J., Zhang, T.Y., Sharron, M., Cen, Y.H., Wang, Z.X., Guo, H.H., Du, J.G., Accavitti, M.A., Doms, R.W. and Peiper, S.C. (1997) Two distinct CCR5 domains can mediate coreceptor usage by human immunodeficiency virus type 1. *J. Virol.*, **71**, 6305.

40 Rabut, G.E., Konner, J.A., Kajumo, F., Moore, J.P. and Dragic, T. (1998) Alanine substitutions of polar and nonpolar residues in the amino-terminal domain of CCR5 differently impair entry of macrophage- and dualtropic isolates of human immunodeficiency virus type 1. *J. Virol.*, **72**, 3464.

41 Königs, C., Pustowka, A., Irving, J., Kessel, C., Klich, K., Wegner, V., Rowley, M.J., Mackay, I.R., Kreuz, W., Griesinger, C. and Dietrich, U. (2007) Peptide mimotopes selected with HIV-1-blocking monoclonal antibodies against CCR5 represent motifs specific for HIV-1 entry. *Immunol. Cell Biol.*, **85**, 511.

42 Cormier, E.G., Persuh, M., Thompson, D.A., Lin, S.W., Sakmar, T.P., Olson, W.C. and Dragic, T. (2000) Specific interaction of CCR5 amino-terminal domain peptides containing sulfotyrosines with HIV-1 envelope glycoprotein gp120. *Proc. Natl Acad. Sci. USA*, **97**, 5762.

43 Cormier, E.G., Tran, D.N., Yukhayeva, L., Olson, W.C. and Dragic, T. (2001) Mapping the determinants of the CCR5 amino-terminal sulfopeptide interaction with soluble human immunodeficiency virus type 1 gp120-CD4 complexes. *J. Virol.*, **75**, 5541.

44 Farzan, M., Vasilieva, N., Schnitzler, C.E., Chung, S., Robinson, J., Gerard, N.P., Gerard, C., Choe, H. and Sodroski, J. (2000) A tyrosine-sulfated peptide based on the N terminus of CCR5 interacts with a CD4-enhanced epitope of the HIV-1 gp120 envelope glycoprotein and inhibits HIV-1 entry. *J. Biol. Chem.*, **275**, 33516.

45 Farzan, M., Chung, S., Li, W., Vasilieva, N., Wright, P.L., Schnitzler, C.E., Marchione, R.J., Gerard, C., Gerard, N.P., Sodroski, J. and Choe, H. (2002) Tyrosine-sulfated peptides functionally reconstitute a CCR5 variant lacking a critical amino-terminal region. *J. Biol. Chem.*, **277**, 40397.

46 Huang, C.C., Lam, S.N., Acharya, P., Tang, M., Xiang, S.H., Hussan, S.S., Stanfield, R.L., Robinson, J., Sodroski, J., Wilson, I.A., Wyatt, R., Bewley, C.A. and Kwong, P.D. (2007) Structures of the CCR5 N terminus and of a tyrosine-sulfated antibody with HIV-1 gp120 and CD4. *Science*, **317**, 1930.

47 Napier, K.B., Wang, Z.X., Peiper, S.C. and Trent, J.O. (2007) CCR5 interactions with the variable 3 loop of gp120. *J. Mol. Model.*, **13**, 29.

48 Agrawal, L., VanHorn-Ali, Z., Berger, E.A. and Alkhatib, G. (2004) Specific inhibition of HIV-1 coreceptor activity by synthetic peptides corresponding to the predicted extracellular loops of CCR5. *Blood*, **103**, 1211.

49 Sumner-Smith, M., Zheng, Y., Zhang, Y.P., Twist, E.M. and Climie, S.C. (1995) Antiherpetic activities of N-alpha-acetyl-nona-D-arginine amide acetate. *Drugs Exp. Clin. Res.*, **21**, 1.

50 Doranz, B.J., Grovit-Ferbas, K., Sharron, M.P., Mao, S.H., Goetz, M.B., Daar, E.S., Doms, R.W. and O'Brien, W.A. (1997) A small-molecule inhibitor directed against the chemokine receptor CXCR4 prevents its use as an HIV-1 coreceptor. *J. Exp. Med.*, **186**, 1395.

51 Daelemans, D., Schols, D., Witvrouw, M., Pannecouque, C., Hatse, S., van Dooren, S., Hamy, Klimkait, F., T., de Clercq, E. and Van Damme, A.M. (2000) A second target for the peptoid Tat/transactivation response element inhibitor CGP64222: inhibition of human immunodeficiency virus replication by blocking CXC-chemokine receptor 4-mediated virus entry. *Mol. Pharmacol.*, **57**, 116.

52 Kazmierski, W.M., Kenakin, T.P. and Gudmundsson, K.S. (2006) Peptide, peptidomimetic and small-molecule drug discovery targeting HIV-1 host-cell attachment and entry through gp120, gp41, CCR5 and CXCR4. *Chem. Biol. Drug Des.*, **67**, 13.

53 DeMarco, S.J., Henze, H., Lederer, A., Moehle, K., Mukherjee, R., Romagnoli, B., Robinson, J.A., Brianza, F., Gombert, F.O., Lociuro, S., Ludin, C., Vrijbloed, J.W., Zumbrunn, J., Obrecht, J.P., Obrecht, D., Brondani, V., Hamy, F. and Klimkait, T. (2006) Discovery of novel, highly potent and selective beta-hairpin mimetic CXCR4 inhibitors with excellent anti-HIV activity and pharmacokinetic profiles. *Bioorg. Med. Chem.*, **14**, 8396.

54 Moncunill, G., Armand-Ugón, M., Clotet-Lodina, I., Pauls, E., Ballana, E., Llano, A., Romagnoli, B., Vrijbloed, J.W., Gombert, F.O., Clotet, B., De Marco, S. and Esté, J.A. (2008) Anti-HIV activity and resistance profile of the CXC chemokine receptor 4 antagonist POL3026. *Mol. Pharmacol.*, **73**, 1264.

55 Wild, C.T., Shugars, D.C., Greenwell, T.K., McDanal, C.B. and Matthews, T.J. (1994) Peptides corresponding to a predictive alpha-helical domain of human immunodeficiency virus type 1 gp41 are potent inhibitors of virus infection. *Proc. Natl Acad. Sci. USA*, **91**, 9770.

56 Kliger, Y. and Shai, Y. (2000) Inhibition of HIV-1 entry before gp41 folds into its fusion-active conformation. *J. Mol. Biol.*, **295**, 163.

57 Wild, C., Greenwell, T. and Matthews, T. (1993) A synthetic peptide from HIV-1 gp41 is a potent inhibitor of virus-mediated cell-cell fusion. *AIDS Res. Hum. Retroviruses*, **9**, 1051.

58 Kilby, J.M., Hopkins, S., Venetta, T.M., DiMassimo, B., Cloud, G.A., Lee, J.Y., Alldredge, L., Hunter, E., Lambert, D., Bolognesi, D., Matthews, T., Johnson, M.R., Nowak, M.A., Shaw, G.M. and Saag, M.S. (1998) Potent suppression of HIV-1 replication in humans by T-20, a peptide inhibitor of gp41-mediated virus entry. *Nat. Med.*, **4**, 1302.

59 Chinnadurai, R., Münch, J. and Kirchhoff, F. (2005) Effect of naturally-occurring gp41 HR1 variations on susceptibility of HIV-1 to fusion inhibitors. *AIDS*, **19**, 1401.

60 Gallo, S.A., Sackett, K., Rawat, S.S., Shai, Y. and Blumenthal, R. (2004) The stability of the intact envelope glycoproteins is a major determinant of sensitivity of HIV/SIV to peptidic fusion inhibitors. *J. Mol. Biol.*, **340**, 9.

61 Gustchina, E., Hummer, G., Bewley, C.A. and Clore, G.M. (2005) Differential inhibition of HIV-1 and SIV envelope-mediated cell fusion by C34 peptides derived from the C-terminal heptad repeat of gp41 from diverse strains of HIV-1, HIV-2, and SIV. *J. Med. Chem.*, **48**, 3036.

62 Zahn, R.C., Hermann, F.G., Kim, E.Y., Rett, M.D., Wolinsky, S.M., Johnson, R.P., Villinger, F., von Laer, D. and Schmitz, J.E. (2008) Efficient entry inhibition of human and nonhuman primate immunodeficiency virus by cell surface-expressed gp41-derived peptides. *Gene Ther.*, **15**, 1210.

63 Cervia, J.S. and Smith, M.A. (2003) Enfuvirtide (T-20): a novel human immunodeficiency virus type 1 fusion inhibitor. *Clin. Infect. Dis.*, **37**, 1102.

64 Lazzarin, A., Clotet, B., Cooper, D., Reynes, J., Arastéh, K., Nelson, M., Katlama, C., Stellbrink, H.J., Delfraissy, J.F., Lange, J., Huson, L., DeMasi, R., Wat, C., Delehanty, J., Drobnes, C., Salgo, M. and Group, T.S. (2003) Efficacy of enfuvirtide in patients infected with drug-resistant HIV-1 in Europe and Australia. *N. Engl. J. Med.*, **348**, 2186.

65 Rimsky, L.T., Shugars, D.C. and Matthews, T.J. (1998) Determinants of human immunodeficiency virus type 1 resistance to gp41-derived inhibitory peptides. *J. Virol.*, **72**, 986.

66 Chan, D.C., Chutkowski, C.T. and Kim, P.S. (1998) Evidence that a prominent cavity in the coiled coil of HIV type 1 gp41 is an attractive drug target. *Proc. Natl Acad. Sci. USA*, **95**, 15613.

67 Dwyer, J.J., Hasan, A., Wilson, K.L., White, J.M., Matthews, T.J. and Delmedico, M.K. (2003) The hydrophobic pocket contributes to the structural stability of the N-terminal coiled coil of HIV gp41 but is not required for six-helix bundle formation. *Biochemistry*, **42**, 4945.

68 Greenberg, M.L., Davison, D., Jin, L., Mosier, S., Melby, T., Sista, P., Demasi, R., Miralles, D., Cammack, N. and Matthews, T.J. (2002) In vitro antiviral activity of T-1249. *Antivir. Ther.*, **7**, S10.

69 Lalezari, J.P., Bellos, N.C., Sathasivam, K., Richmond, G.J., Cohen, C.J., Myers, R.A.J., Henry, D.H., Raskino, C., Melby, T., Murchison, H., Zhang, Y., Spence, R., Greenberg, M.L., Demasi, R.A., Miralles, G.D. and Group, T.-S. (2005) T-1249 retains potent antiretroviral activity in patients who had experienced virological failure while on an enfuvirtide-containing treatment regimen. *J. Infect. Dis.*, **191**, 1155.

70 Lohrengel, S., Hermann, F., Hagmann, I., Oberwinkler, H., Scrivano, L., Hoffmann, C., von Laer, D. and Dittmar, M.T. (2005) Determinants of human immunodeficiency virus type 1 resistance to membrane-anchored gp41-derived peptides. *J. Virol.*, **79**, 10237.

71 Chan, D.C., Fass, D., Berger, J.M. and Kim, P.S. (1997) Core structure of gp41 from the HIV envelope glycoprotein. *Cell*, **89**, 263.

72 Liu, S., Lu, H., Niu, J., Xu, Y., Wu, S. and Jiang, S. (2005) Different from the HIV fusion inhibitor C34, the anti-HIV drug Fuzeon (T-20) inhibits HIV-1 entry by targeting multiple sites in gp41 and gp120. *J. Biol. Chem.*, **280**, 11259.

73 Heil, M.L., Decker, J.M., Sfakianos, J.N., Shaw, G.M., Hunter, E. and Derdeyn, C.A. (2004) Determinants of human immunodeficiency virus type 1 baseline susceptibility to the fusion inhibitors enfuvirtide and T-649 reside outside the peptide interaction site. *J. Virol.*, **78**, 7582.

74 Schneider, S.E., Bray, B.L., Mader, C.J., Friedrich, P.E., Anderson, M.W., Taylor, T.S., Boshernitzan, N., Niemi, T.E., Fulcher, B.C., Whight, S.R., White, J.M., Greene, R.J., Stoltenberg, L.E. and Lichty, M. (2005) Development of HIV fusion inhibitors. *J. Pept. Sci.*, **11**, 744.

75 Dwyer, J.J., Wilson, K.L., Davison, D.K., Freel, S.A., Seedorff, J.E., Wring, S.A., Tvermoes, N.A., Matthews, T.J., Greenberg, M.L. and Delmedico, M.K.

(2007) Design of helical, oligomeric HIV-1 fusion inhibitor peptides with potent activity against enfuvirtide-resistant virus. *Proc. Natl Acad. Sci. USA*, **104**, 12772.

76 Otaka, A., Nakamura, M., Nameki, D., Kodama, E., Uchiyama, S., Nakamura, S., Nakano, H., Tamamura, H., Kobayashi, Y., Matsuoka, M. and Fujii, N. (2002) Remodeling of gp41-C34 peptide leads to highly effective inhibitors of the fusion of HIV-1 with target cells. *Angew. Chem. Int. Ed. Engl.*, **41**, 2937.

77 He, Y., Xiao, Y., Song, H., Liang, Q., Ju, D., Chen, X., Lu, H., Jing, W., Jiang, S. and Zhang, L. (2008) Design and evaluation of sifuvirtide, a novel HIV-1 fusion inhibitor. *J. Biol. Chem.*, **283**, 11126.

78 Wild, C., Oas, T., McDanal, C., Bolognesi, D. and Matthews, T. (1992) A synthetic peptide inhibitor of human immunodeficiency virus replication: correlation between solution structure and viral inhibition. *Proc. Natl Acad. Sci. USA*, **89**, 10537.

79 Eckert, D.M. and Kim, P.S. (2001) Mechanisms of viral membrane fusion and its inhibition. *Annu. Rev. Biochem.*, **70**, 777.

80 Lu, M., Blacklow, S.C. and Kim, P.S. (1995) A trimeric structural domain of the HIV-1 transmembrane glycoprotein. *Nat. Struct. Biol.*, **2**, 1075.

81 Bewley, C.A., Louis, J.M., Ghirlando, R. and Clore, G.M. (2002) Design of a novel peptide inhibitor of HIV fusion that disrupts the internal trimeric coiled-coil of gp41. *J. Biol. Chem.*, **277**, 14238.

82 Root, M.J., Kay, M.S. and Kim, P.S. (2001) Protein design of an HIV-1 entry inhibitor. *Science*, **11**, 11.

83 Münch, J., Ständker, L., Adermann, K., Schulz, A., Schindler, M., Chinnadurai, R., Pöhlmann, S., Chaipan, C., Biet, T., Peters, T., Meyer, B., Wilhelm, D., Lu, H., Jing, W., Jiang, S., Forssmann, W.G. and Kirchhoff, F. (2007) Discovery and optimization of a natural HIV-1 entry inhibitor targeting the gp41 fusion peptide. *Cell*, **129**, 263.

84 Kehoe, J.W. and Kay, B.K. (2005) Filamentous phage display in the new millennium. *Chem. Rev.*, **105**, 4056.

85 Wiesehan, K. and Willbold, D. (2003) Mirror-image phage display: aiming at the mirror. *Chembiochem*, **4**, 811.

86 Ferrer, M. and Harrison, S.C. (1999) Peptide ligands to human immunodeficiency virus type 1 gp120 identified from phage display libraries. *J. Virol.*, **73**, 5795.

87 Biorn, A.C., Cocklin, S., Madani, N., Si, Z., Ivanovic, T., Samanen, J., Van Ryk, D.I., Pantophlet, R., Burton, D.R., Freire, E., Sodroski, J. and Chaiken, I.M. (2004) Mode of action for linear peptide inhibitors of HIV-1 gp120 interactions. *Biochemistry*, **43**, 1928.

88 Wang, F.Y., Zhang, T.Y., Luo, J.X., He, G.A., Gu, Q.L. and Xiao, F. (2006) Selection of CC chemokine receptor 5-binding peptide from a phage display peptide library. *Biosci. Biotechnol. Biochem.*, **70**, 2035.

89 Boggiano, C., Jiang, S., Lu, H., Zhao, Q., Liu, S., Binley, J. and Blondelle, S.E. (2006) Identification of a D-amino acid decapeptide HIV-1 entry inhibitor. *Biochem. Biophys. Res. Commun.*, **347**, 909.

90 Königs, C., Rowley, M.J., Thompson, P., Myers, M.A., Scealy, M., Davies, J.M., Wu, L., Dietrich, U., Mackay, C.R. and Mackay, I.R. (2000) Monoclonal antibody screening of a phage-displayed random peptide library reveals mimotopes of chemokine receptor CCR5: implications for the tertiary structure of the receptor and for an N-terminal binding site for HIV-1 gp120. *Eur. J. Immunol.*, **30**, 1162.

91 O'Connor, K.H., Königs, C., Rowley, M.J., Irving, J.A., Wijeyewickrema, L.C., Pustowka, A., Dietrich, U. and Mackay, I.R. (2005) Requirement of multiple phage displayed peptide libraries for optimal mapping of a conformational antibody epitope on CCR5. *J. Immunol. Methods*, **299**, 21.

92 Huang, J.H., Yang, H.W., Liu, S., Li, J., Jiang, S. and Chen, Y.H. (2007) The mechanism by which molecules containing the HIV gp41 core-binding motif HXXNPF inhibit HIV-1 envelope

glycoprotein-mediated syncytium formation. *Biochem. J.*, **403**, 565.

93 Huang, J.H., Liu, Z.Q., Liu, S., Jiang, S. and Chen, Y.H. (2006) Identification of the HIV-1 gp41 core-binding motif—HXXNPF. *FEBS Lett.*, **580**, 4807.

94 Eckert, D.M., Malashkevich, V.N., Hong, L.H., Carr, P.A. and Kim, P.S. (1999) Inhibiting HIV-1 entry: discovery of D-peptide inhibitors that target the gp41 coiled-coil pocket. *Cell*, **99**, 103.

95 Welch, B.D., Van Demark, A.P., Heroux, A., Hill, C.P. and Kay, M.S. (2007) Potent D-peptide inhibitors of HIV-1 entry. *Proc. Natl Acad. Sci. USA*, **104**, 16828.

96 Korber, B.T.M., Brander, C., Haynes, B.F., Koup, R., Moore, J.P., Walker, B.D. and Watkins, D.I. (2006/2007) *HIV Molecular Immunology Database*. Los Alamos National Laboratory, Los Alamos, New Mexico, USA. Available at: http://www.hiv.lanl.gov/content/immunology.

97 Vincent, N., Tardy, J.C., Livrozet, J.M., Lucht, F., Frésard, A., Genin, C. and Malvoisin, E. (2005) Depletion in antibodies targeted to the HR2 region of HIV-1 glycoprotein gp41 in sera of HIV-1-seropositive patients treated with T20. *J. Acquir. Immune. Defic. Syndr.*, **38**, 254.

98 Walmsley, S., Henry, K., Katlama, C., Nelson, M., Castagna, A., Reynes, J., Clotet, B., Hui, J., Salgo, M., DeMasi, R. and Delehanty, J. (2003) Enfuvirtide (T-20) cross-reactive glycoprotein 41 antibody does not impair the efficacy or safety of enfuvirtide. *J. Infect. Dis.*, **188**, 1827.

99 Trottier, B., Walmsley, S., Reynes, J., Piliero, P., O'Hearn, M., Nelson, M., Montaner, J., Lazzarin, A., Lalezari, J., Katlama, C., Henry, K., Cooper, D., Clotet, B., Arastéh, K., Delfraissy, J.F., Stellbrink, H.J., Lange, J., Kuritzkes, D., Eron, J.J.J., Cohen, C., Kinchelow, T., Bertasso, A., Labriola-Tompkins, E., Shikhman, A., Atkins, B., Bourdeau, L., Natale, C., Hughes, F., Chung, J., Guimaraes, D., Drobnes, C., Bader-Weder, S., Demasi, R., Smiley, L. and Salgo, M.P. (2005) Safety of enfuvirtide

in combination with an optimized background of antiretrovirals in treatment-experienced HIV-1-infected adults over 48 weeks. *J. Acquir. Immune. Defic. Syndr.*, **40**, 413.

100 McPhee, J.B.G., Scott, M.G. and Hancock, R.E. (2005) Design of host defence peptides for antimicrobial and immunity enhancing activities. *Comb. Chem. High Throughput Screen.*, **8**, 257.

101 Schumacher, T.N.M., Mayr, L.M., Minor, D.L., Milhollen, M.A., Burgess, M.W. and Kim, P.S. (1996) Identification of D-peptide ligands through mirror-image phage display. *Science*, **271**, 1854.

102 Mygind, P.H., Fischer, R.L., Schnorr, K.M., Hansen, M.T., Sönksen, C.P., Ludvigsen, S., Raventós, D., Buskov, S., Christensen, B., De, M.L., Taboureau, O., Yaver, D., Elvig-Jørgensen, S.G., Sørensen, M.V., Christensen, B.E., Kjaerulff, S., Frimodt-Moller, N., Lehrer, R.I., Zasloff, M. and Kristensen, H.H. (2005) Plectasin is a peptide antibiotic with therapeutic potential from a saprophytic fungus. *Nature*, **437**, 975.

103 Zhu, P., Olson, W.C. and Roux, K.H. (2001) Structural flexibility and functional valence of CD4-IgG2 (PRO 542): potential for cross-linking human immunodeficiency virus type 1 envelope spikes. *J. Virol.*, **75**, 6682.

104 Libyh, M.T., Goossens, D., Oudin, S., Gupta, N., Dervillez, X., Juszczak, G., Cornillet, P., Bougy, F., Reveil, B., Philbert, F., Tabary, T., Klatzmann, D., Rouger, P. and Cohen, J.H. (1997) A recombinant human scFv anti-Rh(D) antibody with multiple valences using a C-terminal fragment of C4-binding protein. *Blood*, **90**, 3978.

105 Shinya, E., Dervillez, X., Edwards-Levy, F., Duret, V., Brisson, E., Ylisastigui, L., Levy, M.C., Cohen, J.H. and Klatzmann, D. (1999) In-vivo delivery of therapeutic proteins by genetically-modified cells: comparison of organoids and human serum albumin alginate-coated beads. *Biomed. Pharmacother.*, **53**, 471.

106 Dahlbäck, B. and Stenflo, J. (1981) High molecular weight complex in human plasma between vitamin K-dependent protein S and complement component

C4b-binding protein. *Proc. Natl Acad. Sci. USA*, **78**, 2512.

107 Oudin, S., Libyh, M.T., Goossens, D., Dervillez, X., Philbert, F., Reveil, B., Bougy, F., Tabary, T., Rouger, P., Klatzmann, D. and Cohen, J.H. (2000) A soluble recombinant multimeric anti-Rh(D) single-chain Fv/CR1 molecule restores the immune complex binding ability of CR1-deficient erythrocytes. *J. Immunol.*, **164**, 1505.

108 Dervillez, X., Hüther, A., Schuhmacher, J., Griesinger, C., Cohen, J.H., von Laer, D. and Dietrich, U. (2006) Stable expression of soluble therapeutic peptides in eukaryotic cells by multimerisation: application to the HIV-1 fusion inhibitory peptide C46. *ChemMedChem*, **1**, 330.

109 Kopetzki, E., Jekle, A., Ji, C., Rao, E., Zhang, J., Fischer, S., Cammack, N., Sankuratri, S. and Heilek, G. (2008) Closing two doors of viral entry: intramolecular combination of a coreceptor- and fusion inhibitor of HIV-1. *Virol. J.*, **5**, 56.

110 Pusch, O., Kalyanaraman, R., Tucker, L.D., Wells, J.M., Ramratnam, B. and Boden, D. (2006) An anti-HIV microbicide engineered in commensal bacteria: secretion of HIV-1 fusion inhibitors by lactobacilli. *AIDS*, **20**, 1917.

111 Baltimore, D. (1988) Gene therapy. Intracellular immunization. *Nature*, **335**, 395.

112 Lund, O., Lund, O.S., Gram, G., Nielsen, S.D., Schonning, K., Nielsen, J.O., Hansen, J.E. and Mosekilde, E. (1997) Gene therapy of T helper cells in HIV infection: mathematical model of the criteria for clinical effect. *Bull. Math. Biol.*, **59**, 725.

113 Malim, M.H., Bohnlein, S., Hauber, J. and Cullen, B.R. (1989) Functional dissection of the HIV-1 Rev trans-activator – derivation of a trans-dominant repressor of Rev function. *Cell*, **58**, 205.

114 Pearson, L., Garcia, J., Wu, F., Modesti, N., Nelson, J. and Gaynor, R. (1990) A transdominant tat mutant that inhibits tat-induced gene expression from the human immunodeficiency virus long terminal repeat. *Proc. Natl Acad. Sci. USA*, **87**, 5079.

115 Bevec, D., Jaksche, H., Oft, M., Wohl, T., Himmelspach, M., Pacher, A., Schebesta, M., Koettnitz, K., Dobrovnik, M., Csonga, R., Lottspeich, F. and Hauber, J. (1996) Inhibition of HIV-1 replication in lymphocytes by mutants of the Rev cofactor eIF-5A. *Science*, **271**, 1858.

116 Zhou, P., Goldstein, S., Devadas, K., Tewari, D. and Notkins, A.L. (1997) Human CD4+ cells transfected with IL-16 cDNA are resistant to HIV-1 infection: inhibition of mRNA expression. *Nat. Med.*, **3**, 659.

117 Cremer, I., Vieillard, V. and De Maeyer, E. (2000) Retrovirally mediated IFN-beta transduction of macrophages induces resistance to HIV, correlated with up-regulation of RANTES production and down-regulation of C-C chemokine receptor-5 expression. *J. Immunol.*, **164**, 1582.

118 Sanhadji, K., Leissner, P., Firouzi, R., Pelloquin, F., Kehrli, L., Marigliano, M., Calenda, V., Ottmann, M., Tardy, J.C., Mehtali, M. and Touraine, J.L. (1997) Experimental gene therapy: the transfer of Tat-inducible interferon genes protects human cells against HIV-1 challenge in vitro and in vivo in severe combined immunodeficient mice. *AIDS*, **11**, 977.

119 Lauret, E., Vieillard, V., Rousseau, V., De Maeyer-Guignard, J. and De Maeyer, E. (1994) Exploring interferon beta for gene therapy of HIV infection. *Res. Immunol.*, **145**, 674.

120 Levy-Mintz, P., Duan, L., Zhang, H., Hu, B., Dornadula, G., Zhu, M., Kulkosky, J., Bizub-Bender, D., Skalka, A.M. and Pomerantz, R.J. (1996) Intracellular expression of single-chain variable fragments to inhibit early stages of the viral life cycle by targeting human immunodeficiency virus type 1 integrase. *J. Virol.*, **70**, 8821.

121 Sanhadji, K., Grave, L., Touraine, J.L., Leissner, P., Rouzioux, C., Firouzi, R., Kehrli, L., Tardy, J.C. and Mehtali, M. (2000) Gene transfer of anti-gp41 antibody and CD4 immunoadhesin strongly reduces the HIV-1 load in humanized severe combined immunodeficient mice. *AIDS*, **14**, 2813.

122 Shaheen, F., Duan, L., Zhu, M., Bagasra, O. and Pomerantz, R.J. (1996) Targeting human immunodeficiency virus type 1 reverse transcriptase by intracellular expression of single-chain variable fragments to inhibit early stages of the viral life cycle. *J. Virol.*, **70**, 3392.

123 Hildinger, M., Dittmar, M.T., Schult-Dietrich, P., Fehse, B., Schnierle, B.S., Thaler, S., Stiegler, G., Welker, R. and von Laer, D. (2001) Membrane-anchored peptide inhibits human immunodeficiency virus entry. *J. Virol.*, **75**, 3038.

124 Egelhofer, M., Brandenburg, G., Martinius, H., Schult-Dietrich, P., Melikyan, G., Kunert, R., Baum, C., Choi, I., Alexandrov, A. and von Laer, D. (2004) Inhibition of human immunodeficiency virus type 1 entry in cells expressing gp41-derived peptides. *J. Virol.*, **78**, 568.

125 Schambach, A., Schiedlmeier, B., Kuhlcke, K., Verstegen, M., Margison, G.P., Li, Z., Kamino, K., Bohne, J., Alexandrov, A., Hermann, F.G., von Laer, D. and Baum, C. (2006) Towards hematopoietic stem cell-mediated protection against infection with human immunodeficiency virus. *Gene Ther.*, **13**, 1037.

126 Melikyan, G.B., Egelhofer, M. and von Laer, D. (2006) Membrane-anchored inhibitory peptides capture human immunodeficiency virus type 1 gp41 conformations that engage the target membrane prior to fusion. *J. Virol.*, **80**, 3249.

127 Hermann, F.G., Martinius, H., Egelhofer, M., Giroglou, T., Tonn, T., Roth, S.D., Zahn, R., Schult-Dietrich, P., Alexandrov, A., Dietrich, U., Baum, C. and von Laer, D. (2009) Protein scaffold and expression level determine antiviral activity of membrane-anchored antiviral peptides. *Hum. Gene Ther.* DOI 10.1089/hgt.2006.158.

128 Hermann, F.G., Egerer, L., Brauer, F., Gerum, C., Schwalbe, H., Dietrich, U. and von Laer, D. (2009) Mutations in gp120 contribute to resistance of HIV-1 against the membrane–anchored C-peptide maC46. *J. Virol.* DOI. 10.1128/JVF.00666–08.

129 van Lunzen, J., Glaunsinger, T., Stahmer, I., von Baehr, V., Baum, C., Schilz, A., Kuehlcke, K., Naundorf, S., Martinius, H., Hermann, F., Giroglou, T., Newrzela, S., Müller, I., Brauer, F., Brandenburg, G., Alexandrov, A. and von Laer, D. (2007) Transfer of autologous gene-modified T cells in HIV-infected patients with advanced immunodeficiency and drug-resistant virus. *Mol. Ther.*, **15**, 1024.

130 von Laer, D., Baum, C., Schambach, A., Kuehlcke, K., Zahn, R., Newrzela, S., van Lunzen, J., Johnson, R.P. and Schmitz, J.E. (2008) Gene therapeutic approaches for immune modulation in AIDS. *Antiinflamm. Antiallergy Agents Med. Chem.*, **6**, 121.

131 Hufert, F.T., van Lunzen, J., Janossy, G., Bertram, S., Schmitz, J., Haller, O., Racz, P. and von Laer, D. (1997) Germinal centre CD4+ T cells are an important site of HIV replication in vivo. *AIDS*, **11**, 849.

132 Hufert, F.T., von Laer, D., Schramm, C., Tarnok, A. and Schmitz, H. (1989) Detection of HIV-1 DNA in different subsets of human peripheral blood mononuclear cells using the polymerase chain reaction. *Arch. Virol.*, **106**, 341.

133 von Laer, D., Kern, P., Hufert, F.T., Schwander, S., Dietrich, M. and Schmitz, H. (1990) Low percentage of blood and bone marrow monocytes infected with the human immunodeficiency virus (HIV-1) in vivo. *Exp. Hematol.*, **18**, 693.

134 Hacein-Bey-Abina, S., Le Deist, F., Carlier, F., Bouneaud, C., Hue, C., De Villartay, J.P., Thrasher, A.J., Wulffraat, N., Sorensen, R., Dupuis-Girod, S., Fischer, A., Davies, E.G., Kuis, W., Leiva, L. and Cavazzana-Calvo, M. (2002) Sustained correction of X-linked severe combined immunodeficiency by ex vivo gene therapy. *N. Engl. J. Med.*, **346**, 1185.

135 Fischer, A., Hacein-Bey-Abina, S., Lagresle, C., Garrigue, A. and Cavazana-Calvo, M. (2005) Gene therapy of severe combined immunodeficiency disease:

proof of principle of efficiency and safety issues. Gene therapy, primary immunodeficiencies, retrovirus, lentivirus, genome. *Bull. Acad. Natl Med.*, **189**, 779.

136 Bordignon, C., Notarangelo, L.D., Nobili, N., Ferrari, G., Casorati, G., Panina, P., Mazzolari, E., Maggioni, D., Rossi, C. and Servida, P. (1995) Gene therapy in peripheral blood lymphocytes and bone marrow for ADA- immunodeficient patients. *Science*, **270**, 470.

137 Aiuti, A., Vai, S., Mortellaro, A., Casorati, G., Ficara, F., Andolfi, G., Ferrari, G., Tabucchi, A., Carlucci, F., Ochs, H.D., Notarangelo, L.D., Roncarolo, M.G. and Bordignon, C. (2002) Immune reconstitution in ADA-SCID after PBL gene therapy and discontinuation of enzyme replacement. *Nat. Med.*, **8**, 423.

138 Muul, L.M., Tuschong, L.M., Soenen, S.L., Jagadeesh, G.J., Ramsey, W.J., Long, Z., Carter, C.S., Garabedian, E.K., Alleyne, M., Brown, M., Bernstein, W., Schurman, S.H., Fleisher, T.A., Leitman, S.F., Dunbar, C.E., Blaese, R.M. and Candotti, F. (2003) Persistence and expression of the adenosine deaminase gene for 12 years and immune reaction to gene transfer components: long-term results of the first clinical gene therapy trial. *Blood*, **101**, 2563.

139 Kawamura, N., Ariga, T., Ohtsu, M., Kobayashi, I., Yamada, M., Tame, A., Furuta, H., Okano, M., Egashira, M., Niikawa, N., Kobayashi, K. and Sakiyama, Y. (1999) In vivo kinetics of transduced cells in peripheral T cell-directed gene therapy: role of CD8+ cells in improved immunological function in an adenosine deaminase (ADA)-SCID patient. *J. Immunol.*, **163**, 2256.

140 von Laer, D., Hasselmann, S. and Hasselmann, K. (2006) Gene therapy for HIV infection, what does it need to make it work? *J. Gene Med.*, **8**, 658.

141 Morgan, R.A., Looney, D.J., Muenchau, D.D., Wong-Staal, F., Gallo, R.C. and Anderson, W.F. (1990) Retroviral vectors expressing soluble CD4: a potential gene therapy for AIDS. *AIDS Res. Hum. Retroviruses*, **6**, 183.

142 Gay, W., Lauret, E., Boson, B., Larghero, J., Matheux, F., Peyramaure, S., Rousseau, V., Dormont, D., De Maeyer, E. and Le Grand, R. (2004) Low autocrine interferon beta production as a gene therapy approach for AIDS: infusion of interferon beta-engineered lymphocytes in macaques chronically infected with SIVmac251. *Retrovirology*, **1**, 29.

143 Loh, Y.P., Kim, T., Rodriguez, Y.M. and Cawley, N.X. (2004) Secretory granule biogenesis and neuropeptide sorting to the regulated secretory pathway in neuroendocrine cells. *Mol. Neurosci.* **22**, 63.

6
Intracellular Expression of Peptides

Christian Wichmann, Yvonne Becker, and Manuel Grez

6.1
Introduction

The delivery of peptides to cells represents a promising tool to study cellular functions. Although the technologies and methodologies for the delivery of peptides to target cells have improved considerably during the past few years (see the earlier chapters of this book), peptide delivery mediated by protein transduction domains has still not reached the efficacy of viral vector delivery. Peptide delivery by protein transduction is largely dependent on membrane permeability, endosomal release and intracellular stability. In contrast, the intracellular expression of peptides may offer particular advantages, and in many cases results in significant physiological effects. Both, viral and nonviral DNA delivery systems have been commonly used for the intracellular expression of peptides. These technologies allow for a highly efficient transfer of peptide-coding sequences into the cells and enable peptide synthesis inside the cells by the cellular expression machinery. They also include the possibility of post-translational modifications of the expressed peptides which may be required for specific target recognition and proper intracellular function. Intracellular expression by viral and nonviral vectors should further be considered as a valuable tool for functional studies of intracellularly acting peptides before starting the time-consuming and expensive task of the synthesis or *in vitro* production of recombinant peptides. This allows a quick assessment of the biological properties of selected peptides after expression in the target cell. A variety of viral and nonviral delivery systems conferring stable or transient expression are available; in this chapter the current status of the viral delivery of peptides will briefly be summarized.

6.2
Peptide Design and Expression Cassettes

While the intracellular expression of peptides can result in rapid degradation, it is possible to avoid this situation by fusing the peptide to a stable scaffold protein.

Peptides as Drugs. Discovery and Development. Edited by Bernd Groner
Copyright © 2009 WILEY-VCH Verlag GmbH & Co. KGaA, Weinheim
ISBN: 978-3-527-32205-3

Among the most commonly used scaffolds are the enhanced green fluorescent protein (eGFP), the *Escherichia coli* thioredoxin A protein (TrxA) [1], or scaffolds derived from staphylococcal nuclease [2] or ankyrin repeats [3]. Among these scaffolds, eGFP is currently the only one which, in addition to stabilizing the peptides, serves as a valuable marker for peptide expression and cellular localization in cell lines and *in vivo* [4]. In order to ensure proper function, the peptide sequences must be separated from the eGFP protein by a poly linker sequence, thereby allowing for flexibility and correct interaction with their targets. Repeats of small side-chain amino acids such as glycine, serine or alanine are well suited for linker sequences [5]. The desired peptide sequence can be added either N- or C-terminally to the eGFP scaffold protein, resulting in a stable fusion protein. Alternatively, the peptide sequence can be inserted into the reading frame of an engineered circular eGFP scaffold [6]. Paschke *et al.* demonstrated the feasibility of introducing and presenting small peptides – or even peptide libraries – within several loops of an optimized eGFP-scaffold protein, without disturbing eGFP or peptide function. For any given scaffold protein, interference between the scaffold and the cellular functions under study should be excluded – that is, the scaffold must be neutral. The optimal positional order of the linker and nature of the fusion protein must be evaluated in functional assays. Furthermore, the fusion protein (if required) may be targeted to the correct location within the cell by the introduction of an intracellular targeting signal. For instance, peptides designed to interfere with transcription factors should be equipped with a nuclear localization signal.

Viral expression vectors can be modified to express two proteins from one transcript. These bi-cistronic viral vectors contain an internal ribosome entry site (IRES) which directs the coexpression of the gene of interest and an additional marker gene. The marker gene allows the detection of the transgene-expressing cells, for example through fluorescence measurement (Figure 6.1). The most commonly used IRES sequence was derived from the encephalomyocarditis virus (ECMV), and consists of about 500 base pairs [7]. However, one disadvantage of this system is the unequal expression levels of both cistrons, depending on their position with respect to the IRES element. Usually, the cistron located upstream of the IRES element is expressed at higher levels compared to that located downstream. In order to avoid unequal expression levels, both proteins can be separated by a small self-cleaving peptide, T2A, derived from picornavirus [8]. Through a ribosomal skipping mechanism this 19-amino acid-long peptide allows for the equal translation of two or more cistrons derived from only one transcript [9]. One drawback of this strategy is that small amounts of uncleaved polypeptides may remain inside the cells with unknown properties and physiological effects.

Another means of circumventing unequal expression levels of two cistrons is to use two independent promoters to drive the expression of each peptide or protein. This strategy has been shown to allow for high expression levels of multiple transgenes, as demonstrated in hematopoietic stem cells [10]. Bi-directional promoters that allow the transcription initiation of two transgenes in opposite directions have

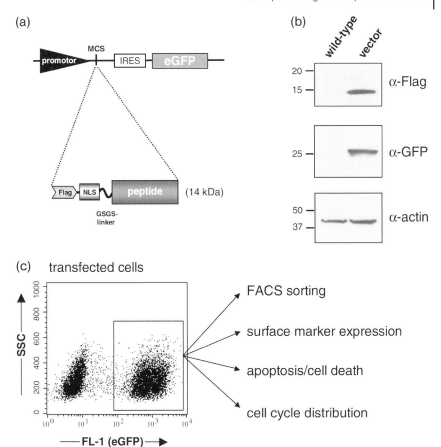

Figure 6.1 Expression cassette and peptide design. (a) Schematic representation of a standard expression cassette. The cDNA of interest is cloned into the multiple cloning site (MCS) of the expression vector. The expression cassette can be integrated into retro- or adenoviral vector backbones for the production of viral particles. Here, a nuclear localization site (NLS), linked by a glycine-serine repeat, targets the intracellular expressed peptides into the nucleus. The IRES element enables the coexpression of a second open reading frame, in this case the eGFP;

(b) The FLAG-tag allows for the convenient detection of expressed peptides by Western blotting; (c) Delivery and expression of viral transgenes is monitored by FACS analysis of transfected cells. The transduced cell population (right), coexpressing the eGFP, is well separated from the untransduced population (left). Upon peptide expression, transduced cells (i.e., eGFP-positive cells) can be examined for physiological alterations. Enrichment of eGFP-positive cells by FACS sorting is also feasible.

also been used to express two gene products independently from each other; in this way, fairly equal amounts of two peptides or proteins have been obtained [11]. In any case it is advisable to include an epitope-tag (Flag-tag, c-Myc-tag, His-tag, others) in the peptide or protein expressed in order to monitor proper expression and intracellular localization.

6.3
Stable Delivery and Expression of Peptides: Gamma-Retro- and Lentiviral Vectors

For the stable delivery of peptides, the gamma-retroviral/lentiviral delivery systems represent attractive tools for the sustained and longlasting intracellular expression of a desired peptide. For a large number of cells, gene transfer efficiencies are much higher when retroviral vectors, instead of conventional non-viral DNA transfection methods, are used. Depending on the type of target cell, gene transfer efficiencies of up to 90% can be achieved by retroviral vector delivery. A wide variety of cell types, as well as primary cells and embryonic stem cells, can be efficiently transduced by retroviral vectors while DNA transfection efficiencies in these cell types are rather low. Even after several rounds of infection, most retro/lentivirally transduced cells still contain a single copy of the gene of interest. This single transgene is stably inherited, usually without variability or loss of expression. In comparison, the tandem DNA insertions arising after plasmid DNA transfection or microinjection are often subject to deletions and rearrangements. Retroviral transduction is one of the easiest and most reliable techniques to stably express a peptide. The target cells merely have to be incubated with the virus-containing cell culture media. A high transduction efficiency and genetic stability of the infected cells facilitate the selection of stable cell lines with the required expression characteristics. A further benefit of retroviral vectors is that the same vector construct can be used to transduce multiple, diverse hosts.

Depending on the targeted cell type, two retroviral vector systems can be used. The gamma-retroviral vector system, as exemplified by vectors derived from the Moloney murine leukemia virus (Mo-MLV) genome and its derivatives, are the most common retroviral vector delivery systems used today. The reason for this is their well-known biological properties, their innate property to integrate into the genome of the host cells, the simplicity of their vector construction, and the large amount of vector particles that can be generated. One major drawback of gamma-retroviral vectors is their inability to infect nondividing cells. In contrast, lentiviral vectors, which are mostly derived from the HIV genome, have the capability to infect both dividing and nondividing cells [12, 13].

The most conducive argument for retroviral gene delivery is the convenient handling, and the well-established and efficient procedures (Figure 6.2), which circumvent many problems associated with protein transduction procedures. A mammalian cell line (usually HEK293T cells) is transfected by calcium phosphate-mediated transfection or any other efficient transfection method, with packaging constructs encoding the core and envelope viral proteins along with the retroviral vector construct. This procedure yields large amounts of infectious, replication-incompetent vector particles.

Alternatively, there are producer cell lines available which already express the viral proteins necessary for the proper packaging of retroviral vectors. After transfection, the genomic vector RNA, together with the viral membrane and capsid proteins, assemble into retroviral particles which are released into the medium.

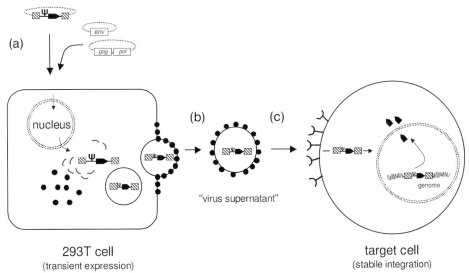

Figure 6.2 Production of retroviral particles and transduction of target cells. (a) The retroviral expression plasmid and the appropriate helper constructs coding for *gag*, *pol*, and *env* proteins are cotransfected into adherent cells. Upon transient transfection of the plasmid DNA, retroviral vector RNA is packaged into viral particles which are then released into the medium; (b) At 24 h after transfection, the virus particle-containing medium is collected and filtered; (c) Viral particles, which usually are concentrated on retronectin-coated plates, are incubated together with the target cells for transduction. Cell entry of viral particles is mediated through receptors on the cell surface. Within the cells, the viral RNA strand is reverse-transcribed and stably integrated into the genome of the target cells.

Thereafter, the target cells are cultured for transduction together with the collected and filtered cell culture supernatant containing the retroviral vector particles. If required, the vector supernatants can be frozen and stored for several months. The choice of the producer cell line, vector stability issues, medium additives, serum, type of bioreactor and other factors can influence optimal vector production [14]. Altogether, the production of retroviral vectors, their transduction and intracellular expression can be carried out within a few days. The typical step-wise process for gamma-retroviral particle production and the transduction of suspension cells on retronectin-coated plates is as follows:

- Step 1: Retroviral vector production

  ○ For retroviral particle production, subconfluent adherent cell lines (e.g., HEK293T, HeLa) are cotransfected with the retroviral expression construct and the appropriate helper plasmids; alternatively producer cell lines, stably expressing *gag*, *pol*, and *env* (e.g., Phoenix A, E) can be used.

  ○ At 6 h after transfection, the medium should be exchanged for one that is adequate for the target cells.

○ After 24 h, the viral supernatant should be harvested. This is achieved by centrifuging the viral supernatant at 1500 rpm to pellet the cell debris; the supernatant is then filtered (0.22 μm filter).

○ The virus supernatant is then applicable for transduction, or can be stored at −80 °C for several months.

- Step 2: Preparation of retronectin-coated plates

  ○ At one day before transduction, add 400 μl retronectin solution (50 μg ml^{-1}) to each well of a 24-well plate (non-tissue culture-treated) and incubate overnight at room temperature.

  ○ Next day: Discard the retronectin solution (reusable up to four times), add 1 ml stop solution [1 × phosphate-buffered saline (PBS) + 2% bovine serum albumin (BSA)] and incubate for 30 min at room temperature.

  ○ Discard stop solution, rinse once with HBSS (Hank's buffered salt solution) and once with 1 × PBS.

  ○ The coated plates are then ready for virus upload.

- Step 3: Upload of viral particles

  ○ Quickly defrost the virus supernatant and dilute as necessary.

  ○ Discard the PBS solution from the retronectin-coated wells and add the virus supernatant at the appropriate multiplicity of infection (MOI).

  ○ Centrifuge at 3000 rpm at 4 °C for 30 min.

  ○ Discard the virus supernatant and repeat upload three times, each with the appropriate volume.

- Step 4: Transduction of target cells

  ○ Remove the remaining virus supernatant before adding the cells.

  ○ Count the cells and dilute them to a concentration of 7.5×10^5 cells ml^{-1} in the appropriate culture medium.

  ○ Add 400 μl cell suspension into each well and incubate at 37 °C and 5% CO_2 at least for 8 h.

  ○ Addition of protamine sulfate (4 μg ml^{-1}) might increase the transduction efficiency.

  ○ Prepare a second retronectin-coated, 24-well plate and repeat the upload and transduction procedure for a second, third or fourth transduction (maximum two transductions per day).

  ○ At 8 h after the last transduction, exchange the medium and transfer the transduced cells into a fresh tissue-coated plate without retronectin.

○ Wash the plate three times with $1 \times$ PBS to collect any remaining cells on the plate.

6.4
Gamma-Retroviral Vectors

Gamma-retroviruses are enveloped viruses that carry a 7–12 kb RNA genome which is linear, single-stranded, nonsegmented and of positive polarity. Retroviruses enter the host cell through the attachment of their surface glycoproteins to specific plasma membrane receptors. The association between the glycoprotein and the receptor is a highly specific event, and is required to trigger a conformational change of the viral transmembrane protein, this being a prerequisite for delivery of the virion core into the cytoplasm. Following reverse transcription of the viral RNA into double-stranded linear DNA, the viral genome is delivered into the nucleus in the form of a preintegration complex. Upon integration, the provirus achieves the status of a cellular gene and is expressed by the cellular transcription machinery. Retroviral genomes commonly encode three essential proteins found in the mature virus, namely *gag*, *pol*, and *env*.

Two identical repeats – the long terminal repeats (LTRs) – are placed at both ends of the integrated proviral DNA. These noncoding sequences contain the major regulatory elements for viral gene expression (promoter, enhancer and polyadenylation signals), and can be divided into three elements, namely U3, R, and U5. The promoter region with the regulatory sequences such as the TATA box and the transcription start site is situated at the 5′ LTR, while the polyadenylation signal is found at the boundary between R and U5 of the 3′ LTR (Figure 6.3). In a gamma-retroviral vector, the genes encoding the viral structural and regulatory proteins (*gag*, *pol*, and *env*) are replaced by the transgene of interest. The vector construct carrying the transgene contains merely the sequences needed for integration of the virus into the target cell, the LTR and the Ψ signal for packaging the genomic viral RNA into the viral capsid.

Conventional transcription from retroviral vectors is dependent on promoter/enhancer elements located in the U3 region of the LTR, which impel in almost all the cases a constitutive expression. Although an independently controlled transcriptional unit can be introduced in the backbone, the expression obtained is usually influenced by the activity of the LTR. Strategies have been developed to deal with this problem. One approach is based on the replacement of the constitutive transcriptional control elements (promoter and enhancers) within the U3 region of the retroviral LTR with cell-specific promoter sequences [15–18]. Another alternative is the self-inactivating (SIN) vector configuration. Self-inactivating retroviral vectors are engineered so that transcription of the target gene can only be driven by an internal promoter once the expression cassette has been integrated into the genome of the target cell [19]. SIN vectors are constructed by deleting the enhancer and/or the promoter in the U3 region of the 3′ LTR. Since the 5′ LTR is derived from the 3′ LTR after reverse transcription and cDNA

(a) Proviral structure of the MLV genome (8.8 kb)

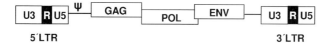

(b) Structure of a gamma-retroviral vector

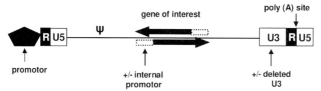

Figure 6.3 Schematic representation of the proviral structure of the MLV genome and gamma-retroviral vectors. (a) In the MLV provirus, *gag*, *pol*, and *env* coding regions are flanked by LTRs. The LTR contains three regions, U3, R, and U5. These regions are necessary for reverse transcription, proviral integration and transcriptional activation. ψ indicates the packaging signal. In the recombinant vector (b), the genomic RNA is transcribed using the 5′ U3 or an internal heterologous promoter.

synthesis, the integrated form of a SIN retroviral vector lacks enhancer and promoter sequences at the 5′ LTR and therefore cannot generate transcripts. No full-length vector RNA is produced in transduced cells. As a consequence, SIN retroviral vectors must include an internal promoter to drive expression of the gene of interest.

Retroviral vectors are safe and effective when standard guidelines are followed. One apparent disadvantage of gamma-retroviral vectors is their failure to transduce nondividing cells. The transport of the proviral DNA into the nucleus – and thus the gene transduction ability of gamma-retroviral vectors – depends heavily on the breakdown of the nuclear membrane during mitosis [20]. This restricts the use of gamma-retroviral vectors to dividing cells.

One important issue to consider when using gamma-retroviral vectors is their *integration potential*. The proviral DNA usually integrates within a 5 kb window around the transcription initiation site of genes. However, in cases where a strong LTR is used to drive gene expression, viral integration close to the transcription initiation sites may result in the unwarranted activation of cellular genes. In those cases in which proto-oncogenes are activated, the retroviral insertion may provide a selective advantage to cells expressing activated proto-oncogenes. This might lead to the expansion of cellular clones due to insertional mutagenesis. Thus, these clones will predominate in the cell population, and any physiological effects attributed to the action of the expressed peptides may result from insertional activation of cellular genes in the vicinity of the proviral integration site [21]. Appropriate controls must be included when using gamma-retroviral vectors to study the effects of peptides on cell physiology. The use of self-inactivating vectors largely decreases the likelihood of insertional mutagenesis [22, 23].

Promoter silencing represents another mechanism which might potentially inter-fere with appropriate retroviral vector expression. The mechanism of transcrip-tional silencing of retroviral expression involves methylation at CpG dinucleotides within the promoter region of the LTR. DNA methylation inhibits transcription largely by the recruitment of repressive chromosomal proteins such as histone deacetylases [24]. In order to rule out gene silencing, the correct expression of the desired peptide must be carefully monitored over time.

During the past few years, gamma-retroviral vectors have been used routinely for the intracellular expression of peptides. For example, a gamma-retroviral vector was used to express a peptide targeted against the coiled-coil oligomerization domain of BCR in BCR/ABL transformed cells [25]. The BCR/ABL oncogene is responsible for the phenotype of Philadelphia chromosome-positive (Ph+) leuke-mias, and exhibits an aberrant ABL-tyrosine kinase activity. Tetramerization of ABL through the N-terminal coiled-coil region of BCR is essential for the ABL-kinase activation. Beissert *et al.* have shown that, upon the intracellular expression of a peptide representing the Helix-2 of the coiled-coil domain of BCR, the auto-phosphorylation of BCR/ABL is significantly reduced, leading to the inhibition of the transformation potential of BCR/ABL.

Similarly, peptides derived from a critical protein–protein interaction domain of the nuclear corepressor molecule N-CoR were cloned into a bi-cistronic gam-ma-retroviral expression vector, together with eGFP. The cloned peptide motifs represent the contact sites between N-CoR and various leukemia-associated trans-location products, among others PML/RARα and AML1/ETO. After retroviral transduction, intracellular expression of these peptides resulted in disruption of the interaction between N-CoR and PML/RARα or AML1/ETO, and in an abroga-tion of the transcriptional block of essential myeloid genes involved in cellular differentiation. Consequently, in the presence of the N-CoR peptides, the fusion oncoproteins lost their leukemogenic potential and myeloid differentiation in peptide expressing cells was restored [26].

6.5
Lentiviral Peptide Delivery

Lentiviruses (LVs) are complex retroviruses that are similar to gamma-retroviruses in their basic genomic organization, but with several additional accessory genes present in the viral genome which play crucial roles in their replication cycle (Figure 6.4). Lentiviral vectors offer a number of advantages over other popular gene delivery systems such as gamma-retroviral and adenoviral delivery systems. Most importantly, lentiviral vectors can stably transduce nondividing cells [27], which widens the option to transfer genes into tissues refractory to gamma-retro-viral transduction. Lentiviral vectors are more robust for long-term gene expres-sion compared to retroviral vectors and escape gene silencing [28]. Lentiviral vectors also do not show toxicity and induce no immune or inflammatory response in the recipient. The infection specificity of lentiviral vectors can be modulated by

(a) HIV-1 proviral DNA (9.6 kb)

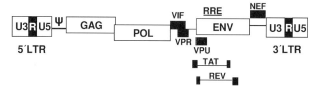

(b) Structure of a lentiviral SIN-vector

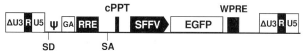

Figure 6.4 Schematic representation of the proviral structure of the HIV genome and lentiviral vectors. (a) Besides the structural and regulatory *gag*, *pol*, and *env* genes, the HIV-1 proviral DNA contains the six additional regulatory genes *vif*, *vpr*, *vpu*, *tat*, *rev* and *nef*, and the RRE element. (b) In the HIV-based SIN-lentiviral vector, the viral *gag*, *pol*, and *env* have been replaced by promoter and transgene sequence, and are flanked by the viral LTRs. The packaging of viral RNA is ensured by the presence of a packaging signal from the 5′ untranslated region of the *gag* ORF. In addition, two *cis*-acting sequences RRE and cPPT are present in the vector. The 3′ LTR contains a large deletion in the U3 region (depicted as ΔU3) to prevent transcription from the LTR. A WPRE element downstream from the transgene is used to improve transport of unspliced viral genomic RNA from the nucleus into the cytoplasm. The SFFV promoter in this example acts as an internal promoter to drive the expression of enhanced GFP (eGFP).

pseudotyping of its envelope protein. The use of the VSV-G envelope, vesicular stomatitis virus G protein, allows for a broad tropism. VSV-G pseudotyping also strongly increases the stability of the viral particles and allows virus concentration by ultracentrifugation, after which the amount of vector particles may be as high as 10^{10} transduction units per milliliter [29].

Although lentiviral vectors are capable of transducing a broad spectrum of cells, transduction efficiencies – for example, in hematopoietic stem cells – are rather low. For this reason, experimental conditions, including extended cytokine stimulation, high vector dosage and centrifugation on fibronectin fragments, can be manipulated to affect cell proliferation and differentiation. In order to avoid these problems, the surfaces of LV particles can be modified to display early-acting cytokines such as thrombopoietin and stem cell factor. These modified LVs exceed the current generation of LVs in transduction efficiencies of the most primitive CD34-positive hematopoietic cells [30]. Unlike gamma-retroviral vectors, lentiviral vectors integrate randomly within a transcription unit, thereby reducing the danger of inadvertent gene activation at the site of viral integration [31].

Lentiviral vectors have been frequently used for the intracellular expression of peptides. For example, a polypeptide of 100 amino acids in length derived from the cyclin A binding sequences of Skp2 was shown to block Skp2-cyclin A protein–

protein interaction when expressed intracellularly [32]. Consequently, cell proliferation was blocked. In this study, the 100-amino acid peptide sequence was fused to eGFP, resulting in a stable eGFP fusion protein from which a number of smaller deletion constructs were tested and a 20-amino acids sequence was found to be able to abrogate Skp2-cyclinA interaction and cause cell cycle arrest. This inhibitory peptide was subsequently expressed from a lentiviral vector in cancer cells. Proper expression within the cell was achieved with the strong cytomegalovirus (CMV) promoter. The peptide also synergizes with another TAT-mediated delivered peptide which blocks the interaction of cyclinA and E2F1, resulting in an enhanced killing of cancer cell lines [33].

A strong intracellular expression of a polypeptide targeting the oligomerization domain of AML1/ETO was achieved with a lentiviral vector harboring enhancer elements from the spleen focus-forming virus (SFFV). A nuclear localization site was attached to the oligomerization motif via a glycine-serine linker to target the polypeptide into the nucleus, where it binds to the aberrant leukemic transcription factor AML1/ETO. Intracellular expression of the polypeptide interfered with AML1/ETO oligomer formation and abrogated the oncogenic potential of AML1/ETO. Upon peptide expression, leukemic cells lost their self-renewal capacity and underwent cellular differentiation [34]. The same lentiviral expression vector was used to express a peptide aptamer with high binding affinity against the intracellular signaling domain of the oncogenic receptor tyrosine kinase ErbB2, which is found to be overexpressed in ~30% of breast cancer cells and confers resistance to chemotherapy and correlates with poor prognosis. This peptide was selected from a 12mer peptide library in a yeast two-hybrid screen using an intracellular domain of the ErbB2 kinase as bait. The lentiviral vector-mediated intracellular expression of this peptide in breast cancer cell lines inhibited ErbB2-activated downstream AKT signaling, and restored sensitivity towards chemotherapy-induced cell death [35].

Besides protein–protein interaction surfaces, RNA molecules may also serve as a targeting structure for intracellularly expressed peptides. As an example, a random phage display library of peptides was screened for high-affinity binders to the HIV ψ-packaging signal represented by specific RNA stem loops. After selection, lentiviral-delivered peptides which competitively block binding of the nucleocapsid *gag* polyprotein inhibited the assembly of functional infectious lentiviral HIV particles. Peptides discovered in this way can serve as lead compounds for novel antiviral drugs for the treatment of HIV infection [36].

Lentiviral vectors, as well as gamma-retroviral vectors, can be adapted to express peptides at different levels. For this, promoter elements which differ in their expression strength are used. For example, use of the SFFV promoter guarantees high expression levels in almost all cells, while the CMV promoter allows for intermediate expression levels. The use of tissue-restricted promoters may also be used to target peptide expression to desired organs or cell types [37]. Finally, gamma-retroviral and -lentiviral expression systems can be combined with an inducible promoter to tightly control the intracellular expression of the peptide [38, 39].

6.6
Vectors for Transient Expression of Peptides: Adenoviruses and Adeno-Associated Viruses

An alternative to retroviral vector-mediated gene transfer is the transient expression of peptides from nonintegrating vectors, the most prominent of which are adenovirus-based vectors. Currently, 51 human adenovirus serotypes have been identified which may be classified into six subgroups (A–F). They infect a broad spectrum of tissues (including the respiratory and gastrointestinal tracts) and cause infections which are usually not severe, with common clinical syndromes ranging from pharyngitis to diarrhea. In addition to its low pathogenicity for humans, adenovirus infection has not been associated with cancer initiation, which makes this virus a safe gene transfer vector. Further advantages of adenovirus as an expression system are the ability to produce high titers (up to 10^{12} infectious particles per ml) combined with high transduction efficiencies of dividing, as well as a broad range of differentiated, nondividing cells. Based on these favorable properties, adenoviral vectors have been used in several clinical trials. Initially, because of their natural tropism for pulmonary epithelial cells, adenoviruses were evaluated as gene transfer vectors for the cystic fibrosis transmembrane conductance regulator (CFTR). They have also been used for *in vivo* human gene transfer into kidney, heart, liver, central nervous system, muscle, and hematopoietic and cancer cells [40–42].

Adenovirus (Ad) is a nonenveloped, icosahedral virus which is 60–90 nm in size. The linear, double-stranded DNA genome of about 36 kb consists of early and late genes. The four early, regulatory genes (E1–4) encode proteins required for viral DNA replication and modulation of the host immune response; the five late, structural genes (L1–5) express the core and capsid proteins (Figure 6.5). On both ends of the viral DNA "inverted terminal repeats" (ITRs) are located which include the origin of replication. Adenoviral vectors are usually derived from serotypes 2 or 5 (Ad2 or Ad5). In order to target the vector to cell types which are refractory to adenovirus infection because of the lack of the primary Ad-receptor (e.g., muscle cells, endothelial cells, hematopoietic cells and many tumor cells), the viral capsid proteins can be modified [43, 44]. This approach expands or even shifts the adenoviral vector tropism, leading to retargeted vectors.

In the "first-generation" vectors, the E1 gene is substituted by the transgene or therapeutic gene, leading to replication-deficient vector particles. For vector production, the E1 function, transactivation of transcription of the early genes, is provided by a producer cell line, for example HEK293 [45], into which the adenoviral-vector is transfected. The recombinant virus can be purified from the cell culture media by means of cesium chloride equilibrium centrifugation or chromatography, and be used to infect the target cells. Since viral genes are still expressed at low levels in transduced cells, one disadvantage of this vector is its immunogenicity. Together with its epichromosomal location, it contributes to transient gene expression [46]. Several studies have pointed out that proper transgene expression lasts from only a few days to some weeks [47, 48]. It has been

(a)   Wild-type Ad5

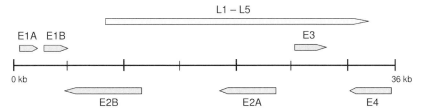

(b)   Transfer vector

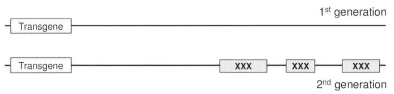

Figure 6.5 Structure of the Ad5 genome and Ad5-derived vectors. (a) The 36 kb genome of wild-type adenovirus 5 (Ad5) encodes four early (E) and five late (L) genes; (b) In the first generation of vectors, the E1 region is substituted by the transgene under the control of a suitable promoter. For the second generation of vectors, the early genes E2A, E3, and E4 are further deleted and expressed in *trans* by the producer cell line to generate replication-incompetent vectors.

observed that adenoviral gene transfer provokes a strong cytotoxic T-cell response that destroys the transduced cells and induces a humoral immunity and IgG and IgA antibodies [49]. Antiviral antibodies neutralize the vector when it is administered for a second time, and this may preclude repeated therapeutic applications. In human trials, a local and systemic inflammatory response has been observed in vascular endothelium and lung tissue after adenoviral administration [50].

In order to overcome problems with inflammation and toxicity – and thereby prolong transgene expression – "second-generation" vectors have been derived in which additional, early genes of the virus are deleted. Several studies have shown the usefulness of these adenoviral vectors. In applications such as tumor therapy and vaccination, the short-term gene expression is usually sufficient for a therapeutic effect, and the immunogenicity associated with first-generation adenoviral vectors might even be supportive. In 2000, Sauter *et al.* [51] demonstrated the potential of vector-mediated antiangiogenic gene therapy as an effective strategy in cancer treatment. A recombinant adenovirus was used for expression of the 20 kDa antiangiogenic peptide endostatin in a mouse tumor model to suppress angiogenesis induced by the vascular endothelial growth factor (VEGF). For this purpose, an Ad5-derived vector was generated in which the E1 region was substituted by the murine endostatin gene and a rat insulin leader sequence. Following systemic administration of the vector, persistent high levels of the peptide in the serum could be detected, resulting in a significant reduction of the volumes and growth rates of lung carcinoma. In addition, the complete prevention of lung metastasis formation was observed.

In a study of the development of new therapeutic agents against poxviruses, peptide mimetics of gamma interferon (IFN-γ) were introduced into an adenoviral vector for intracellular expression. In this Ad5-derived vector, the E1 gene was replaced by the expression cassette consisting of the amino acids (aa) 95–133 of the murine IFN-γ or the aa 95–134 of the human IFN-γ, respectively, driven by the human CMV promoter. The virulence factor B8R protein of poxvirus is known to be a homologue of the extracellular domain of the IFN-γ receptor, and thus is able to bind to IFN-γ, preventing its interaction with the receptor. The peptide mimetics instead bind to the cytoplasmic domain of the receptor, and therefore were able to bypass the inhibitory effect of the poxvirus B8R. The antiviral effect of these peptides against vesicular stomatitis virus and the upregulation of MHC class I molecules were retained even in the presence of the B8R protein, whereas the replication of vaccinia virus was inhibited [52].

As mentioned above, a serious problem with adenoviral vectors can result from their ability to induce a strong immune response leading to inflammation and the generation of neutralizing antibodies. In cases where this interferes with the therapeutic aim, or where repeated administrations of the vector are required, adeno-associated virus (AAV), a human parvovirus, might be a good option. This virus is not associated with human disease and causes only a very mild immune response. To date, 11 AAV serotypes have been described that are able to infect diverse tissue types and dividing as well as nondividing cells. AAV is a replication-defective virus because it requires a coinfection of the host cell with a helper virus, usually adenovirus or herpes simplex virus, in order to proliferate. In the absence of a helper virus, wild-type AAV remains latent in the host genome by stably integrating at a defined site in chromosome 19 in humans [53] and thus allowing prolonged transgene expression.

The nonenveloped, icosahedral AAV is one of the smallest viruses (ca. 22 nm in diameter). The wild-type genome is a linear, single-stranded DNA molecule of 4.7 kb consisting of two open reading frames (ORFs) which code for *rep* and *cap* proteins generated by alternative splicing (Figure 6.6). The four early *rep* proteins control viral replication, as well as integration of the virus into the host genome via the palindromic inverted terminal repeat elements (ITRs) that flank the genome at both ends. The late structural *cap* proteins (VP1–3) form the viral capsid. The most often used AAV-vector is derived from serotype 2 (AAV-2), which naturally infects muscle cells, neurons and hepatocytes. As for other viral vectors, modification of the AAV capsid results in targeted vectors with altered tropism [54].

For the generation of a viral vector, the *rep* and *cap* genes are replaced by the transgene and its associated regulatory sequences, preserving the ITRs and the packaging signal in the vector genome, this is similar to the derivation of the retrovirus-based vectors. The production of the recombinant AAV (rAAV) was originally achieved by using producer cells which were cotransfected with the vector construct and a plasmid expressing the viral *rep* and *cap* genes, and subse-

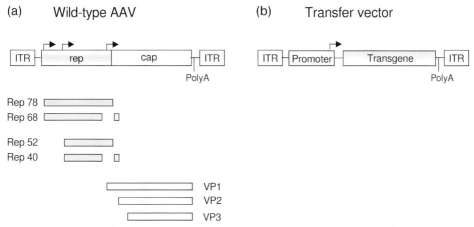

Figure 6.6 Structure of the AAV virus and the vector genome. Both genomes are flanked by inverted terminal repeats (ITRs). The wild-type AAV comprises the two major viral genes which code for different splice variants of the *rep* and *cap* proteins. The arrowheads indicate the three promoters. A PolyA signal confers stability of the mRNA (a). In the recombinant AAV vector, the viral genes are substituted by the transgene under the control of a suitable promoter (b).

quently infecting the cells with wild-type adenovirus. Since this method led to low yields of rAAVs and contamination with adenovirus, recent protocols allow adenofree production of rAAVs by providing the necessary, regulatory, early genes of adenovirus on a third plasmid and using an Ad E1-expressing cell line for production. The rAAVs are then purified by density gradient centrifugation and chromatography (Figure 6.7).

In the absence of a helper virus, the AAV-DNA can either integrate into the host genome or persist in an episomal form. Although integration of the wild-type viral genome usually occurs at a specific site in the human chromosome, the integration may not be site-specific in immortalized cell lines [55]. Accordingly, recombinant AAV do not integrate site-specifically. The random integration of vector sequences has been demonstrated in established cell lines, but only in some cases and at low frequency in primary cultures and *in vivo*. However, episomal concatamers predominate which consist of multiple copies of the AAV genome linked in series. Therefore, the risk of insertional mutagenesis and activation of oncogenes is probably low. rAAV stocks should be used free of contaminating replication-competent AAV [56].

The nonimmunogenic AAVs allow longlasting transgene expression in contrast to adenoviruses, and therefore have been extensively used in gene therapy trials. There are reports of long-term gene expression following the delivery of AAV vectors into muscle, heart, liver and lung tissues [57–60]. In order to treat type 1 diabetes – an autoimmune disease which results from the almost total destruction of insulin-producing β-cells in the pancreas – a recombinant AAV-vector was used to deliver a biologically active single-chain insulin analogue (SIA) under control

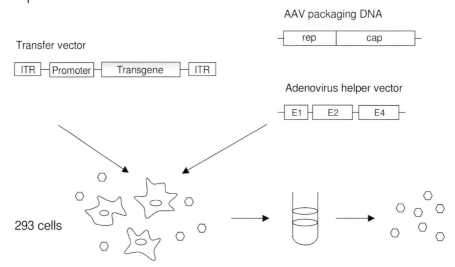

Figure 6.7 Production of recombinant AAV2-vectors. HEK293 cells are transfected in a three-plasmid system with the transfer vector, an AAV packaging plasmid coding for *rep* and *cap*, and a third plasmid which provides the adenovirus helper proteins E1, E2, and E4. The vector particles are then purified from the supernatant by density gradient ultracentrifugation and/or column chromatography (heparin column, FPLC).

of the liver-specific L-type pyruvate kinase (LKP) promoter. The A and B chains of insulin were linked directly by insertion of a heptapeptide. In order to facilitate SIA expression and secretion, the albumin leader sequence was cloned in front and the poly-adenylation signal (polyA) sequence of the simian virus 40 (SV40), as well as its enhancer sequence, were added behind the transgene. In a mouse model of inherited type 1 diabetes and in an inducible diabetic rat model, the insulin analogue was expressed in response to elevated blood glucose levels, leading to a remission of the diabetic phenotype over 8 months [61].

Another study proved the usefulness of rAAV-vectors in the neuroprotective treatment of *Parkinson's disease*. This progressive neurodegenerative disorder predominantly affects dopaminergic neurons in the substantia nigra, a part of the mesencephalon. The 18 kDa glial cell line-derived neurotrophic factor (GDNF) is the most potent neurotrophic factor for dopaminergic neurons, enhancing their survival. At 4 weeks after the induction of a lesion in the striatum of rat brains, an AAV-vector expressing GDNF was injected into the animals. The rAAV-2 vector contained the C-terminal Flag-tagged mouse GDNF cDNA under transcriptional control of the CMV promoter. The SV40 polyA signal sequence was cloned at the C-terminus, and the first intron of human growth hormone inserted between the promoter and the transgene (ITR-CMV-Intron-GDNF/Flag-polyA-ITR). A significant behavioral recovery was observed in the AAV-GDNF-treated animals for up to 4 months after injection of the vector; the delivered GDNF was found in the substantia nigra, while dopamine levels in the lesioned striatum were remarkably higher than in the control group, which received a vector expressing an unspecific control protein. Taken together, these data indicate that even at one month after the onset of progressive degeneration, a delayed delivery of the GDNF gene using AAV vectors is efficient in a rat model of Parkinson's disease [62].

AAV-mediated gene delivery can also reprogram transforming viral gene expression in tumor cells. Expression of the human papillomavirus (HPV)-associated viral oncogenes E6 and E7 is highly upregulated in HPV-positive cervical carcinoma cells. Both, E6 and E7 are responsible for the efficient immortalization of genital keratinocytes, a prerequisite for full cervical carcinogenesis. The 8.7 kDa monocyte chemoattractant peptide-1 (MCP-1) indirectly suppresses E6/E7 gene expression, and is found to be absent in HPV-positive cervical carcinoma cells. AAV-2 vectors carrying the MCP-1 gene were used to transduce high-risk HPV16- or HPV18-positive cervical carcinoma cell lines. For the generation of these vectors, the cDNA coding for human MCP-1 was cloned behind either the CMV or the cytokeratin 14 promoter with the intron of Poly (ADP-ribose) polymerase (PARP) used as a spacer (ITR-polyA-spacer-CMV-MCP1-SV40polyA-ITR). The expression of MCP-1 strongly inhibited the development of tumors derived from HeLa or SiHa cells transduced *in vitro*. Similar results were also achieved after the *in vivo* delivery of AAV2/MCP-1 into SiHa-derived tumors in mice [63].

6.7
Perspective

Depending on the individual experimental requirements, the viral vector systems described here might be considered for the intracellular expression of peptides. Gamma-retroviruses allow persistent gene expression in dividing cells, whereas the stable transduction of nondividing cells can be achieved with lentiviral vectors. In those cases where the delivery of a viral vector to a certain organ or cell type *in vitro* and *in vivo* is required, modifications within the virus envelope protein allow for specific cell targeting. If transient expression of the peptide is sufficient, or even desired, then nonintegrating vectors represent powerful tools for peptide expression at high levels, and this approach might become very attractive in the future for the treatment of tumors and their metastases. With adenoviral as well as adeno-associated viral vectors, the efficient transduction of most tissues already can be achieved. For a targeted tumor therapy, replicative, oncolytic viral vectors – which replicate and kill only tumor cells – are being developed [64, 65]. In future, the use of viral vectors for peptide expression, in combination with specific cell targeting, will result in a valuable tool for the analysis of protein function in cellular processes and their physiological role, and for therapeutic approaches by disrupting protein–protein interactions in cancer cells.

Acknowledgments

The authors acknowledge support from research grants from the José Carreras Leukämie-Stiftung (grant DJCLS R 05/07), graduate school Biologicals (gk1172), the NGFN Cancer Network (grant 01GS0450), and the Deutsche Krebshilfe (grant 102362, TP7).

References

1 Colas, P., Cohen, B., Jessen, T., Grishina, I., McCoy, J. et al. (1996) Genetic selection of peptide aptamers that recognize and inhibit cyclin-dependent kinase 2. Nature, 380, 548–50.

2 Norman, T.C., Smith, D.L., Sorger, P.K., Drees, B.L., O'Rourke, S.M. et al. (1999) Genetic selection of peptide inhibitors of biological pathways. Science, 285, 591–5.

3 Binz, H.K., Amstutz, P., Kohl, A., Stumpp, M.T., Briand, C. et al. (2004) High-affinity binders selected from designed ankyrin repeat protein libraries. Nat. Biotechnol., 22, 575–82.

4 Zernicka-Goetz, M., Pines, J., McLean Hunter, S., Dixon, J.P., Siemering, K.R. et al. (1997) Following cell fate in the living mouse embryo. Development, 124, 1133–7.

5 Robinson, C.R. and Sauer, R.T. (1998) Optimizing the stability of single-chain proteins by linker length and composition mutagenesis. Proc. Natl Acad. Sci. USA, 95, 5929–34.

6 Paschke, M., Tiede, C. and Hohne, W. (2007) Engineering a circularly permuted GFP scaffold for peptide presentation. J. Mol. Recognit., 20, 367–78.

7 Gallardo, H.F., Tan, C. and Sadelain, M. (1997) The internal ribosomal entry site of the encephalomyocarditis virus enables reliable coexpression of two transgenes in human primary T lymphocytes. Gene Ther., 4, 1115–19.

8 Ryan, M.D., King, A.M. and Thomas, G.P. (1991) Cleavage of foot-and-mouth disease virus polyprotein is mediated by residues located within a 19 amino acid sequence. J. Gen. Virol., 72 (Pt 11), 2727–32.

9 Szymczak, A.L., Workman, C.J., Wang, Y., Vignali, K.M., Dilioglou, S. et al. (2004) Correction of multi-gene deficiency in vivo using a single "self-cleaving" 2A peptide-based retroviral vector. Nat. Biotechnol., 22, 589–94.

10 Yu, X., Zhan, X., D'Costa, J., Tanavde, V.M., Ye, Z. et al. (2003) Lentiviral vectors with two independent internal promoters transfer high-level expression of multiple transgenes to human hematopoietic stem-progenitor cells. Mol. Ther., 7, 827–38.

11 Sammarco, M.C. and Grabczyk, E. (2005) A series of bidirectional tetracycline-inducible promoters provides coordinated protein expression. Anal. Biochem., 346, 210–16.

12 Lewis, P., Hensel, M. and Emerman, M. (1992) Human immunodeficiency virus infection of cells arrested in the cell cycle. EMBO J., 11, 3053–8.

13 Lewis, P.F. and Emerman, M. (1994) Passage through mitosis is required for oncoretroviruses but not for the human immunodeficiency virus. J. Virol., 68, 510–16.

14 Merten, O.W. (2004) State-of-the-art of the production of retroviral vectors. J. Gene Med., 6 (Suppl. 1), S105–24.

15 Moore, K.A., Scarpa, M., Kooyer, S., Utter, A., Caskey, C.T. et al. (1991) Evaluation of lymphoid-specific enhancer addition or substitution in a basic retrovirus vector. Hum. Gene Ther., 2, 307–15.

16 Ferrari, G., Salvatori, G., Rossi, C., Cossu, G. and Mavilio, F. (1995) A retroviral vector containing a muscle-specific enhancer drives gene expression only in differentiated muscle fibers. Hum. Gene Ther., 6, 733–42.

17 Diaz, R.M., Eisen, T., Hart, I.R. and Vile, R.G. (1998) Exchange of viral promoter/ enhancer elements with heterologous regulatory sequences generates targeted

hybrid long terminal repeat vectors for gene therapy of melanoma. *J. Virol.*, **72**, 789–95.

18 Jager, U., Zhao, Y. and Porter, C.D. (1999) Endothelial cell-specific transcriptional targeting from a hybrid long terminal repeat retrovirus vector containing human prepro-endothelin-1 promoter sequences. *J. Virol.*, **73**, 9702–9.

19 Yu, S.F., von Ruden, T., Kantoff, P.W., Garber, C., Seiberg, M. *et al.* (1986) Self-inactivating retroviral vectors designed for transfer of whole genes into mammalian cells. *Proc. Natl Acad. Sci. USA*, **83**, 3194–8.

20 Roe, T., Reynolds, T.C., Yu, G. and Brown, P.O. (1993) Integration of murine leukemia virus DNA depends on mitosis. *EMBO J.*, **12**, 2099–108.

21 Baum, C. (2007) Insertional mutagenesis in gene therapy and stem cell biology. *Curr. Opin. Hematol.*, **14**, 337–42.

22 Modlich, U., Bohne, J., Schmidt, M., von Kalle, C., Knoss, S. *et al.* (2006) Cell-culture assays reveal the importance of retroviral vector design for insertional genotoxicity. *Blood*, **108**, 2545–53.

23 Zychlinski, D., Schambach, A., Modlich, U., Maetzig, T., Meyer, J. *et al.* (2008) Physiological promoters reduce the genotoxic risk of integrating gene vectors. *Mol Ther.*, **16** (4), 718–25.

24 Bestor, T.H. (2000) Gene silencing as a threat to the success of gene therapy. *J. Clin. Invest.*, **105**, 409–11.

25 Beissert, T., Hundertmark, A., Kaburova, V., Travaglini, L., Mian, A.A. *et al.* (2008) Targeting of the N-terminal coiled coil oligomerization interface by a helix-2 peptide inhibits unmutated and imatinib-resistant BCR/ABL. *Int. J. Cancer*, **122**, 2744–52.

26 Racanicchi, S., Maccherani, C., Liberatore, C., Billi, M., Gelmetti, V. *et al.* (2005) Targeting fusion protein/corepressor contact restores differentiation response in leukemia cells. *EMBO J.*, **24**, 1232–42.

27 Naldini, L., Blomer, U., Gallay, P., Ory, D., Mulligan, R. *et al.* (1996) In vivo gene delivery and stable transduction of nondividing cells by a lentiviral vector. *Science*, **272**, 263–7.

28 Pfeifer, A. (2004) Lentiviral transgenesis. *Transgenic Res.*, **13**, 513–22.

29 Reiser, J. (2000) Production and concentration of pseudotyped HIV-1-based gene transfer vectors. *Gene Ther.*, **7**, 910–13.

30 Verhoeyen, E., Wiznerowicz, M., Olivier, D., Izac, B., Trono, D. *et al.* (2005) Novel lentiviral vectors displaying "early-acting cytokines" selectively promote survival and transduction of NOD/SCID repopulating human hematopoietic stem cells. *Blood*, **106**, 3386–95.

31 Montini, E., Cesana, D., Schmidt, M., Sanvito, F., Ponzoni, M. *et al.* (2006) Hematopoietic stem cell gene transfer in a tumor-prone mouse model uncovers low genotoxicity of lentiviral vector integration. *Nat. Biotechnol.*, **24**, 687–96.

32 Ji, P., Goldin, L., Ren, H., Sun, D., Guardavaccaro, D. *et al.* (2006) Skp2 contains a novel cyclin A binding domain that directly protects cyclin A from inhibition by p27Kip1. *J. Biol. Chem.*, **281**, 24058–69.

33 Ji, P., Sun, D., Wang, H., Bauzon, F. and Zhu, L. (2007) Disrupting Skp2-cyclin A interaction with a blocking peptide induces selective cancer cell killing. *Mol. Cancer Ther.*, **6**, 684–91.

34 Wichmann, C., Chen, L., Heinrich, M., Baus, D., Pfitzner, E. *et al.* (2007) Targeting the oligomerization domain of ETO interferes with RUNX1/ETO oncogenic activity in t(8,21)-positive leukemic cells. *Cancer Res.*, **67**, 2280–9.

35 Kunz, C., Borghouts, C., Buerger, C. and Groner, B. (2006) Peptide aptamers with binding specificity for the intracellular domain of the ErbB2 receptor interfere with AKT signaling and sensitize breast cancer cells to Taxol. *Mol. Cancer Res.*, **4**, 983–98.

36 Dietz, J., Koch, J., Kaur, A., Raja, C., Stein, S. *et al.* (2008) Inhibition of HIV-1 by a peptide ligand of the genomic RNA packaging signal Psi. *ChemMedChem*, 749–55.

37 Zheng, C. and Baum, B.J. (2008) Evaluation of promoters for use in tissue-specific gene delivery. *Methods Mol. Biol.*, **434**, 205–19.

38 Hofmann, A., Nolan, G.P. and Blau, H.M. (1996) Rapid retroviral delivery of tetracycline-inducible genes in a single

autoregulatory cassette. *Proc. Natl Acad. Sci. USA*, **93**, 5185–90.

39 Zhou, B.Y., Ye, Z., Chen, G., Gao, Z.P., Zhang, Y.A. *et al.* (2007) Inducible and reversible transgene expression in human stem cells after efficient and stable gene transfer. *Stem Cells*, **25**, 779–89.

40 Moullier, P., Friedlander, G., Calise, D., Ronco, P., Perricaudet, M. *et al.* (1994) Adenoviral-mediated gene transfer to renal tubular cells in vivo. *Kidney Int.*, **45**, 1220–5.

41 Ragot, T., Vincent, N., Chafey, P., Vigne, E., Gilgenkrantz, H. *et al.* (1993) Efficient adenovirus-mediated transfer of a human minidystrophin gene to skeletal muscle of mdx mice. *Nature*, **361**, 647–50.

42 Simons, J.W., Mikhak, B., Chang, J.F., DeMarzo, A.M., Carducci, M.A. *et al.* (1999) Induction of immunity to prostate cancer antigens: results of a clinical trial of vaccination with irradiated autologous prostate tumor cells engineered to secrete granulocyte-macrophage colony-stimulating factor using ex vivo gene transfer. *Cancer Res.*, **59**, 5160–8.

43 Wickham, T.J., Roelvink, P.W., Brough, D.E. and Kovesdi, I. (1996) Adenovirus targeted to heparan-containing receptors increases its gene delivery efficiency to multiple cell types. *Nat. Biotechnol.*, **14**, 1570–3.

44 Gonzalez, R., Vereecque, R., Wickham, T.J., Vanrumbeke, M., Kovesdi, I. *et al.* (1999) Increased gene transfer in acute myeloid leukemic cells by an adenovirus vector containing a modified fiber protein. *Gene Ther.*, **6**, 314–20.

45 Graham, F.L., Smiley, J., Russell, W.C. and Nairn, R. (1977) Characteristics of a human cell line transformed by DNA from human adenovirus type 5. *J. Gen. Virol.*, **36**, 59–74.

46 Yang, Y., Nunes, F.A., Berencsi, K., Furth, E.E., Gonczol, E. *et al.* (1994) Cellular immunity to viral antigens limits E1-deleted adenoviruses for gene therapy. *Proc. Natl Acad. Sci. USA*, **91**, 4407–11.

47 Jaffe, H.A., Danel, C., Longenecker, G., Metzger, M., Setoguchi, Y. *et al.* (1992) Adenovirus-mediated in vivo gene transfer and expression in normal rat liver. *Nat. Genet.*, **1**, 372–8.

48 Engelhardt, J.F., Simon, R.H., Yang, Y., Zepeda, M., Weber-Pendleton, S. *et al.* (1993) Adenovirus-mediated transfer of the CFTR gene to lung of nonhuman primates: biological efficacy study. *Hum. Gene Ther.*, **4**, 759–69.

49 Van Ginkel, F.W., Liu, C., Simecka, J.W., Dong, J.Y., Greenway, T. *et al.* (1995) Intratracheal gene delivery with adenoviral vector induces elevated systemic IgG and mucosal IgA antibodies to adenovirus and beta-galactosidase. *Hum. Gene Ther.*, **6**, 895–903.

50 Channon, K.M. and George, S.E. (1997) Improved adenoviral vectors: cautious optimism for gene therapy. *Q. J. Med.*, **90**, 105–9.

51 Sauter, B.V., Martinet, O., Zhang, W.J., Mandeli, J. and Woo, S.L. (2000) Adenovirus-mediated gene transfer of endostatin in vivo results in high level of transgene expression and inhibition of tumor growth and metastases. *Proc. Natl Acad. Sci. USA*, **97**, 4802–7.

52 Ahmed, C.M., Burkhart, M.A., Subramaniam, P.S., Mujtaba, M.G. and Johnson, H.M. (2005) Peptide mimetics of gamma interferon possess antiviral properties against vaccinia virus and other viruses in the presence of poxvirus B8R protein. *J. Virol.*, **79**, 5632–9.

53 Kotin, R.M., Siniscalco, M., Samulski, R.J., Zhu, X.D., Hunter, L. *et al.* (1990) Site-specific integration by adeno-associated virus. *Proc. Natl Acad. Sci. USA*, **87**, 2211–15.

54 Buning, H., Ried, M.U., Perabo, L., Gerner, F.M., Huttner, N.A. *et al.* (2003) Receptor targeting of adeno-associated virus vectors. *Gene Ther.*, **10**, 1142–51.

55 Kearns, W.G., Afione, S.A., Fulmer, S.B., Pang, M.C., Erikson, D. *et al.* (1996) Recombinant adeno-associated virus (AAV-CFTR) vectors do not integrate in a site-specific fashion in an immortalized epithelial cell line. *Gene Ther.*, **3**, 748–55.

56 Tenenbaum, L., Lehtonen, E. and Monahan, P.E. (2003) Evaluation of risks related to the use of adeno-associated virus-based vectors. *Curr. Gene Ther.*, **3**, 545–65.

57 Xiao, X., Li, J. and Samulski, R.J. (1996) Efficient long-term gene transfer into muscle tissue of immunocompetent mice by adeno-associated virus vector. *J. Virol.,* **70**, 8098–108.

58 Snyder, R.O., Miao, C.H., Patijn, G.A., Spratt, S.K., Danos, O. *et al.* (1997) Persistent and therapeutic concentrations of human factor IX in mice after hepatic gene transfer of recombinant AAV vectors. *Nat. Genet.,* **16**, 270–6.

59 Woo, Y.J., Zhang, J.C., Taylor, M.D., Cohen, J.E., Hsu, V.M. *et al.* (2005) One year transgene expression with adeno-associated virus cardiac gene transfer. *Int. J. Cardiol.,* **100**, 421–6.

60 Flotte, T.R., Zeitlin, P.L., Reynolds, T.C., Heald, A.E., Pedersen, P. *et al.* (2003) Phase I trial of intranasal and endobronchial administration of a recombinant adeno-associated virus serotype 2 rAAV2)-CFTR vector in adult cystic fibrosis patients: a two-part clinical study. *Hum. Gene Ther.,* **14**, 1079–88.

61 Lee, H.C., Kim, S.J., Kim, K.S., Shin, H.C. and Yoon, J.W. (2000) Remission in models of type 1 diabetes by gene therapy using a single-chain insulin analogue. *Nature,* **408**, 483–8.

62 Wang, L., Muramatsu, S., Lu, Y., Ikeguchi, K., Fujimoto, K. *et al.* (2002) Delayed delivery of AAV-GDNF prevents nigral neurodegeneration and promotes functional recovery in a rat model of Parkinson's disease. *Gene Ther.,* **9**, 381–9.

63 Kunke, D., Grimm, D., Denger, S., Kreuzer, J., Delius, H. *et al.* (2000) Preclinical study on gene therapy of cervical carcinoma using adeno-associated virus vectors. *Cancer Gene Ther.,* **7**, 766–77.

64 Alemany, R., Balague, C. and Curiel, D.T. (2000) Replicative adenoviruses for cancer therapy. *Nat. Biotechnol.,* **18**, 723–7.

65 Tai, C.K. and Kasahara, N. (2008) Replication-competent retrovirus vectors for cancer gene therapy. *Front. Biosci.,* **13**, 3083–95.

7
The Internalization Mechanisms and Bioactivity of the Cell-Penetrating Peptides

Mats Hansen, Elo Eriste, and Ülo Langel

7.1
Introduction

In 1994, a family of short cationic peptides was introduced, collectively termed the cell-penetrating peptides (CPPs) [1]. These peptides have attracted great interest within the research community due to their unique ability to penetrate the plasma membrane and to deliver a variety of cargos into the cytoplasmic or even nuclear compartments of the cell. The efficient delivery of proteins, DNA, siRNA and small hydrophobic molecules, conjugated to different CPPs, has been reported by several research groups, although the exact internalization pathway of CPPs and CPP–cargo conjugates continues to be the subject of extensive discussions. What initially appeared as an energy-independent internalization pathway in early studies, has later been proven to be an artifact based on experimental peculiarities. The uptake mechanism, in the meantime, has been shown to be of an endocytic nature [2–12]. The results of more recent studies have suggested that two or more endocytic routes may be employed simultaneously, and that different peptides may prefer different uptake pathways [13, 14]. The involvement of heparan sulfates in the internalization of CPPs has also been reported on several occasions, with heparan sulfates perhaps acting as nonspecific receptors for CPPs [15–17].

7.2
Discovery and Classification of CPPs

The history of CPPs dates back to the late 1980s, when it was first observed that living cells were able to internalize an 86-amino acid fragment from the HIV-1 TAT protein [18]. Deletion studies revealed that amino acids 48–60 were necessary and sufficient for transduction, and that replacing three arginine residues with alanines greatly reduced the activity [19]. Several years after the discovery of TAT transduction, it was demonstrated that the 60-amino acid homeodomain of the

Peptides as Drugs. Discovery and Development. Edited by Bernd Groner
Copyright © 2009 WILEY-VCH Verlag GmbH & Co. KGaA, Weinheim
ISBN: 978-3-527-32205-3

Antennapedia protein of *Drosophila* was also able to translocate through cell membranes [1]. This indicated that the translocation of TAT protein was not an isolated case, and raised interest in the phenomenon of cell-penetration in general. Subsequent site-directed mutation studies of the Antennapedia protein led to the discovery that its third helix was necessary and sufficient for membrane translocation, and provided details of the CPP of 16 amino acids, which today often referred to as penetratin (Pen) [20].

The large number of cell types and organisms where CPPs can be found, suggests that protein uptake is a biologically relevant process. When analyzing G-protein-coupled receptors with a computer-aided CPP prediction algorithm, it was found that the majority of CPP sequences in these receptors were located in the third intracellular loop [21]. This was an interesting finding, and raised questions regarding the possible role of CPPs in these protein sequences. It has been suggested that transcription factors and homeoproteins–molecules which often contain CPP sequences–were responsible for cellular signaling in early multicellular organisms [22], and might have retained this function throughout evolution [23, 24]. The same might also be true for seven-transmembrane (7TM) receptors, although no experimental proof has yet been provided.

Several suggestions for the classification of CPPs have been made by different groups (for a review, see Ref. [25]). The term "cell-penetrating peptide" was discussed for a long time before being adopted by many in the field and, indeed, alternative terms such as "Trojan peptide", "protein transduction domain" (PTD) or "membrane translocating sequences" (MTSs) may still be found in the scientific literature. The most common and most logical way to classify CPPs, however, is by their origin. Such a classification, which is shown in Table 7.1, comprises natural, chimeric and designed CPPs. *Natural* CPPs are derived from naturally occurring proteins, *chimeric* CPPs are engineered and combine domains of two (or more) proteins, while *designed* CPPs are tailored to be efficient delivery vectors.

7.3
Internalization Mechanisms of Cell-Penetrating Peptides

Despite their popular use as delivery vectors, the mechanisms behind the internalization of CPPs remain unclear. This question has been extensively studied since the discovery of CPPs, and a wide variety of tools is available to address this question. One of the most frequently used methods to assess the involvement of endocytosis in CPP uptake has been the application of fluorescein-labeled CPP to cells at +4 °C. At temperatures below +10 °C, endocytosis is greatly diminished, due to restraints in the flexibility of the plasma membrane [39, 40]. A lower temperature, however, will only cause an inhibition of internalization, with binding of proteins to the plasma membrane still being observed [39]. As all endocytic pathways are energy-dependent, it was considered instructive to study endocytic mechanisms in cells depleted of ATP. This can be achieved by treatment with sodium azide and/or 2-deoxyglucose prior to the addition of fluorescein-labeled CPPs.

Table 7.1 A selection of CPPs classified by their origin.

Common name	Sequence	Origin	Reference(s)
Protein-derived			
Tat(48-60)	GRKKRRQRRRPPQ[a]	HIV-1 TAT(48-60)	[26]
Pen	RQIKIWFQNRRMKWKK	Antennapedia homeodomain	[1]
pVEC	LLILRRIRKQAHAHSK-NH$_2$	Murine vascular endothelial cadherin	[27]
bPrPp	MVKSKIGSWILVLFVAMWSDVGLCKKRPKP-NH$_2$	Mouse prion protein	[28]
pIsl	RVIRVWFQNKRCKDKK-NH$_2$	Rat transcription factor Islet-1	[29]
VP22	DAATATRGRSAARPTERPRAPARSASRPRRPVE	Herpes simplex virus envelope protein	[30]
M918	MVTVLFRRLRIRRASGPPRVRV-NH$_2$	p14ARF	[31]
Chimeric			
TP	GWTLNSAGYLLGKINLKALAALAKKIL-NH$_2$	Galanin(1-12)-Lys-mastoparan	[32]
TP10	AGYLLGKINLKALAALAKKIL-NH$_2$	Deletion analogue of TP	[33]
MPGA^{NLS}	GALFLGFLGAAGSTMGAWSQPKSKRKV-cysteamide	Cationic NLS+Hydrophobic tail	[34]
Synthetic/Designed			
MAP	KLALKLALKAALKLA-NH$_2$	Model amphipathic peptide	[35]
Pep-1	KETWWETWWTEWSQPKKKRKV-cysteamide	Cationic NLS + Hydrophobic tail	[36]
Oligo Arg	RRRRRRRR-NH$_2$[b]	Ultimate arginine-rich peptide	[37, 38]

a Originally synthesized as free acid with N- and C-terminal Cys.
b Various lengths of Arg stretches between 6 and 9 have been used.

The pretreatment of cells with inhibitors of endocytosis has also been widely employed to define the endocytic pathway involved in CPP-mediated protein uptake. While providing a convenient tool for studying the endocytic pathways, it should be emphasized that the specificity of endocytosis inhibitors is usually limited to one particular protein or protein complex involved in the endocytosis pathway. Therefore, a combination of different inhibitors should be considered for more informative results. Another commonly applied method to study the internalization of CPPs is coapplication with pathway-specific tracer molecules. Here, the overlapping signals from two different channels provide information about the contribution of different internalization routes although, again, it should be borne in mind that the internalization of tracers may not exclusively favor one particular pathway.

An alternative experimental approach to investigate the internalization route is the manipulation of candidate genes and their products. Several proteins have been identified as being crucial for clathrin-mediated endocytosis (CME) or caveolin-dependent endocytosis; examples include the Rab family proteins and AP2 (dynamin). The dominant-negative mutant form of dynamin has been used to distinguish macropinocytosis from other internalization routes [13]. Additionally, and alternatively, genetic knockout mice (e.g., caveolin-1 knockout) or RNAi techniques can be employed.

7.4
Models of CPP Uptake

The initial studies with penetratin and Tat(48-60) showed that these peptides would be internalized within minutes, and were not found to be concentrated in any endosomal structures. Moreover, lowering the incubation temperature did not decrease the uptake to any notable extent [1, 26]. Later studies showed that the internalization of other CPPs, such as TP [32], MPG [41] and MAP [35], followed the same pattern; furthermore, the internalization was similar for both L- and D-enantiomers of the studied peptides [42–44]. These observations led to the conclusion that the internalization pathway of CPPs is apparently nonendocytic, and that no membrane receptor is involved in the process.

As a result, several theories were proposed to explain the possible internalization routes. Initially, it was believed that some type of direct penetration through the plasma membrane was driving the uptake of CPPs [1, 26], but this theory could not explain the delivery of various cargos into the cytoplasm, as it would cause significant membrane disturbance that would not correlate with the low cytotoxicity associated with CPPs. Similar arguments were raised when the CPP-mediated protein uptake was associated with peptide-induced pore formation. Such pore formation model suggested that the peptide chains would multimerize after membrane insertion, and that this would lead to the development of pores through which the CPP could rapidly internalize into the cytoplasm [45]. This model was consistent with the internalization of some amphipathic and more cytotoxic peptides, such as MAP and TP, but did not explain the internalization of relatively large cargo complexes.

The first model of internalization was the "inverted micelle", which was initially proposed by Derossi *et al.* and advanced to explain the internalization mechanism of Pen [20]. In this model, the basic peptide first interacts with negatively charged phospholipids in the plasma membrane. The hydrophobic tryptophan residues then insert into the lipid bilayer, rearranging it and forming a membrane-embedded inverted micelle. The hydrophilic cavity inside the micelle accommodates the peptide that subsequently will be released into cytoplasm upon micelle disruption [20]. This model can, at least potentially, explain the peptide and peptide-cargo internalization studies that have demonstrated the importance of tryptophan residues in the Pen sequence [1, 46, 47]. However, although these investigations support the inverted micelle model, they also suggest that other basic CPPs – such as polyarginines and Tat (48-60), which lack the hydrophobic residues – most likely internalize via different mechanisms.

7.5
The Current View of CPP Uptake

The internalization of CPPs via an endocytosis-independent route was commonly accepted, until two reports demonstrated the artificial redistribution of fluorescently labeled peptides upon fixation [8, 48]. In addition, it was shown that CPPs bind strongly to the plasma membrane, and that repeated washing steps after incubation might be insufficient to remove all of the extracellularly bound peptide, which in turn led to an overestimation of the uptake. In order to avoid these artifacts, trypsination of the cells after incubation and washing was suggested [8], and subsequent observations led to the re-evaluation of mechanisms underlying CPP uptake. Today, the prevalent view is that CPPs are mainly internalized via endocytosis, although the exact endocytic route remains a subject of much debate.

Cell-surface proteoglycans play important roles in the uptake of arginine-rich CPPs. In 2002, Suzuki *et al.* demonstrated the importance of heparan sulfates in the uptake of octa-arginine and Tat (48-60) [16]. Binding to heparan sulfates and the subsequent endocytic uptake was later shown also for other arginine-rich CPPs, such as nona-arginine [49], Tat (47-57) [50], and Tat (48-60) [7].

In a functional assay, it was shown that a recombinant fusion protein comprising Tat (48-60) and Cre recombinase (Tat-Cre) internalizes via macropinocytosis [11], and this was further confirmed by the effect of 5-(N-ethyl-N-isopropyl) amiloride (EIPA), a specific inhibitor of macropinocytosis. Pretreatment with EIPA decreased Tat-Cre uptake in dose-dependent fashion, while the coexpression of Tat-Cre with a dominant-negative mutant of Dynamin[K44A] had no effect on the Tat-Cre internalization, indicating that neither caveolin nor clathrin-mediated endocytosis was involved in the process [11]. The same mechanism also applied for fluorescein-labeled Tat (48-60), the uptake of which was reduced by pretreatment with EIPA and cytochalasine D [4]. The Tat-mediated delivery of the Bcl-2 protein was found to be impeded at lower temperatures, while the removal of cholesterol from the cell membrane with nystatin or methyl-β-cyclodextrin also reduced the uptake; this suggested that uptake of the fusion protein was of an endocytic nature and heavily dependent on lipid rafts [9]. Macropinocytosis and actin rearrangement has been suggested as the main uptake route also for polyarginines [51, 52].

The results of other studies have suggested that the endocytosis of Tat (48-60) is dependent on CME, rather than on macropinocytosis, as recently demonstrated by Richard *et al.* [7]. Authors observed that the uptake of fluoresceinyl-Tat (48-60) was strongly inhibited by the CME-specific endocytosis inhibitor chlorpromazine, and also by potassium depletion. However, uptake in HepG2, Jurkat T and HeLa cells, which did not express caveolin-1, remained unaltered [7]. A partial dependence of CME in combination with macropinocytosis has also been shown for TP and TP10 conjugated to avidin [53].

The majority of reports to date have indicated that the endocytic component is involved in CPP uptake, with some peptides (e.g., Pep1 and MPG) appearing to be internalized via nonendocytic pathways [41, 54]. Although the divergent results reported by different groups remain difficult to reconcile, taken together they indicate that different peptides may utilize different routes of endocytosis, and that it might occur in a parallel, perhaps compensating, fashion. Moreover, the routes may be different for different CPPs, and also be a function of their cargo, as was demonstrated for Tat (48-60) [10, 55]. It was also shown the different peptides may use not only different endocytosis pathways, but the uptake is also dependent on the applied concentrations [13].

7.6
CPPs as Cargo Delivery Vehicles

Since they were first reported, the number of known CPP sequences has grown rapidly, with tens of new peptide sequences being added to the list each year. These novel CPPs are very often derived from known proteins, and are both delimited and optimized, such that those peptide sequences, still capable of penetrating the plasma membrane and carrying a cargo, are well defined.

Cell penetration is not limited to a particular cell type; rather, it occurs with equal efficiency in mammalian cells, yeast [56], bacteria [57], and plant protoplasts [58]. This wide variety of possible target cells makes CPPs attractive candidates for drug delivery and, indeed, a large number of reports have been made outlining the efficient delivery of various small- and macromolecular cargos into the cytoplasmic compartment. Such cargos have included DNA, RNA, siRNA, proteins, peptides, low-molecular-weight cytostatics and gold nanoparticles. Somewhat surprisingly, there appear to be few limits to the classes of molecules that can be introduced into cells!

7.7
Delivery of Proteins

The delivery of proteins with assistance from CPPs has been extensively studied, with the efficient uptake of different functional proteins conjugated to CPPs having been reported both *in vitro* and *in vivo* (for reviews, see Refs [59, 60]). In 1994, Fawell and colleagues demonstrated for the first time that peptides, derived from HIV-1 TAT protein, namely Tat (1-72) and Tat (37-72), could carry covalently linked β-galactosidase into HeLa cells in culture, and that the introduced enzyme was active intracellularly [61]. When the cells were treated with enzyme-peptide conjugates, an intensive membrane binding was observed after short (0–20 min) incubation times, and the membrane-bound protein remained accessible to trypsin. However, prolonged incubation times, ranging from 30 min up to 6 h, resulted in the cytoplasmic appearance of conjugates, where they became trypsin-insensitive. Quantification of the enzymatic activity of β-galactosidase revealed an approximate 20% internalization of the conjugate [61], and similar results were observed when internalization of the conjugates with horseradish peroxidase was measured. Shorter sequences of HIV-1 TAT protein Tat (37-58) and Tat (47-58) were also shown to be capable of promoting the uptake, although the efficiency of the process was cargo-dependent [61].

7.8
CPPs in Gene Delivery

The delivery of plasmid DNA and different oligonucleotides by CPPs provides a tool for gene regulation studies. The transfection of mammalian cells with plasmid DNA is often achieved by the recruitment of lipid vectors, polyethylenimine, microinjection, or electroporation, all of which methods suffer from appreciable cytotoxicity and result in limited yields for gene delivery. In recent years, several studies have described the delivery of plasmid DNA with assistance from CPPs (for a review, see Ref. [62]). This results in an efficient transduction of, for example, the genes encoding green fluorescent protein (GFP) [63], luciferase [34, 64, 65], and β-galactosidase [66].

7.9
Delivery of Oligonucleotides

The use of antisense techniques as a pharmaceutical tool has the ability to down-regulate the expression of any desired gene product. Antisense techniques are based on sequence-specific oligonucleotides (ON) which, after reaching the cyto-plasm, form hybrids with complementary mRNA. This hybridization sterically hinders the recruitment of the translational machinery, or may lead to degradation of the double-stranded mRNA by RNaseH [67]. While the downregulation with different antisense ONs may be highly efficient and selective, the suitability for therapeutical applications of this method is often limited by the poor uptake of ONs. However, such uptake can be significantly increased when the ONs are coupled to a CPP sequence [34].

In order to prevent the rapid cytoplasmic degradation of ONs, a variety of different chemical modifications have been introduced to alter the ribose phosphate backbone. This results in the production of DNA analogues such as peptide nucleic acid (PNA), locked nucleic acid (LNA) and phosphorodiamidite morpholino-oligonucleotides (PMO), all of which are known to form stable complexes with DNA and RNA. PNA is an ON where the original negatively charged deoxyribose phosphate backbone of DNA has been replaced by neutral N-(2-aminoethyl)-glycine units linked by peptide bonds [68]. Although greatly improving the annealing to its complementary strand of nucleic acid, the overall neutral charge of PNA renders it virtually impermeable to the cell. Lipid-based delivery vectors, based on charge interactions, are incapable of transporting the PNA molecules through the plasma membrane, and therefore CPPs are often employed as transport vectors for PNA (for reviews, see Refs [69, 70]). An early example of this was the 21mer PNA which, when coupled via a disulfide bond to penetratin or transportan (TP), efficiently blocked the expression of the galanin receptor in human Bowes melanoma cells [71]. Since then, a myriad of other ONs, in combination with various CPPs, have been used for the regulation of gene expression (recently reviewed in Refs [62, 72]).

An elegant assay to assess the efficacy of CPPs for intracellular delivery has been introduced by Astriab-Fischer *et al.* [73]. In this assay, an ON sequence which redirects splicing of the luciferase gene transcript is coupled to the CPP. Upon application of the ON–CPP complex to HeLa/705 cells, the expression of luciferase gene can be modulated. This cell line, which originally was developed by Kang, *et al.* is stably transfected with a luciferase gene variant interrupted by the human β-globin intron 2 [74]. A single T→G mutation at nucleotide 705 activates aberrant splice sites in the intron, causing noncomplete splicing of the entire luciferase gene. The introduction of the complementary ON sterically blocks this splice site, the entire intron 2 is removed from the gene, and correct splicing of luciferase gene is restored [74].

During recent years, gene regulation with small interfering RNA (siRNA) molecules has undergone intensive study, although the internalization of siRNA with assistance from CPPs has been addressed in only very few reports. In 2003, Simeoni *et al.* were the first to report on the successful delivery of siRNA targeting glyceraldehyde-3-phosphate dehydrogenase (GAPDH) mRNA by coincubating siRNA with a modified MPG peptide [41]. Since then, both noncovalent [75, 76] and covalent [70, 77, 78] conjugation of siRNA with different peptides have been reported *in vitro*.

Recently, a series of experiments was described in which the expression of p38 MAP kinase in mouse lung was regulated by siRNA conjugated to Tat (48-60) and penetratin [77]. Although the expression of the respective mRNA was reduced *in vitro*, administration of the conjugates *in vivo* did not have any appreciable effect on mRNA levels. Interestingly, it was observed that the Tat (48-60) and penetratin peptides themselves exhibited activities and reduced mRNA expression [77]. This suggests a direct involvement of these CPPs in gene regulation, and should signal caution to those investigators employing CPPs as delivery vehicles *in vivo*.

7.10
Cytotoxicity of Cell-Penetrating Peptides

All CPPs are cationic peptides which can not only be taken up by cells but also deliver linked cargo molecules. This procedure requires that the CPPs interact with the plasma membrane, perhaps causing membrane disturbances. Some peptides, for example pVEC, are derived directly from membrane proteins [27], whereas others such as transportans originate from membrane lytic proteins [32]; still others are designed to have high amphipathic properties, which could lead to membrane disturbances [35]. When such molecules are considered for therapeutic applications such as gene therapy or cancer treatment, their toxicity is of central importance for the development process. Notably, it is critical for their therapeutic applications, although nonspecific toxic side effects might also cause artifacts. The toxicities of applied peptides are often assessed in studies with CPPs, but the results are not necessarily included in published reports. Furthermore, very few studies have compared the toxicity of different classes of CPPs under the same conditions as are used for the linked peptide sequences [79–82].

Fluorophores such as carboxyfluorescein or tetramethylrhodamine are routinely conjugated to CPPs to follow internalization of the peptides. Whilst providing a convenient detection method, fluorophores may however contribute to the toxic effects of the peptides. As shown recently by El Andaloussi *et al.*, the attachment of carboxyfluorescein to CPP increases the toxicity of the peptide [80], while the position of the label in the peptide sequence also appears to have some influence on the toxicity of the peptide, as might apply for other biologically relevant cargos [80]. It has been shown that different fluorescent dyes, when conjugated to proteins, exhibit different phototoxicities [83]. In this study, four commonly used fluorescent dyes, when conjugated to albumin, were used to examine phototoxicity towards rat erythrocytes. Fluorescein isothiocyanate (FITC)-labeled albumin was shown to exhibit light-induced toxicity after only a 10 min period of illumination, while other commercially available dyes, namely BODIPY-FL, Texas Red and tetramethylrhodamine isothiocyanate (TRITC), showed phototoxicity after an exposure time of 30 min or longer [83]. To date, as no studies have been reported describing these effects on CPPs, it is reasonable to assume that phototoxicity might be generally associated with short peptides linked to fluorescent dyes.

In a recent report, Cardozo *et al.* showed that the cytotoxicity of Tat (48-57) and penetratin was higher for CPP conjugates with longer cargo peptides when compared to unlabeled or shorter conjugates. Moreover, unconjugated peptides, at concentrations of up to $100 \mu M$ Tat (48-57) and $30 \mu M$ (Pen), did not trigger any significant cell death [79]. However, the authors compared the toxic effects of different cargos, rather than the shorter and longer versions of the same cargo.

When comparing different rhodamine-labeled CPPs and their conjugates with peptides, Jones *et al.* found that the cargo did not generally alter the toxicity profile. However, Tat (48-60) seemed to be an exception, showing a higher toxicity at 100 μM concentration as compared to the unconjugated peptide. Similar toxicity profiles were obtained for the tested peptides in three different cell lines, while the rhodamine label was also found to cause a significant increase in peptide toxicity [81].

An increased cytotoxicity of fluorescently labeled CPP was also observed by Dupont and colleagues, whereby carboxyfluorescein attached to the Pen peptide significantly increased membrane disturbance in MDCK cells at a concentration of 20 μM, whereas no membrane leakage was observed for unlabeled penetratin or the biotin-labeled peptide [84].

7.11
In Vivo Drug Delivery with CPPs

Although the number of reports of established and novel CPPs for *in vitro* applications continues to increase rapidly, this is not yet the case for delivery *in vivo* [85], with the lack of selective tissue uptake being a limiting factor. CPP-linked molecules are taken up at the site of their administration, and local application can be beneficial if, for example, intratumoral effects are desired. While the local administration of cyclosporine linked to polyarginine has been shown to be highly efficient [38], systemic application also appears promising, with intraperitonally injected Tat-β-galactosidase conjugates being detected in all of the tissues studied [86]. A similar distribution of Tat-β-galactosidase conjugates was also observed for other administration routes, including the portal vein, and intravenous and oral routes [87].

During the past few years, an increasing number of studies have demonstrated the usefulness of CPPs for *in vivo* drug delivery [88–90]. Initially, CPP was conjugated to β-galactosidase, yet in the meantime other reporter systems have been both developed and applied. A selection of studies showing various targets and their elicited biological responses is provided in Table 7.2.

As mentioned above, Fawell and colleagues demonstrated in 1994, that Tat (1-72) and Tat (37-72) could carry covalently conjugated β-galactosidase into HeLa cells in culture, following which an intracellular enzymatic activity could be documented [61]. *In vivo*, the distribution of the enzyme conjugate after intravenous administration in mice revealed very high activities in the liver, heart and spleen, lower activities in skeletal muscle and lung, very little activity in the kidney, and no activity in the brain [61]. The distribution pattern was very similar to that reported by Cai *et al.* [87].

Another study reported an efficient uptake of the anti-apoptotic protein Bcl-xL protein linked with Tat (47-57) in rat primary cortical neuronal culture; here, uptake occurred within 15 min of incubation, and attenuated the staurosporin-

Table 7.2 Targets and biological responses used in different CPP delivery studies *in vivo*.

Cargo	CPP	Organism	Effect	Reference
β-Galactosidase	Tat	BALB/C mouse	β-Galactosidase enzyme activity in various tissues	[61]
BCL-xL	Tat	C57BL/6 mouse	Inhibition of staurosporin-induced neural apoptosis	[91]
Uch-L1	Tat	APP/PS1 mouse	Rescue of synaptic function. Improvement in contextual memory	[92]
β-Galactosidase	Tat	BALB/C mouse	β-Galactosidase enzyme activity in various tissues	[87]
β-Galactosidase	Smac/ DIA BLO CTP	BALB/C mouse	β-Galactosidase enzyme activity in liver and lymph nodes	[93]
p53C′	Tat	A/J mouse	Reduced tumor growth	[94]
NF-κB	Pen	Wistar rat	Improvement of acute pancreatitis	[95]
siRNA	Tat, Pen	mouse	Downregulation of p38 MAPK	[78]
siRNA	Tat, Pen	BALB/C mouse	Downregulation of p38 MAPK	[77]
NADPH oxidase	Tat	C57Bl/6Tac mouse	Attenuation of angiotensin-induced O_2-levels and systolic blood pressure	[96]
IKK2	Pen	mouse	Acute inflammatory response	[97]
XIAP (BIR3-RING)	Pen	SD rat	Neuroprotective effect; inhibition of caspase activation	[98]
XIAP (BIR3-RING)	Pen	SD rat	Reduced neural apoptosis, inhibition of caspase-3 processing	[99]
Tyrosine hydroxylase	Tat	SD rat	Improved behavioral effects on PD model rats	[100]
Tumor-homing peptide	TP10, pVEC	BALB/C mouse	Accumulation of the homing peptide into MDA-MB-435 tumors	[101]
PNA	Pep-3	Athymic nude mouse	Tumor growth inhibition; tumor cyclin B1 downregulation	[102]
Plasmid DNA	Tat	C57BL/6	eGFP expression in tumors	[103]

NF-κB, nuclear factor κB; CTP, cytoplasmic transduction peptide; siRNA, small interfering RNA; IKK2, inhibitor of κB kinase β; XIAP, X-linked inhibitor of apoptosis protein; SD, Sprague–Dawley; PD, Parkinson's disease.

induced apoptosis in dose-dependent manner [91]. When injected intraperitoneally into mice, the fusion protein was detectable in various brain regions after 4 h; the induction of cerebral infarction was reduced on average by 40%, and the fusion protein suppressed caspase-3 activation when administered 2 h before the onset of ischemia [91].

Recently, the rescue of synaptic function and an improvement in contextual memory was observed following the intraperitoneal administration of an ubiquitin hydrolase (Uch-L1) fusion protein linked to Tat (57-48) to mice with Alzheimer's disease [92].

7.12
CPPs for Targeted Delivery

In order to overcome the problems of poor selectivity of CPPs *in vivo*, targeted delivery is currently under consideration, the proposal being to include a tissue-specific targeting domain with the CPP–drug conjugate. This could increase the selectivity of the conjugate, while decreasing any undesirable side effects. It was shown recently that this strategy would hold promise when a cyclic tumor-homing motif, CPGPEGAGC, conjugated to the CPP, caused a preferential localization of the CPP in MDA-MB-435 cell-induced tumors in nude Balb/c mice. CPP without the homing sequence can be found in multiple organs, as well as in the tumor tissues [101].

Another suggestion for increasing the specificity of CPPs is based on the incorporation of an enzymatically cleavable inactivation sequence in the CPP–cargo conjugate. Several tumors have been shown to secrete matrix metalloproteinases 2 and 9, both of which may serve as selective activators of inactivated CPPs. In fact, this approach has been proven particularly useful for polycationic CPP sequences that can be inactivated by polyanionic peptide sequences [104]. Several other studies have also demonstrated the efficient delivery of CPPs into tumor cells by similarly inactivated CPPs, both *in vitro* [105–107] and *in vivo* [107].

7.13
Conclusions

Small, positively charged peptides – generally known as CPPs – that are capable of delivering pharmaceutically relevant molecules through the plasma membrane *in vitro* and *in vivo*, have opened interesting options for basic research and pharmaceutical applications. Today, the intracellular delivery of molecules via CPPs is of major importance for research groups in a wide variety of areas. While the cargos to be coupled to the CPP for delivery may range from small fluorescent molecules to large proteins, all can be efficiently internalized. Although, at present, the exact mechanism of internalization of CPPs and their conjugates remains unclear, and may vary between different materials, the value of this approach in many different fields has been established unequivocally.

Acknowledgments

These studies were supported by Swedish Research Council VR-NT; Stockholm Center for Biomembrane Research and Estonian target financing project SF0180027s08.

Abbreviations

7TM	seven-transmembrane
CPP	cell-penetrating peptide
CME	clathrin-mediated endocytosis
PTD	protein transduction domain
MTS	membrane-translocating sequence
HIV-1	human immunodeficiency virus 1
NF-κB	nuclear factor κB
CTP	cytoplasmic transduction peptide
siRNA	small interfering RNA
IKK2	inhibitor of κB kinase β
XIAP	X-linked inhibitor of apoptosis protein

References

1 Derossi, D., Joliot, A.H., Chassaing, G. and Prochiantz, A. (1994) The third helix of the Antennapedia homeodomain translocates through biological membranes. *J. Biol. Chem.*, **269**, 10444–50.

2 El-Andaloussi, S., Johansson, H.J., Lundberg, P. and Langel, Ü. (2006) Induction of splice correction by cell-penetrating peptide nucleic acids, *J. Gene Med.*, **8**, 1262–73.

3 Geisler, I. and Chmielewski, J. (2007) Probing length effects and mechanism of cell penetrating agents mounted on a polyproline helix scaffold. *Bioorg. Med. Chem. Lett.*, **17**, 2765–8.

4 Kaplan, I.M., Wadia, J.S. and Dowdy, S.F. (2005) Cationic TAT peptide transduction domain enters cells by macropinocytosis. *J. Control. Release*, **102**, 247–53.

5 Lundberg, M., Wikström, S. and Johansson, M. (2003) Cell surface adherence and endocytosis of protein transduction domains. *Mol. Ther.*, **8**, 143–50.

6 Massodi, I., Bidwell, G.L., 3rd and Raucher, D. (2005) Evaluation of cell penetrating peptides fused to elastin-like polypeptide for drug delivery. *J. Control. Release*, **108**, 396–408.

7 Richard, J.P., Melikov, K., Brooks, H., Prevot, P., Lebleu, B. and Chernomordik, L.V. (2005) Cellular uptake of unconjugated TAT peptide involves clathrin-dependent endocytosis and heparan sulfate receptors. *J. Biol. Chem.*, **280**, 15300–6.

8 Richard, J.P., Melikov, K., Vivés, E., Ramos, C., Verbeure, B., Gait, M.J., Chernomordik, L.V. and Lebleu, B. (2003) Cell-penetrating peptides. A reevaluation of the mechanism of cellular uptake. *J. Biol. Chem.*, **278**, 585–90.

9 Soane, L. and Fiskum, G.T.A. (2005) T-mediated endocytotic delivery of the loop deletion Bcl-2 protein protects neurons against cell death. *J. Neurochem.*, **95**, 230–43.

10 Tünnemann, G., Martin, R.M., Haupt, S., Patsch, C., Edenhofer, F. and Cardoso, M.C. (2006) Cargo-dependent mode of uptake and bioavailability of TAT-containing proteins and peptides in living cells. *FASEB J.*, **20**, 1775–84.

11 Wadia, J.S., Stan, R.V. and Dowdy, S.F. (2004) Transducible TAT-HA fusogenic peptide enhances escape of TAT-fusion proteins after lipid raft macropinocytosis. *Nat. Med.*, **10**, 310–15.

12 Vivés, E., Richard, J.P., Rispal, C. and Lebleu, B. (2003) TAT peptide internalization: seeking the mechanism of entry. *Curr. Protein Pept. Sci.*, **4**, 125–32.

13 Duchardt, F., Fotin-Mleczek, M., Schwarz, H., Fischer, R. and Brock, R. (2007) A comprehensive model for the cellular uptake of cationic cell-penetrating peptides. *Traffic*, **8**, 848–66.

14 Jones, A.T. (2007) Macropinocytosis: searching for an endocytic identity and role in the uptake of cell penetrating peptides. *J. Cell. Mol. Med.*, **11**, 670–84.

15 Sandgren, S., Cheng, F. and Belting, M. (2002) Nuclear targeting of macromolecular polyanions by an HIV-Tat derived peptide. Role for cell-surface proteoglycans. *J. Biol. Chem.*, **277**, 38877–83.

16 Suzuki, T., Futaki, S., Niwa, M., Tanaka, S., Ueda, K. and Sugiura, Y. (2002) Possible existence of common internalization mechanisms among arginine-rich peptides. *J. Biol. Chem.*, **277**, 2437–43.

17 Tyagi, M., Rusnati, M., Presta, M. and Giacca, M. (2001) Internalization of HIV-1 tat requires cell surface heparan sulfate proteoglycans. *J. Biol. Chem.*, **276**, 3254–61.

18 Green, M. and Loewenstein, P.M. (1988) Autonomous functional domains of chemically synthesized human immunodeficiency virus tat trans-activator protein. *Cell*, **55**, 1179–88.

19 Vivés, E., Granier, C., Prevot, P. and Lebleu, B. (1997) Structure-activity relationship study of the plasma membrane translocating potential of a short peptide from HIV-1 Tat protein. *Lett. Pept. Sci.*, **4**, 429–36.

20 Derossi, D., Calvet, S., Trembleau, A., Brunissen, A., Chassaing, G. and Prochiantz, A. (1996) Cell internalization of the third helix of the Antennapedia homeodomain is receptor-independent. *J. Biol. Chem.*, **271**, 18188–93.

21 Hällbrink, M., Kilk, K., Elmquist, A., Lundberg, P., Lindgren, M., Jiang, Y., Pooga, M., Soomets, U. *et al.* (2005) Prediction of cell-penetrating peptides. *Int. J. Peptide Res. Ther.*, **11**, 249–59.

22 Prochiantz, A. (2008) Protein and peptide transduction, twenty years later a happy birthday. *Adv. Drug Deliv. Rev.*, **60**, 448–51.

23 Joliot, A. and Prochiantz, A. (2008) Homeoproteins as natural Penetratin cargoes with signaling properties. *Adv. Drug Deliv. Rev.*, **60**, 608–13.

24 Prochiantz, A. and Joliot, A. (2003) Can transcription factors function as cell-cell signalling molecules? *Nat. Rev. Mol. Cell Biol.*, **4**, 814–19.

25 Langel, Ü. (ed.) (2002) *Cell-penetrating Peptides, Processes and Applications*, CRC Press, Boca Raton.

26 Vivés, E., Brodin, P. and Lebleu, B. (1997) A truncated HIV-1 Tat protein basic domain rapidly translocates through the plasma membrane and accumulates in the cell nucleus. *J. Biol. Chem.*, **272**, 16010–17.

27 Elmquist, A., Lindgren, M., Bartfai, T. and Langel, Ü. (2001) VE-cadherin-derived cell-penetrating peptide, pVEC, with carrier functions. *Exp. Cell Res.*, **269**, 237–44.

28 Magzoub, M., Sandgren, S., Lundberg, P., Oglecka, K., Lilja, J., Wittrup, A., Göran Eriksson, L.E., Langel, Ü. *et al.* (2006) N-terminal peptides from unprocessed prion proteins enter cells by macropinocytosis. *Biochem. Biophys. Res. Commun.*, **348**, 379–85.

29 Kilk, K., Magzoub, M., Pooga, M. Eriksson, L.E., Langel, Ü. and Gräslund,

A. (2001) Cellular internalization of a cargo complex with a novel peptide derived from the third helix of the islet-1 homeodomain. Comparison with the penetratin peptide. *Bioconjug. Chem.*, **12**, 911–16.

30 Elliott, G. and O'Hare, P. (1997) Intercellular trafficking and protein delivery by a herpesvirus structural protein. *Cell*, **88**, 223–33.

31 El-Andaloussi, S., Johansson, H.J., Holm, T. and Langel, Ü. (2007) A novel cell-penetrating peptide, M918, for efficient delivery of proteins and peptide nucleic acids. *Mol. Ther.*, **15**, 1820–6.

32 Pooga, M., Hällbrink, M., Zorko, M. and Langel, Ü. (1998) Cell penetration by transportan. *FASEB J.*, **12**, 67–77.

33 Soomets, U., Lindgren, M., Gallet, X., Hällbrink, M., Elmquist, A., Balaspiri, L., Zorko, M., Pooga, M. *et al.* (2000) Deletion analogues of transportan. *Biochim. Biophys. Acta*, **1467**, 165–76.

34 Morris, M.C., Vidal, P., Chaloin, L., Heitz, F. and Divita, G. (1997) A new peptide vector for efficient delivery of oligonucleotides into mammalian cells. *Nucleic Acids Res.*, **25**, 2730–6.

35 Oehlke, J., Scheller, A., Wiesner, B., Krause, E., Beyermann, M., Klauschenz, E., Melzig, M. and Bienert, M. (1998) Cellular uptake of an alpha-helical amphipathic model peptide with the potential to deliver polar compounds into the cell interior non-endocytically. *Biochim. Biophys. Acta*, **1414**, 127–39.

36 Morris, M.C., Depollier, J., Mery, J., Heitz, F. and Divita, G. (2001) A peptide carrier for the delivery of biologically active proteins into mammalian cells. *Nat. Biotechnol.*, **19**, 1173–6.

37 Futaki, S., Suzuki, T., Ohashi, W., Yagami, T., Tanaka, S., Ueda, K. and Sugiura, Y. (2001) Arginine-rich peptides. An abundant source of membrane-permeable peptides having potential as carriers for intracellular protein delivery. *J. Biol. Chem.*, **276**, 5836–40.

38 Rothbard, J.B., Garlington, S., Lin, Q., Kirschberg, T., Kreider, E., McGrane, P.L., Wender, P.A. and Khavari, P.A. (2000) Conjugation of arginine oligomers to cyclosporin A facilitates

topical delivery and inhibition of inflammation. *Nat. Med.*, **6**, 1253–7.

39 Weigel, P.H. and Oka, J.A. (1981) Temperature dependence of endocytosis mediated by the asialoglycoprotein receptor in isolated rat hepatocytes. Evidence for two potentially rate-limiting steps. *J. Biol. Chem.*, **256**, 2615–17.

40 Thorén, P.E., Persson, D., Isakson, P., Goksör, M., Önfelt, A. and Nordén, B. (2003) Uptake of analogs of penetratin, Tat(48-60) and oligoarginine in live cells. *Biochem. Biophys. Res. Commun.*, **307**, 100–7.

41 Simeoni, F., Morris, M.C., Heitz, F. and Divita, G. (2003) Insight into the mechanism of the peptide-based gene delivery system MPG: implications for delivery of siRNA into mammalian cells. *Nucleic Acids Res.*, **31**, 2717–24.

42 Elmquist, A. and Langel, Ü. (2003) In vitro uptake and stability study of pVEC and its all-D analog. *Biol. Chem.*, **384**, 387–93.

43 Wender, P.A., Mitchell, D.J., Pattabiraman, K., Pelkey, E.T., Steinman, L. and Rothbard, J.B. (2000) The design synthesis and evaluation of molecules that enable or enhance cellular uptake: peptoid molecular transporters. *Proc. Natl Acad. Sci. USA*, **97**, 13003–8.

44 Brugidou, J., Legrand, C., Méry, J. and Rabié, A. (1995) The retro-inverso form of a homeobox-derived short peptide is rapidly internalised by cultured neurones: a new basis for an efficient intracellular delivery system. *Biochem. Biophys. Res. Commun.*, **214**, 685–93.

45 Zemel, A., Fattal, D.R. and Ben-Shaul, A. (2003) Energetics and self-assembly of amphipathic peptide pores in lipid membranes. *Biophys. J.*, **84**, 2242–55.

46 Dom, G., Shaw-Jackson, C., Matis, C., Bouffioux, O., Picard, J.J., Prochiantz, A., Mingeot-Leclercq, M.P., Brasseur, R. *et al.* (2003) Cellular uptake of Antennapedia Penetratin peptides is a two-step process in which phase transfer precedes a tryptophan-dependent translocation. *Nucleic Acids Res.*, **31**, 556–61.

47 Letoha, T., Gaal, S., Somlai, C., Czajlik, A., Perczel, A. and Penke, B. (2003) Membrane translocation of penetratin and its derivatives in different cell lines. *J. Mol. Recognit.*, **16**, 272–9.

48 Lundberg, M. and Johansson, M. (2001) Is VP22 nuclear homing an artifact? *Nat. Biotechnol.*, **19**, 713.

49 Fuchs, S.M. and Raines, R.T. (2004) Pathway for polyarginine entry into mammalian cells. *Biochemistry*, **43**, 2438–44.

50 Ziegler, A. and Seelig, J. (2004) Interaction of the protein transduction domain of HIV-1 TAT with heparan sulfate: binding mechanism and thermodynamic parameters. *Biophys. J.*, **86**, 254–63.

51 Nakase, I., Tadokoro, A., Kawabata, N., Takeuchi, T., Katoh, H., Hiramoto, K., Negishi, M., Nomizu, M. *et al.* (2007) Interaction of arginine-rich peptides with membrane-associated proteoglycans is crucial for induction of actin organization and macropinocytosis. *Biochemistry*, **46**, 492–501.

52 Nakase, I., Niwa, M., Takeuchi, T., Sonomura, K., Kawabata, N., Koike, Y., Takehashi, M., Tanaka, S. *et al.* (2004) Cellular uptake of arginine-rich peptides: roles for macropinocytosis and actin rearrangement. *Mol. Ther.*, **10**, 1011–22.

53 Säälik, P., Elmquist, A., Hansen, M., Padari, K., Saar, K., Viht, K., Langel, Ü. and Pooga, M. (2004) Protein cargo delivery properties of cell-penetrating peptides. A comparative study. *Bioconjug. Chem.*, **15**, 1246–53.

54 Henriques, S.T., Quintas, A., Bagatolli, L.A., Homble, F. and Castanho, M.A. (2007) Energy-independent translocation of cell-penetrating peptides occurs without formation of pores. A biophysical study with pep-1. *Mol. Membr. Biol.*, **24**, 282–93.

55 Silhol, M., Tyagi, M., Giacca, M., Lebleu, B. and Vivés, E. (2002) Different mechanisms for cellular internalization of the HIV-1 Tat-derived cell penetrating peptide and recombinant proteins fused to Tat. *Eur. J. Biochem.*, **269**, 494–501.

56 Holm, T., Netzereab, S. Hansen, M., Langel, Ü. and Hällbrink, M. (2005) Uptake of cell-penetrating peptides in yeasts. *FEBS Lett.*, **579**, 5217–22.

57 Nekhotiaeva, N., Elmquist, A., Rajarao, G.K., Hällbrink, M., Langel, Ü. and Good, L. (2004) Cell entry and antimicrobial properties of eukaryotic cell-penetrating peptides. *FASEB J.*, **18**, 394–6.

58 Mäe, M., Myrberg, H., Jiang, Y., Paves, H., Valkna, A. and Langel, Ü. (2005) Internalisation of cell-penetrating peptides into tobacco protoplasts. *Biochim. Biophys. Acta*, **1669**, 101–7.

59 Foerg, C. and Merkle, H.P. (2008) On the biomedical promise of cell penetrating peptides: limits versus prospects. *J. Pharm. Sci.*, **97**, 144–62.

60 Wadia, J.S. and Dowdy, S.F. (2005) Transmembrane delivery of protein and peptide drugs by TAT-mediated transduction in the treatment of cancer. *Adv. Drug. Deliv. Rev.*, **57**, 579–96.

61 Fawell, S., Seery, J., Daikh, Y., Moore, C., Chen, L.L., Pepinsky, B. and Barsoum, J. (1994) Tat-mediated delivery of heterologous proteins into cells. *Proc. Natl Acad. Sci. USA*, **91**, 664–8.

62 Järver, P., Langel, K., El-Andaloussi, S. and Langel, Ü. (2007) Applications of cell-penetrating peptides in regulation of gene expression. *Biochem. Soc. Trans.*, **35**, 770–4.

63 Morris, M.C., Chaloin, L., Mery, J., Heitz, F. and Divita, G. (1999) A novel potent strategy for gene delivery using a single peptide vector as a carrier. *Nucleic Acids Res.*, **27**, 3510–17.

64 Sandgren, S., Wittrup, A., Cheng, F., Jonsson, M., Eklund, E., Busch, S. and Belting, M. (2004) The human antimicrobial peptide LL-37 transfers extracellular DNA plasmid to the nuclear compartment of mammalian cells via lipid rafts and proteoglycan-dependent endocytosis. *J. Biol. Chem.*, **279**, 17951–6.

65 Tung, C.H., Mueller, S. and Weissleder, R. (2002) Novel branching membrane translocational peptide as gene delivery vector. *Bioorg. Med. Chem.*, **10**, 3609–14.

66 Ignatovich, I.A., Dizhe, E.B., Pavlotskaya, A.V., Akifiev, B.N., Burov, S.V., Orlov, S.V. and Perevozchikov, A.P. (2003) Complexes of plasmid DNA with basic domain 47-57 of the HIV-1 Tat protein are transferred to mammalian cells by endocytosis-mediated pathways. *J. Biol. Chem.*, **278**, 42625–36.

67 Crooke, S.T. (2004) Progress in antisense technology. *Annu. Rev. Med.*, **55**, 61–95.

68 Nielsen, P.E., Egholm, M., Berg, R.H. and Buchardt, O. (1991) Sequence-selective recognition of DNA by strand displacement with a thymine-substituted polyamide. *Science*, **254**, 1497–500.

69 Abes, R., Arzumanov, A.A., Moulton, H.M., Abes, S., Ivanova, G.D., Iversen, P.L., Gait, M.J. and Lebleu, B. (2007) Cell-penetrating-peptide-based delivery of oligonucleotides: an overview. *Biochem. Soc. Trans.*, **35**, 775–9.

70 Turner, J.J., Jones, S., Fabani, M.M., Ivanova, G., Arzumanov, A.A. and Gait, M.J. (2007) RNA targeting with peptide conjugates of oligonucleotides, siRNA and PNA. *Blood Cells Mol. Dis.*, **38**, 1–7.

71 Pooga, M., Soomets, U., Hällbrink, M., Valkna, A., Saar, K., Rezaei, K., Kahl, U., Hao, J.X. *et al.* (1998) Cell penetrating PNA constructs regulate galanin receptor levels and modify pain transmission in vivo. *Nat. Biotechnol.*, **16**, 857–61.

72 Mäe, M. and Langel, Ü. (2006) Cell-penetrating peptides as vectors for peptide, protein and oligonucleotide delivery. *Curr. Opin. Pharmacol.*, **6**, 509–14.

73 Astriab-Fisher, A., Sergueev, D., Fisher, M., Shaw, B.R. and Juliano, R.L. (2002) Conjugates of antisense oligonucleotides with the Tat and antennapedia cell-penetrating peptides: effects on cellular uptake, binding to target sequences, and biologic actions. *Pharm. Res.*, **19**, 744–54.

74 Kang, S.H., Cho, M.J. and Kole, R. (1998) Up-regulation of luciferase gene expression with antisense oligonucleotides: implications and applications in functional assay development. *Biochemistry*, **37**, 6235–9.

75 Lundberg, P., El-Andaloussi, S., Sütlü, T., Johansson, H. and Langel, Ü. (2007) Delivery of short interfering RNA using endosomolytic cell-penetrating peptides. *FASEB J.*, **21**, 2664–71.

76 Meade, B.R. and Dowdy, S.F. (2008) Enhancing the cellular uptake of siRNA duplexes following noncovalent packaging with protein transduction domain peptides. *Adv. Drug Deliv. Rev.*, **60**, 530–6.

77 Moschos, S.A., Jones, S.W., Perry, M.M., Williams, A.E., Erjefalt, J.S., Turner, J.J., Barnes, P.J., Sproat, B.S. *et al.* (2007) Lung delivery studies using siRNA conjugated to TAT(48-60) and penetratin reveal peptide induced reduction in gene expression and induction of innate immunity. *Bioconjug. Chem.*, **18**, 1450–9.

78 Moschos, S.A., Williams, A.E. and Lindsay, M.A. (2007) Cell-penetrating-peptide-mediated siRNA lung delivery. *Biochem. Soc. Trans.*, **35**, 807–10.

79 Cardozo, A.K., Buchillier, V., Mathieu, M., Chen, J., Ortis, F., Ladrière, L., Allaman-Pillet, N., Poirot, O. *et al.* (2007) Cell-permeable peptides induce dose- and length-dependent cytotoxic effects. *Biochim. Biophys. Acta*, **1768**, 2222–34.

80 El-Andaloussi, S., Järver, P., Johansson, H.J. and Langel, Ü. (2007) Cargo-dependent cytotoxicity and delivery efficacy of cell-penetrating peptides: a comparative study. *Biochem. J.*, **407**, 285–92.

81 Jones, S.W., Christison, R., Bundell, K., Voyce, C.J., Brockbank, S.M., Newham, P. and Lindsay, M.A. (2005) Characterisation of cell-penetrating peptide-mediated peptide delivery. *Br. J. Pharmacol.*, **145**, 1093–102.

82 Sugita, T., Yoshikawa, T., Mukai, Y., Yamanada, N., Imai, S., Nagano, K., Yoshida, Y., Shibata, H. *et al.* (2008) Comparative study on transduction and toxicity of protein transduction domains. *Br. J. Pharmacol.*, **153**, 1143–52.

83 Rumbaut, R.E. and Sial, A.J. (1999) Differential phototoxicity of fluorescent dye-labeled albumin conjugates. *Microcirculation*, **6**, 205–13.

84 Dupont, E., Prochiantz, A. and Joliot, A. (2007) Identification of a signal peptide for unconventional secretion. *J. Biol. Chem.*, **282**, 8994–9000.

85 Vivés, E. (2005) Present and future of cell-penetrating peptide mediated delivery systems: "is the Trojan horse

too wild to go only to Troy? *J. Control. Release*, **109**, 77–85.

86 Schwarze, S.R., Ho, A., Vocero-Akbani, A. and Dowdy, S.F. (1999) In vivo protein transduction: delivery of a biologically active protein into the mouse. *Science*, **285**, 1569–72.

87 Cai, S.R., Xu, G., Becker-Hapak, M., Ma, M., Dowdy, S.F. and McLeod, H.L. (2006) The kinetics and tissue distribution of protein transduction in mice. *Eur. J. Pharm. Sci.*, **27**, 311–19.

88 Moulton, H.M., Fletcher, S., Neuman, B.W., McClorey, G., Stein, D.A., Abes, S., Wilton, S.D., Buchmeier, M.J. *et al.* (2007) Cell-penetrating peptide-morpholino conjugates alter pre-mRNA splicing of DMD (Duchenne muscular dystrophy) and inhibit murine coronavirus replication in vivo. *Biochem. Soc. Trans.*, **35**, 826–8.

89 Schwarze, S.R. and Dowdy, S.F. (2000) In vivo protein transduction: intracellular delivery of biologically active proteins, compounds and DNA. *Trends Pharmacol. Sci.*, **21**, 45–8.

90 Tilstra, J., Rehman, K.K., Hennon, T., Plevy, S.E., Clemens, P. and Robbins, P.D. (2007) Protein transduction: identification, characterization and optimization. *Biochem. Soc. Trans.*, **35**, 811–15.

91 Cao, G., Pei, W., Ge, H., Liang, Q., Luo, Y., Sharp, F.R., Lu, A., Ran, R. *et al.* (2002) In vivo delivery of a Bcl-xL fusion protein containing the TAT protein transduction domain protects against ischemic brain injury and neuronal apoptosis. *J. Neurosci.*, **22**, 5423–31.

92 Gong, B., Cao, Z., Zheng, P., Vitolo, O.V., Liu, S., Staniszewski, A., Moolman, D., Zhang, H. *et al.* (2006) Ubiquitin hydrolase Uch-L1 rescues beta-amyloid-induced decreases in synaptic function and contextual memory. *Cell*, **126**, 775–88.

93 Kim, D., Jeon, C., Kim, J.H., Kim, M.S., Yoon, C.H., Choi, I.S., Kim, S.H. and Bae, Y.S. (2006) Cytoplasmic transduction peptide (CTP): new approach for the delivery of biomolecules into cytoplasm in vitro and in vivo. *Exp. Cell Res.*, **312**, 1277–88.

94 Snyder, E.L., Meade, B.R., Saenz, C.C. and Dowdy, S.F. (2004) Treatment of terminal peritoneal carcinomatosis by a transducible p53-activating peptide. *PLoS Biol.*, **2**, E36.

95 Letoha, T., Kusz, E., Papai, G., Szabolcs, A., Kaszaki, J., Varga, I., Takács, T., Penke, B. *et al.* (2006) In vitro and in vivo nuclear factor-kappaB inhibitory effects of the cell-penetrating penetratin peptide. *Mol. Pharmacol.*, **69**, 2027–36.

96 Rey, F.E., Cifuentes, M.E., Kiarash, A., Quinn, M.T. and Pagano, P.J. (2001) Novel competitive inhibitor of NAD(P)H oxidase assembly attenuates vascular O(2)(–) and systolic blood pressure in mice. *Circ. Res.*, **89**, 408–14.

97 May, M.J., D'Acquisto, F., Madge, L.A., Glockner, J., Pober, J.S. and Ghosh, S. (2000) Selective inhibition of NF-kappaB activation by a peptide that blocks the interaction of NEMO with the IkappaB kinase complex. *Science*, **289**, 1550–4.

98 Li, T., Fan, Y., Luo, Y., Xiao, B. and Lu, C. (2006) In vivo delivery of a XIAP (BIR3-RING) fusion protein containing the protein transduction domain protects against neuronal death induced by seizures. *Exp. Neurol.*, **197**, 301–8.

99 Fan, Y.F., Lu, C.Z., Xie, J., Zhao, Y.X. and Yang, G.Y. (2006) Apoptosis inhibition in ischemic brain by intraperitoneal PTD-BIR3-RING (XIAP). *Neurochem. Int.*, **48**, 50–9.

100 Wu, S.P., Fu, A.L., Wang, Y.X., Yu, L.P., Jia, P.Y., Li, Q., Jin, G.Z. and Sun, M.J. (2006) A novel therapeutic approach to 6-OHDA-induced Parkinson's disease in rats via supplementation of PTD-conjugated tyrosine hydroxylase. *Biochem. Biophys. Res. Commun.*, **346**, 1–6.

101 Myrberg, H., Zhang, L., Mäe, M. and Langel, Ü. (2008) Design of a tumor-homing cell-penetrating peptide. *Bioconjug. Chem.*, **19**, 70–5.

102 Morris, M.C., Gros, E., Aldrian-Herrada, G., Choob, M., Archdeacon, J., Heitz, F. and Divita, G. (2007) A non-covalent peptide-based carrier for in vivo delivery of DNA mimics. *Nucleic Acids Res.*, **35**, e49.

103 Torchilin, V.P., Levchenko, T.S., Rammohan, R., Volodina, N., Papahadjopoulos-Sternberg, B. and D'Souza, G.G. (2003) Cell transfection in vitro and in vivo with nontoxic TAT peptide-liposome-DNA complexes. *Proc. Natl Acad. Sci. USA*, **100**, 1972–7.

104 Jiang, T., Olson, E.S., Nguyen, Q.T., Roy, M., Jennings, P.A. and Tsien, R.Y. (2004) Tumor imaging by means of proteolytic activation of cell-penetrating peptides. *Proc. Natl Acad. Sci. USA*, **101**, 17867–72.

105 Goun, E.A., Shinde, R., Dehnert, K.W., Adams-Bond, A., Wender, P.A., Contag, C.H. and Franc, B.L. (2006) Intracellular cargo delivery by an octaarginine transporter adapted to target prostate cancer cells through cell surface protease activation. *Bioconjug. Chem.*, **17**, 787–96.

106 Pipkorn, R., Waldeck, W., Spring, H., Jenne, J.W. and Braun, K. (2006) Delivery of substances and their target-specific topical activation. *Biochim. Biophys. Acta*, **1758**, 606–10.

107 Bullok, K.E., Maxwell, D., Kesarwala, A.H., Gammon, S., Prior, J.L., Snow, M., Stanley, S. and Piwnica-Worms, D. (2007) Biochemical and in vivo characterization of a small, membrane-permeant, caspase-activatable far-red fluorescent peptide for imaging apoptosis. *Biochemistry*, **46**, 4055–65.

8

Production and Purification of Monomeric Recombinant Peptide Aptamers: Requirements for Efficient Intracellular Uptake and Target Inhibition

Corina Borghouts and Astrid Weiss

8.1
Introduction

Special classes of molecules are required to interfere with specific protein interactions. The protein surfaces that mediate the interactions are usually large, lack well-defined binding pockets, and are therefore difficult to target with conventional small-molecular-weight compounds. In mammals, central biological processes (e.g., the immune system) are based on specifically binding peptides, which help to protect and cure the host from diseases. Analogously, naturally occurring protein interaction domains or selected peptide ligands are being considered as potential drugs which can act as competitive inhibitors of protein–protein interactions. This biological potential has motivated research groups to develop peptides as antimicrobials, anticancer agents, cytoprotective, anti-inflammatory or diagnostic agents, and has led to the establishment of peptides as nonconventional drugs. Many different cellular functions, including enzyme activities, adaptor proteins and transcription factors, have been targeted by specifically interacting peptide molecules. At present, more than 130 different proteins and peptides have been approved for clinical use by the US Food and Drug Administration (FDA), and many more are currently under development. Considering that recombinantly expressed insulin entered the market only 25 years ago, this can be seen as a remarkable progress (for a review, see Ref. [1]).

Unlike gene therapeutic applications, peptides do not permanently alter the properties of cells through genetic modification, but instead have temporary effects and thus act more like conventional drugs. Furthermore, peptides can affect their targets in many different modes. For example, they can alter or inhibit protein–protein interactions, inhibit aberrantly activated signaling components, or even inhibit DNA-binding domains, ultimately affecting target gene expression patterns. Peptides open additional avenues for therapy and complement small-molecular weight intracellular therapeutics. For instance, many of the targeted therapeutics in cancer which have been introduced over the past years are kinase inhibitors. Peptides – that can bind and inhibit many other functional domains –

can be highly specific and carry less risk of adverse side effects. Peptides can also be developed that are able to amplify or restore signals, and thus can counteract, for example, the loss of tumor suppressor gene functions.

The development and application of peptides, however, remains limited, mainly due to the poor efficiency of these large hydrophilic molecules to cross biological membranes. The first indication that it might be possible to solve this problem came with the observation that proteins such as the *Drosophila* Antennapedia transcription factor or the HIV-1 Tat transactivating protein were able to cross cellular membranes from the outside of the cell and find their way to the nucleus. Such experiments have led to the discovery of a wide range of cell-penetrating peptides (CPPs). The attachment of a CPP to a peptide sequence allows the exogenous introduction of bioactive peptides into the cytosolic environment. Cellular target specificity can be improved by incorporating novel targeting moieties, for example homing peptides, which can use the molecular receptors–for example, of the vasculature–to achieve specific delivery to organs or tumors [2]. Recently, the first therapeutic CPP agent–TAT linked to a peptide inhibitor of protein kinase C (PKC)–was approved for Phase I/II clinical testing in the treatment of cardiac ischemia [3, 4].

The future of peptides as drugs and CPP-mediated protein delivery will depend on the progress made in understanding the mechanism of delivery, as well as in improvements in the activity of the cargo. The activity of the delivered protein requires optimal protein production and purification conditions, the choice of an appropriate scaffold, and selection of the most effective protein transduction domain (PTD). The advantages and disadvantages of the available systems, the different purification parameters, and the options for constructing transducible therapeutic peptides will be summarized in this chapter. This area of research defines the prerequisites for the exploitation of PTD-mediated delivery of intracellular protein therapeutics.

8.2
Protein Production

Numerous protein- and peptide-based therapeutics are currently undergoing development for the treatment of antimicrobial diseases, viral infections, immune system disorders, cardiovascular diseases, neurological disorders and cancer. Recombinant DNA technology is used to produce and purify therapeutic proteins such as glucagon, erythropoietin-α and interferon β1a in a wide range of cells. The production systems for recombinant proteins include bacteria, yeast, insect cells, mammalian cells and even transgenic animals and plants. The system of choice mainly depends on the costs for the production of the desired product and on the requirements for secondary modifications of the protein (see Table 8.1). Recombinantly produced proteins may have several benefits compared to proteins purified from their native source. First, recombinant proteins are

Table 8.1 Comparison of protein expression systems.

Characteristic	Bacteria	Yeast	Insect cells	Mammalian cells	Synthesis
Major advantage(s)	• Very easy to use • Cheap	• Easy to use • Eukaryotic system • Protease-deficient strains available	• Easy scale-up	• High biosafety	• Incorporation of analogues • Easy attachment of labels, etc. • High purity
Expression level	High	High	High	Medium	n.a.
Protein secretion	Yes	Yes	No	Yes	n.a.
Promotors available	T7, tac, P21, P23, P59, P170, cspA, Pzn-zitR	AOX, MOX, FLD1, GAP, AOX2, YPT1, PEX8	Polyhedrin	CMV, SV40, CAG, RSV-LTR, HBV	n.a.
Cell systems used	• E. coli (BL21, Origami Rosetta gami) • L. lactis • B. subtilus	• Pichia pastoris (pep4, prb1, pno1 mutants) • Hansenula polymorpha	• Sf9 • Sf21 • Ld652Y	• Huh7, HepG2 • COS-7, HeLa • CHO, 239 • NIH3T3, A549, etc.	n.a.
Post-translational modifications	No	Yes, but not identical to mammalian cells	Yes	Yes	Yes
Cost	Low	Low	Low	Medium	High
Other disadvantages	• Codon optimization of eukaryotic proteins • Accumulation in inclusion bodies • Protein refolding	• Secreted proteins are diluted in large volumes of culture medium	• Less convenient • Virus purification and concentration	• Less convenient • Virus purification and concentration	• Limited peptide size • Expensive

n.a., not applicable.

often produced more cost-effectively and, potentially, in unlimited quantities. This approach also allows the production of novel proteins, for example those selected from random peptide libraries, and the modification of proteins to improve their function, activity, or specificity. Finally, recombinant technology permits the production of proteins that combine desirable functional domains in a single polypeptide.

8.2.1
Bacterial Systems

Various prokaryotic expression systems have been used for the production of a proteins of interest (e.g., *Escherichia coli*, *Lactococcus lactis*, *Bacillus subtilis*). These cells are usually preferred because growth of the cultures is inexpensive, and they rapidly divide and quickly accumulate in the medium, which is important for scale-up of the protein production process. BL21 *E. coli* strains and derivatives (Novagen, USA) have been optimized for this purpose; these lack lon and OmpT proteases and have been most widely used. Many other bacterial strains are available, with different characteristics to enable the expression of almost every protein; for example, Rosetta-gami strains overxpressing rare tRNAs and Origami2 strains for enhanced disulfide bond formation in the cytoplasm [5, 6]. *Bacillus* species have been used to produce various enzymes. These strains are endotoxin free–a prerequisite for proteins to be administered to humans–and mutant *Bacillus* strains have been developed (e.g., WB800) that are devoid of extra-cellular proteases, thus preventing proteolysis of the secreted protein-of-interest [7]. *Lactobacillus lactis* (e.g., strain IL1403) is today becoming an attractive option for protein expression as it secretes only one major protein (Usp45), thus simplifying the purification procedures of the secreted proteins [8]. For these bacterial strains, strong promoters (P21, P23, and P59) are available to produce recombinant proteins [8, 9]. Additionally, inducible promoters for the production of toxic proteins have been described, and include the nisin-inducible promoter (NICE-system), the pH-sensitive P170 promoter, or the zinc-regulated promoter P_{zn}-*zitR* [10–12].

In order to achieve optimal production of a protein, several aspects must be considered before choosing a system. The overexpression of some proteins in *E. coli* adversely affects the host through their catalytic properties, or it may cause toxicity to the host. Such toxic effects might be suppressed by lowering the growth temperature (15–23 °C). Growth at a lower temperature also enhances the stability and correct folding of the recombinant proteins, because the expression of chaperones in *E. coli* is increased, whereas proteases are poorly active at lower temperatures [13, 14]. As the expression level of the recombinant proteins is usually reduced at a lower temperature, vectors with a cspA promoter have been designed to circumvent this problem [15].

Apart from the type of promoter, two additional factors that will influence the expression level of the protein are the composition of the medium (e.g., LB, SOC, Teriffic Broth, M9) and the cell density [16]. Limitations in optimal nutrients in the medium during induction of the recombinant protein often lead to insoluble proteins in inclusion bodies. Furthermore, the correct folding of a protein might require the presence of specific cofactors such as metal ions (Mg^{2+}, Mn^{2+}, Zn^{2+}). By experimentally optimizing the media formulation, the expression level, solubility and yield of recombinant proteins can be increased.

The expression level of a protein is influenced by the *coding sequence*. Most amino acids are encoded by more than one codon, and each organism has a different codon usage depending on the expression level of the corresponding tRNA. Therefore, it is usually necessary to optimize the codons for expression in *E. coli*. In order to obtain abundantly expressed recombinant proteins, the low-usage codons (in *E. coli*, for example AGG, AGA, CGA, CGG, AUA, CUA, CCC and UCG) should be avoided [17]. These can be exchanged to high-usage codons by site-directed mutagenesis or cloning procedures. Neither modification of the medium nor growth of the cells at lower temperatures has a significant role in shifting the codon usage levels. Commercially available *E. coli* strains have extra genomic copies of several rare tRNA genes [e.g., argU (AGG/AGA), glyT (GAA) and ileX (AUA)]. These strains (e.g., BL21-codon+ or Rosetta-gami cells) are able to efficiently translate AT- or GC-rich genes, thus reducing the chances of obtaining truncated products.

Insoluble proteins expressed in *E. coli* accumulate in inclusion bodies, while soluble recombinant proteins can be obtained in different compartments. Usually, expression in the cytoplasm is preferred, as the production yields are high. For those proteins which require disulfide bond formation, the periplasm is the preferred site of accumulation. *E. coli* strains are available with mutations in the thioredoxin reductase (*trxB*) and glutathione (GSH) reductase (*gor*) genes [18]. In this way, thioredoxin and glutathione are in the oxidized form and are able to reduce cysteines, leading to disulfide bond formation. It is also possible to fuse the protein-of-interest to thioredoxin to improve both disulfide bond formation and folding of the protein [19]. Proteins may also accumulate in the growth medium, although this requires the protein to be fused to a secretion signal such as ompA [20]. The proteins translocate to the periplasm and then "leak" into the medium. Because most *E. coli* strains do not express proteins involved in translocation through the outer membrane, the expression of two secretion factors (secA and secY) improves the secretion of at least some proteins [21].

One disadvantage of bacterial expression is the lack of a post-translational modification machinery equivalent to that found in mammalian cells. Phosphorylation or glycosylation often affect the activities of the expressed proteins. The post-translational modifications of proteins regulate many biological processes, including metabolism, signal transduction and gene expression. To mimic the situation found in mammalian cells, it is possible to coexpress the required kinase and its substrate from two separate vectors or a single plasmid in *E. coli* to obtain phosphorylated proteins [22]. Additionally, other protein-modifying enzymes such as methylases and acetylases can be coexpressed to obtain recombinant proteins that closely resemble eukaryotic proteins. Prokaryotic organisms lack the cellular organelles required for glycosylation by enzymes such as glycosyltransferase and glycosidases; however, it was recently found that bacteria are capable of nonenzymatic glycosylation (glycation) [23]. In this so-called Millard reaction, aldoamines and ketoamines are converted into terminal adducts, which are then bound irreversibly to the target molecules and designated as advanced glycation end (ACE) products. Unfortunately, the details of this process are still not completely understood. Another option to incorporate glycosylated amino acids into proteins is to use modified amino acids in the translation process [24].

8.2.2
Yeast Systems

The expression of foreign proteins in yeast cells combines the ease, simplicity and low costs of bacterial expression systems with the authenticity of the far more expensive and less convenient animal tissue culture systems. As eukaryotes, the yeasts provide an environment for post-translational processing. Although *Saccharomyces cerevisiae* was one of the first yeast strains to be used for protein production, the yields in this strain remain relatively low, even if high-copy plasmids and regulatable promoters are employed. Mytholotrophic yeasts such as *Pichia pastoris* and *Hansenula polymorpha* retain all the advantages of *S. cerevisiae*, but provide a reliable means of achieving greatly elevated yields. These strains are able to grow on medium containing methanol as the sole carbon source [25]. Under these conditions, the expression of the alcohol oxidase (AOX) gene is turned on, and the enzyme can constitute some 30% of the total protein. The AOX promoter (or MOX promoter in *H. polymorpha*) is used for expression of the protein-of-interest in very high yields [26]. Expression is undetectable when the cells are grown on glucose or ethanol, and is highly induced if the cells are shifted to a medium containing methanol. A second regulatable promotor used in *Pichia* is the FLD1 (formaldehyde dehydrogenase) promoter [27]. The advantage of this promoter is that it is activated not only by methanol in the medium but also by methylamine. This allows the induction of foreign protein expression in the presence of glucose or glycerol in the medium [28]. The less widely used constitutive GAP (glyceraldehyde 3-phosphate dehydrogenase) promoter can also be used to obtain high levels of nontoxic foreign proteins in *P. pastoris*; a combination of the AOX and GAP promoters was also shown to be highly productive [29, 30]. If only low amounts of recombinant proteins are required, then the AOX2, YPT1, and PEX8 promoters are optionally available [31, 32].

In order to improve the quality and yield of exogenously expressed proteins in *Pichia*, protease-deficient strains are in general being used (e.g., with a *pep4* and/or *prb1* genotype). In *pep4* mutants, the proteinase A and carboxypeptidase Y activity is eliminated, whereas in *prb1* mutants proteinase B activity is lost. Secreted proteins (e.g., by fusion of the protein with a secretion signal such as the α-factor prepro-signal) can also be degraded by extracellular proteases, membrane-bound proteases, and also by intracellular proteases released by lysed cells. However, it is possible to prevent this by varying the pH of the growth medium, making it suboptimal for the extracellular protease but suitable for the recombinant protein [33].

Other strategies include the addition of protease inhibitors or amino acid-rich nutrients (e.g., casamino acids, peptone) in the medium, all of which act as competing substrates for the proteases. Lowering the temperature might stabilize and enhance folding of the recombinant protein and reduce the activity of the protease [34]. Finally, in order to increase the yield of recombinant proteins the copy number of the expression cassette can be increased. With the AOX1 or GAP promoters, encouraging results have been obtained by increasing the copy number of the heterologous gene expression cassettes [35, 36].

Unlike bacteria, yeast cells are able to perform most of the post-translational modifications usually observed in higher eukaryotes, including disulfide bond formation, O- and N-linked glycosylation and processing of signal sequences. O-Glycosylation implies the enzymatic transfer of *N*-acetyl galactosamine to the hydroxyl groups of serine and threonine, followed by other carbohydrates (e.g., galactose). This process is usually important for the proteins of the extracellular matrix or for those proteins involved in cell–cell contact. For N-linked glycosylations, a 14-sugar precursor is attached to asparagines, and for this process a consensus recognition sequence (Asn-X-Ser/Thr/Cys) has been described [37]. This process is important for the folding of some eukaryotic proteins. Both, O- and N-linked glycosylation of many mammalian proteins is important for their function, and it might be desirable to closely mimic the original glycosylation patterns on the recombinant proteins. The glycosylation potential of *Pichia* offers advantages when compared to bacterial expression. However, it should be noted that in *Pichia*, O-linked glycosylations are composed of mannose residues, whereas in mammals various other sugars are used for this process. Furthermore, it is possible that *Pichia* glycosylates the protein at other sites, or glycosylates proteins which are normally nonglycosylated. An undesired positioning of the glycosides might have detrimental consequences for the function of the recombinant protein. An additional problem stems from the fact, that *Pichia*-derived recombinant proteins, which are glycosylated, are able to induce an immune response in humans. Site-specific mutagenesis of the recombinant protein might help to obtain more humanized glycosylation patterns. A mutant of a *P. pastoris* strain with a disruption in the *PNO1* gene (encoding a protein involved in phosphomannosylation of N-linked oligosaccharides) was shown to reduce glycosylation of the recombinant proteins [38], however this method does not guarantee a sufficiently humanized glycosylation pattern. Consequently, one research group removed the endogenous glycosylation pathway in *Pichia*, and replaced it with five eukaryotic key enzymes for the production of humanized glycoproteins [39]. This strain thus has the potential to produce recombinant proteins that can be used in humans.

The genetic manipulation of *P. pastoris* for the production of various exogenous proteins is simplified by the use of a wide range of selectable markers and promoters. Choosing the correct markers, promoters and culture conditions is essential for obtaining a high yield in this system; the optimal conditions are found to differ for each recombinant protein, with optimization being required not only for the expression constructs but also for protein production and modification processes.

Both, Caraghino and Cregg and Macauley-Patrick and coworkers have presented overviews of proteins that have been successfully expressed in *P. pastoris* [40, 41].

8.2.3
Baculovirus Systems

In addition to bacteria and yeast cells, insect or mammalian cells can be used for the expression of recombinant proteins. In the past, *baculoviruses* have been one of the most popular viral vectors for the expression of recombinant proteins in insect cells. Extremely high levels of gene expression can be obtained, and these viruses show an excellent biosafety profile. In contrast to other commonly used viral vectors, baculoviruses have the unique property of replicating in insect cells while being incapable of initiating a replication cycle and producing infectious viruses in mammalian cells. The use of baculoviruses has led to the successful expression of numerous proteins (17–110 kDa in size), and this approach is used widely in pharmaceutical research for target validation, assay development, antibody generation and structural analysis [42, 43]. One major advantage of the baculovirus–insect cells expression system is the ease of large-scale production.

Most commercially available baculovirus systems are based on the *Autographa californica* multiple nucleopolyhedrosis virus (AcMNPV). Here, the recombinant baculovirus DNA is transfected into insect cells (e.g., Sf9 or Sf21, derived from *Spodoptera frugiperda*), in which replication occurs. The obtained virus particles can be amplified by the infection of fresh insect cells, and can be used for the production of recombinant proteins. The advantage of insect cells over bacteria is the fact that post-translational modifications are comparable to modifications carried out in mammalian cells. In order to even more closely mimic the glycosylation patterns of membrane-bound and secreted mammalian proteins, significant progress has been made by improving both viral vectors and insect host cell lines (for a review, see Refs [44, 45]).

To obtain high expression levels in insects, the dispensable polyhedrin gene present in the double-stranded baculovirus DNA genome (~130 kb in total) is replaced by the gene coding for the recombinant protein. The late polyhedrin promoter is highly active, and is transcribed by a virally encoded RNA polymerase. Transcription can account for up to 25% of the host cell transcript numbers. Numerous derivatives of this promoter with different features are available, because maximal expression does not always yield soluble, active protein. In contrast, if the expression of functional recombinant protein is too low, then production can be increased by the coexpression of chaperones, the addition of DNA elements (e.g., addition of the 5′ leader sequence of the gene of interest), or the use of a baculovirus with a reduced cell lysis capacity [46–48]. Cell lysis usually occurs at 3 to 5 days after infection, and results in proteolytic activity and the release of other factors that may cause degradation of the recombinant protein. Other technical improvements have included the simplified isolation of recombinant viruses, quantification methods, advances in cell culture technology, and the commercial availability of reagents.

The successful use of baculoviruses for recombinant protein expression in mammalian cells was first demonstrated for liver cells well over a decade ago [49]. For this, the baculovirus was modified to contain a promoter active in mammalian cells (e.g., a CMV- or RSV-LTR promoter), commonly referred to as BacMam viruses [50]. Gene delivery can be accomplished by simply adding viral particles isolated from infected insect cells to the culture medium. Soon thereafter, other laboratories reported the delivery to a broad range of other mammalian cell lines (e.g., COS-7 and osteosarcoma cells) and primary cells (e.g., primary rat chondrocytes, primary mouse kidney cells, human mesenchymal stem cells) [51]. However, certain cell types do not efficiently express the gene of interest (e.g., HeLa, CHO, NIH3T3), and various parameters have consequently been explored either to improve the transduction process (including cell density, lowering temperature, the addition of butyrate or EGTA), or to increase the expression level by using other promoter constructs. The system requires further optimization, before microgram quantities of protein per milliliter of culture can be obtained [52–54].

8.2.4
Chemical Synthesis

Recombinant protein expression can be achieved in the above-mentioned cellular systems. Occasionally, it is also possible and desirable to use chemical synthesis to produce the proteins of interest [55]. During the past 15 years, synthetic chemistry has advanced from creating short peptide chains to polypeptides of 40–60 amino acids in length, which realistically represents the efficiency limit of solid-phase peptide synthesis. Subsequently, the process of native chemical ligation was introduced to produce larger proteins, whereby protein segments are joined through native peptide bonds [56]. The native chemical ligation technique employs the principle of a chemoselective reaction between two unprotected peptides in aqueous solution in which a carboxy-terminal thioester undergoes a thiol-exchange with an amino-terminal cysteine sulfhydryl side chain. A subsequent, rapid, intramolecular rearrangement yields a native peptide bond at the site of ligation [55, 57].

Chemical synthesis is an option, if the protein-of-interest is relatively short (i.e., less than 50 aa). The synthesis of larger proteins in greater amounts remains very costly, and therefore recombinant expression is still preferred in these cases. When biologically active proteins cannot be generated by recombinant expression techniques, due to insolubility or misfolding, then chemical synthesis might represent a solution. Furthermore, synthesis has also been employed to answer important structural and functional questions, as well as to screen for inhibitory peptide analogues with improved target binding.

Chemical synthesis embodies a number of advantages over recombinant protein production. For example, the chemist can incorporate D-amino acids, unnatural amino acids, or alternatively attach pseudopeptides, labels, or polymers [58, 59]. Whereas this might increase *in vivo* stability, the addition of polyethylene glycol (PEG) polymers was shown to reduce immunogenicity, to enhance solubility, and also to improve other pharmacological properties [60]. Of course, although such modifications may alter the functionality of the protein, they may also increase the reactivity, bioavailability, and/or longevity. Another advantage of chemical synthesis is the opportunity to add the same glycosylations as are found in the original protein [61]. Finally, the synthesized proteins are free from DNA impurities or endotoxins; this is an important point as a high degree of purity is desirable in the drug development process.

8.3
Protein Purification

For therapeutic use, proteins must be produced in large quantities and purified so as to be free from other proteins, nucleic acids, carbohydrates, lipids or other materials. However, not only must the degree of purity for injectable proteins be 99.99%, but the purification procedure must also be highly reproducible and yield the same amount and quality of protein in independent production cycles. Notably, a method that works exquisitely in the laboratory might not work for large-scale production. While protein similarity is used to purify a protein away from nonprotein contaminants, differences between proteins (i.e., size, shape, charge, hydrophobicity, solubility, activity) are used to purify one protein from another. Although a variety of purification methods can be used, every step must be optimized for every protein (see Figure 8.1). Moreover, during the process of obtaining proteins of high purity, it is essential that their activity is maintained.

The first steps in the purification of proteins will always include sample clarification. This is usually achieved first by centrifugation (to remove any cell debris and lipids), and then by filtration using PVDF or cellulose acetate filters with pore sizes ranging from 1 to $0.22\,\mu m$. If the protein is to be isolated from inclusion bodies, then the bacterial cells must first be mechanically disrupted (e.g., using a French press or with high-pressure homogenization). The addition of detergents such as Triton X-100 and/or low concentrations of chaotropic compounds to the inclusion bodies will allow the removal of membrane proteins and other cell materials [62].

If the protein is tagged [e.g., His-, glutathione S-transferase (GST)-, Streptavidin- or Biotin-tag], then commercially available affinity purification systems can be used. Although tagged proteins can be used for *in vitro* studies, and also for preliminary *in vivo* analyses, they are seldom allowed to be used as part of therapeutic proteins in preclinical and clinical trials.

8.3.1
Ammonium Sulfate Fractionation

Most often, ammonium sulfate fractionation is the first step in protein purification, as it provides a crude purification of proteins away from nonproteins, and also separates some of the proteins from the others. The process is based on the fact that proteins have isoelectric points at which the charges of the amino acid side groups balance each other. Thus, the solubility of the protein depends on the

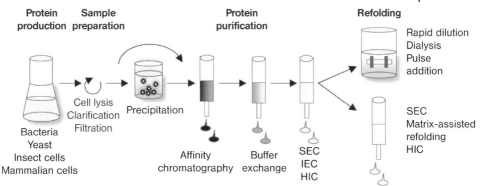

| Protein production | Sample preparation | | Protein purification | | Refolding |

Figure 8.1 Purification scheme of recombinantly expressed proteins. Proteins can be overexpressed intracellularly in various expression systems, with isolation occurring after cell lysis, removal of cell debris by centrifugation, and clarification of the supernatant by filtration. If the proteins are secreted into the medium, purification can be performed directly after removing the cells by centrifugation. The following purification steps include ammonium sulfate precipitation and additional affinity chromatography steps (e.g., via His-tags and/or ion-exchange chromatography, IEC). Buffer exchanges are included between the different purification steps. The final step includes removal of buffer components and refolding of the denatured proteins using dialysis, size-exclusion chromatography (SEC) or hydrophobic interaction chromatography (HIC). See text for further details.

ionic strength and pH of the solution. If the ionic strength is either very high or very low, it can be manipulated by adding ammonium sulfate, such that the proteins will tend to precipitate at their isoelectric point. For an effective precipitation the protein concentration should exceed $1\,mg\,ml^{-1}$. In addition to ammonium sulfate, polymers such as PEG can be used to force proteins out of solution. PEG is inert and, like ammonium sulfate, tends to stabilize proteins. The precipitated proteins can be removed by centrifugation and solubilized in a buffer which is required for the next purification step. For less-soluble proteins, denaturing agents may be required (e.g., $2–8\,M$ urea, $3–6\,M$ guanidine hydrochloride or 2% Triton X-100), but these must be removed by desalting (e.g., on a Sephadex G-25 desalting column) in order to allow refolding of the protein.

8.3.2
Affinity Chromatography

Affinity chromatography can be used late in the purification process, when much of the other material has been removed. As an example, a specific carbohydrate, a specific cofactor or mimics for binding sites, can sometimes be used as affinity matrices. In its most specific form, the immobilized ligand is a substrate or competitive inhibitor of the enzyme to be purified.

Alternatives include the use of *immunoaffinity chromatography*, which is based on the binding of the protein to an immobilized monoclonal antibody. The disadvantages of this method include the fact that antibodies are expensive and cannot be generally employed on a large scale. They also often do not perform as well as might be expected due to nonspecific binding effects. Finally, the binding is usually very strong, and so harsh conditions are required to separate the antibody from the antigen. In general, however, affinity chromatography achieves a higher purification factor (median purification ca. 10-fold) than does ion-exchange chromatography (median ca. threefold).

8.3.3
Buffer Exchange and Desalting

Buffer exchange and desalting play a central role in protein purification, and are used to remove salts and dissolve the protein in the buffer of choice. *Dialysis* is often used in the laboratory, but takes many hours to complete (usually overnight). Moreover, large buffer volumes are required and the sample will be diluted. For large-scale preparations, the selectively permeable membranes can be sandwiched between plates through which the protein solution is pumped and when, under pressure, rapid equilibration occurs. Buffer exchanges always cause a loss of product, and to prevent further loss, any shearing, foaming or rapid changes in ionic strength should be avoided. Alternatively, a Sephadex G-25 column (or PD10 and HiPrep 26/10 desalting columns for larger volumes) can be used, which separates large proteins from salts and other small molecules.

8.3.4
Ion-Exchange Chromatography

Ion-exchange chromatography (IEX) is the most useful purification and concentration method. By choosing different buffers, the same protein can be made to adsorb to both anion exchangers (a matrix with positively charged exchangers but negatively charged, exchangeable counterions) and cation exchangers, depending on the pH. Most proteins are negatively charged at physiological pH values, and therefore most purifications are carried out on anion-exchange columns. When the proteins have been bound to the column, they can be eluted according to their charge. To release the proteins in order of their binding tenacity, the salt concentration should be continuously increased or the pH changed, although extreme pH values should be avoided as they may cause inactivation of the protein. Whilst both methods are used in industrial processes, raising the salt concentration is by far the most common because it is easiest to control. A single anion-exchange column is often insufficient to purify the protein-of-interest, and additional procedures are necessary.

8.3.5
Hydrophobic Interaction Chromatography

Hydrophobic interaction chromatography (HIC) is based on the fact that proteins expose some of their hydrophobic amino acids on the surface under high salt conditions, for example after elution of the protein from an ion-exchange column. This form of chromatography is used to separate proteins according to their hydrophobicity. For this, the column beads are coated with hydrophobic fatty acids (including octyl and phenyl groups) and, after loading, the proteins are eluted with decreasing concentrations of salt in the buffer.

A recent introduction has been Whatman HB1 cellulose, which is designed to interact with proteins by hydrogen bonding. Samples are applied to the matrix in a concentrated (>50% saturated, >2 M) solution of ammonium sulfate, and the proteins are eluted by diluting the ammonium sulfate (this introduces more water, which competes with proteins for the hydrogen-bonding sites). The selectivity of both methods is similar to that of fractional precipitation using ammonium sulfate.

8.3.6
Size-Exclusion Chromatography

At later steps of the purification process, size-exclusion chromatography (SEC) can be used to separate proteins according to their size. The beads in the SEC column are composed of a porous matrix into which small proteins diffuse, whilst any larger proteins are excluded. Simply by loading and washing the column with buffer, the largest proteins will be expelled first, and the smallest last. Unfortunately, however, the sample must be highly concentrated for this process, as only a small percentage of the column volume can be loaded.

8.4
Isolation of Monomeric, Natively Folded Proteins

8.4.1
Correct Refolding versus Aggregation

If proteins are purified under denaturing conditions, this results in a soluble protein which is not in its native conformation. In order to restore a natural conformation, the protein must be incubated under conditions that allow formation of the native structure, although the refolding process may require a few seconds up to several days for completion. During this period, the correct refolding pathway will compete with misfolding and aggregation of the protein. Protein refolding requires intramolecular interactions and follows first order-kinetics. However, protein aggregation involves intermolecular interactions and is, therefore, a kinetic process of second or higher order which is favored at high protein concentrations. In fact, the extent of refolding will be low if high initial protein concentrations are used, independent of the refolding method.

Aggregates are formed by non-native intermolecular hydrophobic interactions between protein folding intermediates, which have not yet buried their hydrophobic amino acid stretches. When the refolding process is beyond these aggregation-prone intermediates, however, the folding pathway is favored and aggregation does not occur. Protein aggregation can also be caused by the formation of nonspecific intramolecular disulfide bonds; these are formed following the solubilization of inclusion bodies, or during the early stages of refolding. These problems can be solved by adding reducing agents such as dithiothreitol (DTT) or β-mercaptoethanol to disrupt the disulfide bonds, if denaturing buffers are used for solubilization of the inclusion bodies, or by the addition of oxidized thiols (e.g., GSH) in the refolding buffer. In addition, it is also possible that proteins might precipitate or are isolated in an inactive form, when native disulfide bonds are not formed correctly upon purification. To prevent the isolation of misfolded protein, it is recommended that thiols are added in both their oxidized and reduced forms in the refolding buffer.

8.4.2
Techniques for Protein Folding

For therapeutic proteins, major efforts are required to identify the ideal conditions for refolding and to obtain the protein in both large quantities and high quality [63–65]. The easiest refolding procedure is based on a dilution of the protein sample in an appropriate refolding buffer. Usually, the protein concentration is reduced to $1–50\,\mu g\,ml^{-1}$ so as to enhance refolding and prevent aggregation. However, although this method is ideal at the laboratory scale it is impossible on an industrial scale, as it would require not only huge refolding vessels but also additional cost-intensive concentration steps after refolding. In order to prevent dilution of the protein, the denatured protein can be added in pulses to the refolding buffer. For a pulse addition, approximately 80% of the protein should be refolded before addition of the next charge of protein in the buffer, but this will require knowledge of the folding kinetics of the protein-of-interest.

Dialysis of the protein is comparable to direct dilution, although here the change from denaturing to native buffer conditions occurs gradually. The disadvantage is that this leaves time for the accumulation of folding intermediates that are, again, prone to aggregation. If more concentrated protein samples are preferred, then SEC can be used [66]. For this, the denatured protein is loaded onto a column which has been equilibrated with refolding buffer, while subsequent elution using the refolding buffer results in a refolded protein in the eluate. In this case, any aggregates are physically separated from the folded proteins in the pores of the resin, if the resin allows efficient separation. To improve this method, an additional small volume of denaturing buffer can be added directly after loading the sample in order to dissolve any aggregates that formed before loading. Furthermore, lower sample concentrations, low elution rates, as well as buffer additives (e.g., arginine), will all improve the refolding of the sample.

An even more advanced method for protein refolding is that of *matrix-assisted protein refolding*. Here, the protein is coupled to the matrix, which prevents intermolecular aggregation from occurring while the buffer is changed from denaturing to native conditions. This method requires binding of the protein to the matrix, as well as elution after folding [67, 68]. Tags (His, GST, 6R) or, for example, charged patches in the protein, can be used for attachment of the protein to the matrix. This method can be used – simultaneously – not only for refolding but also for purification.

As most intermolecular interactions occur among hydrophobic patches in the protein, the use of HIC represents an interesting alternative. During migration through the column, the hydrophobic patches of the protein will bind to the matrix, so that they are not accessible for interactions. The protein will then pass through several steps of absorption and desorption, controlled by the salt concentration in the buffer and the hydrophobicity of the intermediates, resulting finally in elution of the folded proteins [69]. As with matrix-assisted refolding, this method can also be used simultaneously for protein purification.

8.4.3
Factors Influencing Refolding

Physical conditions and chemical factors each have an influence on the folding of proteins. *Temperature* has a dual effect on the folding process: low temperatures support the productive folding pathway because hydrophobic aggregation is suppressed, but increase the time required for refolding and enhancing the formation of aggregates. When attempting to refold a new protein, a temperature of 15 °C has been proposed as a good starting point.

Pressure also influences the refolding process [70]; under a high pressure (up to 3 kbar), oligomeric protein structures can be disrupted, whereas monomeric native-like secondary structures are retained and may even tolerate up to 5 kbar. Upon the gradual release of pressure, intermediates can form but not aggregates. By using this method the proteins can achieve their native state, even at high concentrations.

Protein-stabilizing agents such as glycerol (0.4 to 3 *M*) and other compatible osmolytes (sucrose, sorbitol), low concentrations of denaturing agents (e.g., urea ≤2 *M*), and nonionic surfactants (Triton X-100, Tween 20, CHAPS) have also been identified as useful refolding agents for many proteins. Nowadays, L-arginine is the most commonly used refolding enhancing agent, and is thought – when used at concentrations of 400–800 m*M* – to be able to shield hydrophobic patches in the folding intermediates, which makes them more soluble and less prone to aggregation [71]. Moreover, high-molecular-weight additives such as PEG, and zwitterionic agents such as sulfobetaines, pyridines and pyrroles, have been effectively employed for protein renaturation. Although the mechanisms of action of these compounds are not well understood, the empirical screening of solution additives has led to formulations that substantially increase the refolding yield at atmospheric pressure. However, since not all additives are equally advantageous for all proteins, the benefits of these agents must be determined experimentally for every protein-of-interest.

If disulfide bonds are present in the protein, then purification must be conducted in the presence of reducing agents such as DTT or β-mercaptoethanol, so as to allow

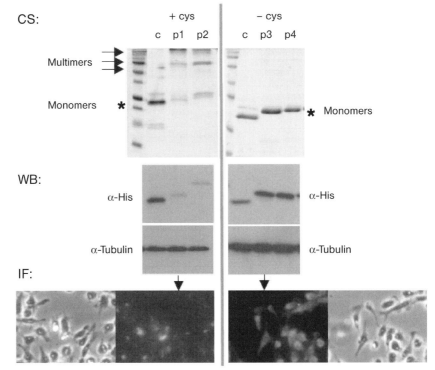

Figure 8.2 Uptake of monomeric recombinantly expressed proteins. Thioredoxin scaffold proteins with (p1–p4) or without (c) different peptide aptamers were expressed in *E. coli* and purified by His-Tag affinity purification using fast protein liquid chromatography. In contrast to p3 and p4, in p1 and p2 the thioredoxin scaffold contains cysteines leading to multimerized proteins, as shown on a Coomassie-stained acrylamide gel (CS) under nonreducing conditions. If these proteins are transduced into cells, Western blots (WB) of the cell lysates show that multimerized peptides cannot be taken up, in contrast to the monomeric forms. Immunofluorescence analysis (IF) confirms this observation. The multimerized proteins can be detected as aggregates on top of the cells, whereas monomeric peptides can be found internalized, distributed evenly in the cytoplasm.

the disruption of non-native disulfide bonds. Naturally, disulfide-bonded proteins in their reduced states are often very unstable and exhibit a high tendency towards aggregation. Hence, to allow non-native disulfide bonds to be reshuffled into native bonds, the refolding buffer should include a redox-shuffling agent [e.g., 2 mM DTT and 6 mM oxidized glutathione (GSSG)]. Instead of using GSH to reduce GSSG, DTT is used so as to prevent high GSH concentrations occurring in the buffer. The reduced thiols should be in excess and the pH slightly alkaline. In fact, an alkaline pH $\geq$7.5 is required to promote thiolate anion formation for the reshuffling of disulfide bonds, allowing rapid disulfide exchange reactions to occur [72]. Occasionally, it is also possible to replace cysteine residues with serine residues, thus minimizing the formation of intermolecular disulfide bonds (see Figure 8.2).

8.5
Increasing Peptide Production, Purification and Efficacy by Using Scaffolds

Short unconstrained peptides (<20 aa) are usually unstable and susceptible to proteolytic degradation [73, 74]. Furthermore, linear peptides have a greater degree of freedom and can exhibit different structural conformations. In this situation, the peptide rather prefers the unbound state, with a higher value of entropy. Binding to its target molecule by noncovalent hydrophobic interactions would be associated with a dramatic decrease in terms of entropy at the cost of free energy of target binding and inhibition.

Peptides can be structurally stabilized in various ways to protect them against degradation, not only during the steps of production and purification, but also during *in vitro* or *in vivo* applications [75]. In order to prevent degradation, peptides can be synthesized with D-amino acids or with chemically modified amino acid homologues. Cyclization of the peptide can also prevent degradation [76]. To enhance structural stability, peptides can be fused on one end to carrier proteins [e.g., green fluorescent protein (GFP) -like tags] or to larger functional domains with distinct properties or structural features [77].

Alternatively, peptides can be inserted into scaffold proteins, such as human thioredoxin (hTrx) [78, 79]. In this way, these so-called "peptide aptamers" are not only stabilized in a three-dimensional (3-D) structure, but the folding and presentation of the peptide sequence is also enhanced. By forcing these peptide aptamers into a constrained conformation, their target binding affinity—and, as a result, their inhibitory function—is increased. In a scaffold protein the aptamer sequence is constrained and forced into a few conformations, or even only one conformation. This also favors target binding under thermodynamic aspects and results in a more efficient inhibition. It has been shown that for some (originally linear) peptide aptamers, the binding affinity could be enhanced 100- to 10 000-fold after insertion into a scaffold protein [80]. Recently, scaffold proteins have attracted much interest in the development of deliverable monomeric recombinant peptide aptamers, and will therefore be detailed in the following sections.

8.5.1
Properties and Requirements of Scaffolds

A general feature of all scaffold proteins is the fact that the domains required for a highly stable protein structure can be distinguished from those required for activity or which are involved in molecular target recognition. If used as scaffold, the active site—or a sequence involved in protein–protein interactions—can be replaced by a peptide sequence, thereby removing any endogenous biological activity. Depending on the scaffold, the peptide is then surrounded by distinct structural elements that define a stable protein conformation. An example of this is the thioredoxin scaffold, the active site of which is solvent-accessible and allows the insertion of foreign sequences by genetic manipulation, without inducing changes to its overall architecture. The aptamer sequence can also be distributed over the surface of a scaffold protein in a nonlinear context, as occurs for the lipocalin scaffolds [81]. The peptides are inserted into four loops of this β-barrel protein to form a 3-D target recognition site. The length, and also the composition, of the peptide inserted into a scaffold might be critical, and varies between the different scaffold proteins. Under optimal conditions the aptamer sequence forms an extended interface for exposure to the target molecule.

Ideally, scaffold proteins are small, biologically inert proteins that allow for modifications. For example, they should be capable of absorbing not only the insertion of peptide aptamer sequences but also the addition of fusion tags, whether for purification or for intracellular purposes, without the structure of the scaffold being disturbed. The efficient production of a scaffold protein, using any of the above-mentioned systems and its simple purification, are additional prerequisites. During the expression and folding process, the aptamer sequence should not alter the scaffold protein conformation. Moreover, the refolding process after purification under denaturing conditions should yield monomeric, soluble proteins with a rigid structure, independent of the aptamer sequence insertion. The protein should be highly stable against shifts in pH, temperature and ionic strength and, if used *in vivo*, it should preferably also display a long serum half-life as well as a low immunogenicity and toxicity.

In the past, a variety of scaffold proteins have been investigated intensively for different purposes, and details of these are listed in Table 8.2, according to their distinct structural properties. Further details of the different scaffolds can be found elsewhere [117–123].

Overall, the properties of all the scaffold proteins vary widely, and the potential advantages and disadvantages must be balanced for each application. The type of scaffold protein depends mainly on the purpose of the designed protein, whether for intracellular or extracellular use, for the targeting of small proteins or macromolecules, or for *in vitro* or *in vivo* use. The structural data of proteins support the selection of a suitable scaffold. Finally, the insertion of a linear aptamer sequence into a scaffold might influence the conformation, and thereby the target binding of the aptamer sequence in a negative way.

8.6
The Use of Cell-Penetrating Peptides for Cellular Uptake of Purified Proteins

The use of peptide-based macromolecules for target validation and as biopharmaceuticals is limited by the techniques available for intracellular delivery. In general, molecules larger than 0.5 kDa exhibit a poor bioavailability, which in turn limits the delivery of many therapeutically active compounds to their intended intracellular targets [124, 125]. However, the results of a number of recent investigations have suggested that this problem might be overcome through the use of CPPs (for a review, see Ref. [126]). It has been shown that purified proteins such as the *Drosophila* Antennapedia transcription factor and the HIV-1 TAT transactivating protein are able to cross cellular membranes [127, 128], since which numerous

Table 8.2 Scaffolds used for presentation of peptide aptamers.

Classification	Scaffold	Reference(s)
(Engineered) Antibodies	Antibodies Minibodies Camelbodies (variable heavy chain antibody fragment VHH, Nanobody) scFv (single chain variable fragment) FN3 (fibronectin type III domain) CTLA-4 (cytotoxic T-lymphocyte associated protein-4)	[82–88]
Kunitz-domains/ protease inhibitors	BPTI (bovine pancreatic trypsin inhibitor) PSTI (pancreatic secretory trypsin inhibitor) APPI (Alzheimer's amyloid β-protein precursor inhibitor) LACI-D1 (human lipoprotein-associated coagulation inhibitor) Tendamistat Ecotin STM (stefin A triple mutant)	[89–95]
Knottins (cysteine knots)	CBD (cellulose-binding domain of cellobiohydrolase I) EETI-II (*Ecballium elaterium* trypsin inhibitor II) ω-Conotoxin Charybdotoxin	[96–99]
Exchanged active sites	NTF2 (buclear transport factor 2) IGPS (indole-3-glycerol-phosphate synthase) Cyclophilin bTrxA (bacterial thioredoxin A) hTrxA (human thioredoxin A) Improved hTrxA Staphylococcal nuclease GST (glutathione S-transferase)	[79, 100–105]
Natural α-helix bundles	Cytochrome b_{562} Staphylococcal protein A (affibodies)	[106, 107]
Artificial α-helix bundles	Zinc-finger	[108]
β-Barrel proteins	Lipocalins, for example RBP (retinol-binding protein)	[109]
Structural domains	Ankyrin-repeats Leucine-repeats Dimerization domain Coiled-coil stem loop	[110–113]
Miscellaneous	GFP (green fluorescent protein) Sp1 LiRP (ligand-regulated peptide)	[114–116]

peptides have been reported to have such cell-penetrating properties. These can be classified as protein-derived CPPs (including protein transduction domains such as Tat, pVP22 and penetratin), as designed CPPs (including the amphiphilic, MAP), as chimeric CPPs (transportan, MPG), as synthetic CPPs (pep-1, KALA, 9R) or as homing peptides (Ly-1, F3). The sequences and characteristics of the different CPPs are detailed in Chapter 7.

The molecular basis of the cellular uptake of CPPs into living cells has long been a controversial topic. The initial concept was that the CPPs could overcome the barrier of the cell membrane by both energy- and receptor-independent direct penetration of the phospholipid bilayer. This model was based on two findings: (i) that internalization occurred not only under physiological temperature conditions but also at 4 °C [127, 129–133]; and (ii) that inhibitors of endocytosis did not significantly alter CPP uptake [134]. Unfortunately, it was a series of artifacts resulting from cell fixation and the inefficient removal of surface-bound proteins that led to this assumption, and these aspects have since undergone critical review [135–138]. After having optimized the methods by including the enzymatic removal or fluorescence quenching of cell surface-bound peptides and the use of live-cell imaging, it became clear that protein transduction did indeed depend on specific interactions between the CPPs and molecules of the cell membrane, which in turn resulted in internalization and endocytic-like vesicle formation (for a review, see Ref. [139]). Intensive studies using different temperatures, together with carefully planned positive and negative controls and RNA interference-mediated knock-down of membrane or vesicle proteins, showed that CPP conjugates were pre-dominantly taken up by an endocytotic process referred to as *lipid raft-dependent macropinocytosis* [136, 140].

8.6.1
Uptake of Proteins by Lipid Raft-Dependent Macropinocytosis

Although some 20 years ago little was known about the exact cellular mechanism of TAT-mediated uptake, two groups investigated the *in vivo* distribution of HIV-TAT-β-galactosidase fusion proteins during the late 1990s [128, 141]. In both studies, the authors demonstrated a successful uptake and wide distribution of TAT-β-galactosidase in the injected animals, which indicated that protein trans-duction might indeed be a valuable tool for therapeutic applications. Interestingly, even today it has still not been possible to define a general uptake mechanism for all CPPs, a conclusion which was in complete agreement with all of the performed studies, although most data point to a process of lipid raft-dependent macropino-cytosis. By using *in vitro* readout systems, such as the TAT-Cre system, Wadia *et al.* were able to show that the transduction of a TAT-Cre fusion protein leads to the excision of a stop codon flanked by two loxP sites in front of a stably integrated EGFP reporter gene. Therefore, successful TAT-Cre protein transduction causes expression of the EGFP protein. By using this system, together with different inhibitors of the macropinocytosis process, it was possible to unravel many of the details of CCP-mediated protein transduction [140].

The first step in protein transduction is the nonspecific electrostatic interaction between positively charged amino acid residues of the CPP (e.g., the guanidinium head groups of arginine) and the negatively charged membrane surface glycosaminoglycans (Figure 8.3) [142]. This is similar to the internalization of growth factors, which also involves heparan sulfate proteoglycans. Soluble heparin can be used as a competitive inhibitor for TAT-mediated protein transduction, as it binds to the TAT sequence and prevents TAT interaction with the cell-surface proteoglycans [142]. Next, a vesicle-like structure is formed and the proteins are taken up by the cell. Compared to phagocytosis (cell-eating), pinocytosis (cell drinking) involves a number of ill-defined pathways, including clathrin- and caveolin-mediated pinocytosis, and clathrin- and caveolin-independent endocytosis and macropinocytosis (Figure 8.3). Macropinocytosis refers to the formation of macropinosomes, which are generated by actin-driven circular protruding ruffles of the plasma membrane close to lipid rafts [143, 144]. The lipid rafts are small, low-density membrane fractions that are enriched in cholesterol and sphingolipids, and which participate in important cellular processes, such as the intracellular sorting of proteins, membrane trafficking, signal transduction and pathogen entry. Although they can be recognized as distinct membrane areas, their components are in dynamic equilibrium with the non-raft membrane [145]. They can enhance or regulate protein–protein interactions, for example in activated immune cells, where clustering of different receptors in the lipid rafts can be observed as platforms for signaling [146].

While phagocytosis, clathrin- and caveolin-mediated endocytosis each involve receptors and transmembrane proteins, macropinocytosis is thought to mediate the unspecific uptake of surrounding solutes. This allows the cells to take up large amounts of extracellular fluid containing not only nutrients but also antigens, pathogens, viruses, apoptotic cell fragments and proteins. It is believed that the CPP fusion proteins are simultaneously internalized in such macropinosomes, because they stick to the membrane near lipid rafts. It is also possible that they are incorporated into the vesicles during growth factor uptake (growth factors and cytokines stimulate macropinocytosis) or receptor cycling. The release of the nutrients and CPP fusion protein possibly occurs upon disruption of the fragile and leaky macropinosomes. This appears to be the rate-limiting step for their delivery into the cells, since it is thought that the escape from macropinosomes and endosomes is an inefficient process. Experiments have shown that this process can be artificially enhanced by combining the CPP fusion protein with a pH-sensitive fusogenic peptide (e.g., HA2 epitope) that destabilizes the macropinosomes [140]. Addition of the lysosomotropic agent chloroquine prevents acidification of the endosome and inhibits the endolysosomal proteases. If used at low concentrations, chloroquine promotes the release of molecules into the cytoplasm, without any detectable endosome rupture.

8.6.2
Points of Consideration for the Use of CPPs

The design of a transducible protein requires the consideration of a variety of points. It has been observed that the cell type influences the efficacy of trans-

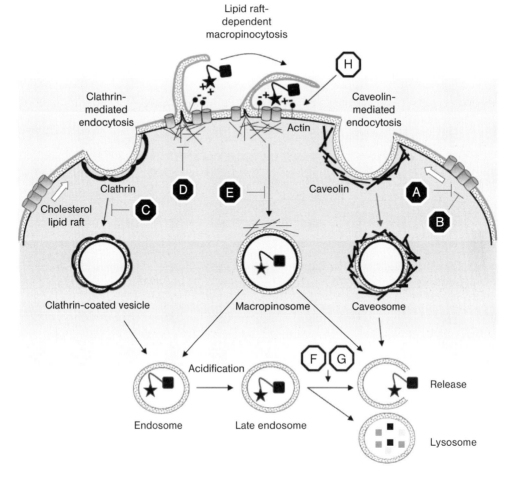

duction. One possible explanation for this is that the genes involved in macropinocytosis (e.g., actin) and in trafficking are differently expressed. Furthermore, the membrane proteins or other components that contribute to the lipid composition might also play a role. In addition, transduction depends on the CPP used (e.g., Tat, 9R or transportan), and is more or less efficient in different target cells. Another question that remains to be answered is whether the structure of the cargo protein influences the transduction process. It is not clear yet, if the CPP fusion protein must be folded into a native conformation; it is also possible that a more unfolded protein is preferred, or that the protein requires a monomeric or a multimeric conformation to enhance the uptake into cells. The present authors' data obtained with peptide aptamers inserted into the hTrx scaffold suggest that a monomeric conformation is very important for uptake in various types of cell (Figure 8.2). The question of whether this is a general rule, or whether it depends on the scaffold and CPP used, remains open. Another point of concern is the release of the transduced peptide from the endopinosomes and macropinosomes

Figure 8.3 Mechanism for protein transduction domain (PTD)-mediated protein transduction. Uptake of macromolecules into cells is mediated by either clathrin-dependent endocytosis, caveolin-dependent endocytosis, or via actin-dependent macropinocytosis. Several agents have been used in the past to investigate the uptake of PTD-linked peptides. By using (A) nystatin, an inhibitor for caveolae formation or (B) beta-cyclodextrin, which depletes cell-surface-associated cholesterol, an involvement of caveolin in the protein transduction process of PTD fusion proteins could be excluded. Chlorpromazine (C), an inhibitor of clathrin-mediated internalization, did not affect the rate of PTD-driven protein uptake. In contrast, studies with cytochalasin D (D), which disrupts actin filaments and prevents actin polymerization, revealed a reduction in protein transduction efficacy. In addition, macropinocytosis inhibitor treatment of the cells with (E) amiloride, which inhibits membrane ruffling, also reduced protein transduction. Therefore, PTD-mediated peptide uptake most likely occurs through lipid raft-dependent macropinocytosis. First, the positively charged PTD interacts with the negatively charged proteoglycans in the cell membrane near actin-driven protruding ruffles (lipid rafts); it was then shown that a high amount of cell-surface heparan sulfates (H) positively influences the PTD-mediated protein uptake. The peptides are then internalized in macropinosomes. Macropinosomes have been described as "leaky vesicles" that continuously release their contents into the cytoplasm. Alternatively, they either acidify and mature into lysosomes, causing degradation of the peptide. Alternatively, they may mature into late endosomes, disrupt, and release their contents in the cytoplasm. This process is enhanced by either chloroquine (F) or the HA2 peptide (H). Chloroquine prevents acidification by inhibiting lysosomal hydrolases, which in turn prevents degradation and ensures release of the trapped protein into the cytosol. The pH-sensitive HA2 domain of the influenza virus hemagglutinin 2 protein destabilizes the macropinosomal membrane, also causing release of the PTD fusion protein.

into the cytosol. although the factors which mediate this process remain to be identified. Usually, chloroquine is used in *in vitro* studies to enhance release, but cannot be applied *in vivo*. Finally, whereas the addition of a CPP might affect structure, purification properties and activity of the fusion protein, in contrast the fusion protein might influence the structure of the CPP, thus affecting its transduction properties. The empirical testing of various parameters is necessary in order to design optimal CPP fusion proteins for intracellular delivery.

8.7
Classification of Therapeutic Peptides

8.7.1
Bioactive Peptides

The identification of natural peptides with therapeutic potential is quite novel, and of major biomedical importance. These molecules can be used as drugs or as lead structures to develop peptidomimetics. They can also be found in various unicellular microorganisms (e.g., Apratoxins in cyanobacteria), as well as in venoms produced by cone snails, spiders, scorpions, and snakes. As each venom can contain up to 100 different peptides, and since such venoms are produced by different species, the total number of active peptides will be extremely high. Venom peptides usually act on mammalian receptors, as well as ion-gated, voltage-gated or ligand-gated channels or to G-protein-linked receptors [147]. Many snake venoms also demonstrate cardiovascular effects [148], perhaps increasing vascular permeability, inducing vasoconstriction or inhibiting angiotensin-converting enzyme activity.

Venom-derived peptides are of major interest in the development of therapeutics for a wide range of neurological conditions [149]. An example is *ziconotide*, a synthetic molecule based on a peptide which is found in a cone snail toxin and interrupts the Ca^{2+}-dependent primary afferent transmission of pain signals [150]. Currently, this peptide is being investigated in clinical studies for the treatment of severe chronic pain [151].

Another interesting peptide, chlorotoxin (CTX), is found in the venom of the scorpion *Leiurus quinquestriatus* [152]. CTX is able to bind to malignant cells, but shows little or no binding to normal tissues. A synthetic version of this peptide has been derived, linked to radioactive iodine-131 (^{131}I -TM-601), and is used in clinical studies in patients with glioblastoma, with encouraging results to date [153]. This material is of particular interest for the development of tumor-targeted therapies.

The *defensins*, or antimicrobial peptides, which also belong to the group of bioactive peptides [154], are produced by vertebrates, invertebrates, plants and certain bacteria, and serve as a first line of defense against microbial pathogens. In mammals, the defensins form part of the innate immune system, and to some extent of the adaptive immune system, and are produced in the granules of phagocytic cells and in epithelial tissues [155]. Defensins are small (3–4.5 kDa), highly cationic peptides, which are characterized by a unique 3-D structure formed by three cysteine disulfide bonds. The results of recent studies have shown that the mechanism of antibiotic activity of defensins involves both the cell membrane (lipopolysaccharides, polysaccharides, phospholipids) and intracellular targets (e.g., activation of autolytic enzymes, inhibition of DNA and protein synthesis) [156, 157]. Interestingly, anti-tumoral activity has also been reported, and in this respect magainin II has been shown to exert cytotoxic effects against a wide range of cancer cell lines, including melanoma, bladder, breast and lung cancers [158, 159]. Whilst it remains unclear how these defensins affect the growth of cancer cells, the mechanisms might include an activation of apoptosis pathways or the inhibition of angiogenesis [160]. Currently, although several defensins are undergoing clinical trials (e.g., Plectasin, P-113, MBI-226 and protegrin-1), none has yet been registered as a drug [161, 162]. It should be pointed out here that the therapeutic use of bioactive peptides also has certain drawbacks, notably that they carry extensive post-translational modifications and numerous disulfide bonds, which in turn implies high production costs and a complex pharmacological formulation.

8.7.2
Peptide Aptamers

Peptide aptamers are short peptides which do not occur naturally but which can be selected from random peptide libraries and are able to bind to a predetermined domain of a target protein (for reviews, see Refs [163–166]). In this respect, they bear a functional resemblance to an antibody. However, a major characteristic of peptide aptamers is insertion of the peptide into a scaffold protein, thus offering conformational stability and ease of recombinant production. In principal, peptide aptamers can be used to bind specifically to intracellular targets that may be crucial components of signalling pathways inside the cell, with the peptide aptamers being used to inhibit any critical disease-associated protein functions. The first peptide aptamer targeting cyclin-dependent kinase 2 (Cdk2) was identified more than 10 years ago by the group of Colas [167], who subsequently defined the "gold standard" for peptide aptamer identification, and used a combinatorial library of constrained 20-residue peptides displayed in the active site of *E. coli* thioredoxin and a yeast-two-hybrid system to select peptide aptamers binding to human Cdk2. A similar course of events has been described in several publications, including target definition and validation, screening with advanced yeast two-hybrid or phage-display systems, aptamer presentation by a scaffold protein, the production and purification of specifically interacting peptide aptamers and, finally, protein transduction for intracellular target binding and the induction of a cellular response.

Several groups have shown that is possible to efficiently isolate specific peptide aptamers which can be used to inhibit targets involved in cancer development and progression, or virus infection and replication (see Figure 8.4 for a detailed overview). An instructive example is a peptide aptamer which targets the transcription factor Stat3. The constitutive activation of Stat3 has been found in leukemias, lymphomas, myeloma, head and neck cancers, breast cancer and melanomas, and has in some cases been shown to be absolutely required for tumor cell survival. Here, peptide aptamers targeting the dimerization or DNA-binding domain of Stat3 were selected with yeast-two-hybrid screenings [169]. For direct transduction experiments with recombinant proteins, the aptamers were expressed in bacteria as fusions with a C-terminal 9 arginine CPP (9R) and a His-tag for Ni^{2+}-affinity purification. This peptide aptamer was able to induce apoptosis and/or arrest proliferation in selected cancer cell lines. The study results showed that it is possible to target not only protein–protein interactions but also DNA–protein interactions with peptide aptamers. Other examples of peptide aptamers targeting crucial signal components in cancer cells include those targeting ErbB2, p53, Ras, XIAP, and Bcl-2 [170–174].

In vitro studies using a variety of cancer cell lines have revealed other useful anticancer effects. For example, it was observed that peptide aptamers could increase the sensitivity of tumor cells towards taxol, and also cause an accumulation of p53 and cell-cycle arrest or an increase in pro-apoptotic activities. Additionally, aptamers have been selected that bind viral proteins such as HPV16-E6 and -E7, the proteins involved in the development of cervical cancer [175, 176], the HIV-1 integrase [177], and the HBV-core protein [178]. All of these aptamers were inserted into the bacterial thioredoxin scaffold, and yeast-two-hybrid screenings were used for identification. Those studies which used HPV16-infected cells expressing the aptamer showed strong inhibitory effects on both growth and viability, without affecting the growth of noninfecting cells. Peptides targeting HIV-1 integrase (IN) caused a shift in the formation from an active IN dimer to an inactive IN tetramer,

(a)

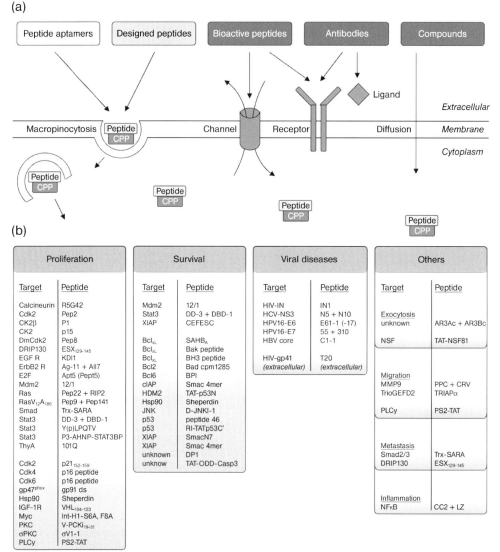

(b)

Figure 8.4 Strategies and targets of therapeutic peptides. (a) Peptide aptamers and designed peptides are able to bind and inhibit intracellular proteins. This requires uptake of the peptides into the cell by lipid raft-dependent macropinocytosis, which is mediated by a CPP domain fused to the peptide. Bioactive peptides and monoclonal antibodies act mostly on extracellular targets such as ion channels (e.g., for chloride), cell-surface receptors (e.g., ErbB2 receptor) or soluble ligands (e.g., TNFα). Small chemical compounds penetrate the plasma membrane by diffusion and interfere with intracellular molecules (e.g., kinase activity); (b) Targets for which peptide aptamers and designed peptides (shaded boxes) have been identified are shown. Further details for each example can be found in excellent reviews [85, 87, 91, 130, 168]. Antitumoral defensins are not included in that scheme because they mainly act on the cellular membrane, perturbing its function and resulting in pore formation, rather than on intracellular target molecules.

thus preventing integration of the reverse-transcribed viral DNA into the host genome. The HBV core protein targeting peptides were seen to inhibit capsid formation and, consequently, HBV replication and virion production.

Despite the encouraging results obtained *in vitro* and in a limited number of *in vivo* experiments, no peptide aptamer has yet been approved for clinical use. Similar to the therapeutic use of bioactive peptides, the development of this strategy is still in its infant stages, and many issues still require thorough investigation. Due to the intracellular targets of the peptide aptamers, this strategy is dependent on progress being made in terms of CPP-mediated delivery.

8.7.3
Designed Peptides

A third category of peptides that is capable of inhibiting certain target protein–protein interactions comprises the designed peptides that mimic the interface amino acid residues of one of the binding partners. This is only possible, if the molecular structure of the target protein has been at least partly resolved, or if the functional domain structure of the interacting proteins has been genetically defined. These strategies have been used in numerous studies, and some examples of the structure-based designer peptides are described here.

Mdm2 is involved in regulation of the activity of the tumor suppressor protein p53. As such, it can bind to p53, marking it for degradation. A peptide derived from p53 (aa 18–23) is known to comprise the minimal Mdm2-binding site, and was used as a starting point. In phage display experiments, the binding properties of this sequence were optimized and reduced to a 8mer peptide. Only a very short sequence of amino acids is actually required for specific binding. Subsequently, the peptide was further optimized by introducing non-natural amino acids, and by constraining its conformation. Finally, the peptide was used as a lead structure to derive a very potent small-molecular-weight compound which was shown to be active as a Mdm2 inhibitor (for reviews, see Refs. [179, 180]).

One peptide which has been approved by the FDA for therapeutic use in the treatment of AIDS is *enfuvirtide* (Fuzeon®). This 36-amino acid peptide (T20) is based on the sequence of the C-terminal heptad repeat (CHR) helix of the HIV envelope glycoprotein gp41 [181]. Its mode of action is to bind to the N-heptad repeat (NHR) coiled-coil region, thus preventing interaction between the CHR and NHR and, in turn, formation of the six-helix bundle that is required for fusion of the viral membrane with the cell membrane. Thus, enfuvirtide is able to inhibit the HIV infection process.

Inhibitory peptides derived from the sequence of interaction partners have also been described for Stat3. This transcription factor, which is found constitutively activated in many cancers, binds to phosphorylated tyrosine residues in the C-terminal region of several growth factor receptors, and a consensus sequence (YXXQ) was identified. A tyrosine-phosphorylated hexapeptide (acetyl-Y(p) LPQTV-amide) was found to effectively inhibit Stat3 dimerization and DNA-binding [182]. This peptide is able to reduce proliferation of cancer cells and induce apoptosis.

Designed peptides may also be used as peptide aptamers. In this case, the peptide derived from an interacting protein is inserted into a scaffold protein. When Zhao and Hoffmann utilized this strategy [183], they inserted a 56-amino acid peptide derived from the Smad anchor for receptor activation (SARA) protein into the bacterial thioredoxin scaffold. This peptide was shown to bind efficiently to Smad2 and Smad3, and also to inhibit not only transforming growth factor-β (TGFβ) -induced gene expression but also an epithelial to mesenchymal transition that might represent a potential therapeutic strategy for blocking cancer metastasis.

8.7.4
Antibodies

Antibodies are the pioneers of therapeutic peptides. In recent years, a variety of antibodies have either undergone (or may still be undergoing) clinical trials, or have been approved (e.g., Erbitux). These antibodies either target the surface receptors that are found to be overexpressed or aberrantly activated in cancer cells [e.g., ErbB2 and trastuzumab (Herceptin), EGFR and panitumumab, VEGFR and bavacizumab], or they target their ligands (e.g., TGFβ). Due to their large size and the complex pattern of disulfide bonds required for their function, they are usually not used to target intracellular proteins. Single-chain antibodies, which are engineered and reduced to the antigen-binding domains, are more suitable for this purpose and are discussed in Chapter 2.

8.8
Production and Administration of Therapeutic Peptides *In Vivo*

Since the approval of recombinant insulin during the 1980s, a remarkable expansion in the number of therapeutic proteins has been observed, with in excess of 130 proteins currently in clinical use and many more undergoing development. The present clinical use of peptides is limited, however, to those agents that have an extracellular mode of action. For those therapeutic proteins with an intracellular mode of action, only preclinical data are available, demonstrating a proof-of-concept that CPP-linked peptides may modify specific intracellular signaling pathways *in vivo*. Some examples of both types of therapeutic strategy are outlined in the following sections.

8.8.1
Extracellular Protein Therapeutics and Peptides with Extracellular Targets

Although protein therapeutics have often been applied in cases of protein deficiency or abnormal protein production, they are also able to negatively interfere with a target protein. Other protein therapeutics have been developed to augment an existing pathway, and the current clinical applications cover a wide range of indications. Typically, proteins are supplied to those patients lacking lactase, or to replace vital blood-clotting factors in hemophiliacs. Other examples include insulin, albumin, laronidase, lactase, idursulfase, lutropin and mecasermin [184, 185].

Lutropin alpha (Luveris®) was developed for the treatment of infertility caused by a luteinizing hormone deficiency [186]. The drug is a recombinant human luteinizing hormone, which binds to the lutropin receptor (hLHR) on the ovarian theca (and granulosa) cells and testicular Leydig cells. This glycoprotein comprises two noncovalently linked, nonidentical protein components, designated the α- and β-subunits. For therapy, Luveris is produced in large-scale cell culture processing by genetically modified Chinese hamster ovary (CHO) cells [187]. The protein is secreted into the culture medium, and then purified via a combination of chromatographic and viral reduction steps. The safety and efficacy of Luveris was examined in six clinical trials that included 170 infertile women with hypogonadotropic hypogonadism, of whom 152 received Luveris and follitropin-alpha (Gonal-F) in 283 treatment cycles. Those patients treated with Luveris exhibited adequate evidence of efficacy for the authorized indication.

Another example of a protein therapeutic targeting extracellular targets is mecasermin (Increlex®). Mecasermin is specifically indicated for the long-term treatment of growth failure in pediatric patients with primary insulin-like growth factor deficiency (IGFD) or with growth hormone gene deletion [188]. This is a recombinantly expressed human insulin-like growth factor-1 (rhIGF-1) which is produced by bacteria (*E. coli*) that have been modified by the addition of the gene for human IGF-1. IGF-1, which binds to the extracellular domain of the IGF-I receptor, is composed of 70 amino acids in a single chain with three intramolecular disulfide bridges, has a molecular weight of 7.6 kDa, and an amino acid sequence which is identical to that of endogenous human IGF-1. The role of this peptide is to restore appropriate statural growth [189]. A variety of other proteins which bind to extracellular targets are being used in this role, the majority of which are antibodies (for a review, see Ref. [1]).

8.8.2
Peptides Targeting Intracellular Targets *In Vivo*

Many peptides, including bioactive peptides, peptide aptamers and designed peptides which bind to intracellular targets have been characterized. However, only a few of these have been applied systemically and analyzed *in vivo*, or have entered clinical trials. The examples described here incorporate the administration of therapeutic peptides fused to a CPP for intracellular uptake.

One of the first reports of an *in vivo* effect of a CPP-linked peptide was made by the group of Paul Robbins [190], who showed that such peptides could indeed be delivered to solid tumors. The peptide was composed of the antimicrobial peptide (KLAKLAK)2 fused by a GG-linker to a CPP. The CPP was a sequence (PTD-5) which was able to effectively deliver β-galactosidase to murine fibrosarcomas by direct injection. Due to its small size, it was possible to chemically synthesize the fusion peptide for therapeutic applications. Subsequently, mice were transplanted with MCA205 fibrosarcoma cells and, after tumor formation, were treated with 50 μl (1 mM) of peptide. The peptide was delivered once daily by intratumoral injections over a 10-day period. The KLAKLAK sequence is known as a mitochondrial membrane disruption domain, and to cause tumor regression in mice by inducing apoptosis. This example confirms that CPP-linked peptides are indeed taken up by tumor cells and are able to induce a cellular response.

Unfortunately, intratumoral injection is not a preferred method for administration, and therefore in 2002 Harada *et al.* carried out a series of experiments in which the peptides were injected into the peritoneum [191]. For these studies, a fusion peptide was constructed that was stable under hypoxic conditions (which often are found in solid tumors) but was degraded in normal cells. The hypoxic regions of a tumor are often more resistant to radiotherapy or chemotherapy than their well-oxygenated counterparts. For this specific purpose, an oxygen-dependent degradation (ODD) domain of the HIF-1α transcription factor was used. The ODD domain was fused to TAT-CPP for intracellular uptake, and to caspase-3 to induce apoptosis in the tumor cells. The fusion protein was produced in *E. coli* (BL21-(DE3)LysS), purified using GSH Sepharose 4B, and treated with Precision-Protease (GE-Healthcare) to remove the GST tag. Mice carrying subcutaneous human pancreatic tumors (CF/PAC-1 cells) were injected intraperitoneally with 100 μl of the protein solution and a dose level of 20 mg kg^{-1}. The protein was injected once and tumor growth monitored subsequently, after which a dose-dependent reduction in tumor mass was observed with increased caspase activity in the hypoxic regions of the lesion.

Although, usually, small-molecule inhibitors are used to inhibit the activity of oncogenic proteins, these molecules cannot be used to restore tumor suppressor functions in cancer cells. Gene therapy might offer a solution in some cases, but a permanent genetic modification of the cancer cells in the body is associated with additional potential problems. Restoring tumor suppressor activity temporarily in cancer cells by deliverable peptides seemed an attractive alternative, and was carried out by Snyder *et al.* [192]. As these peptides are relatively unstable *in vivo* and are quickly degraded and excreted from the body, the investigators stabilized the peptide chemically, by synthesizing it in reverse order and by using D-amino acids. The peptide was derived from the last 22 amino acids of the C-terminus of p53, a peptide which had been shown to restore p53 tumor suppressor functions in cancer cells [193]. The peptide was fused to the TAT-CPP and biotinylated for detection *in vivo*. The synthetic peptide (600 μl, equal to 650 μg) was then administered by intraperitoneal injection to treat those mice bearing subcutaneous mammary carcinomas (TA3/st cells). The result was a wide distribution of the peptide in the body and a reduction in tumor growth.

The effects of an intravenous administration of CPP-linked peptides were investigated by Matsushita *et al.* [194], who derived peptides from the *N*-ethyl-maleimide-sensitive factor (NSF) which plays a critical role in the regulation of exocytosis.

Thrombosis is known to depend in part on the exocytosis of von Willebrand factor by endothelial cells; the factor then interacts with the platelet glycoprotein Ib-IX-V receptor complex to mediate platelet adherence to the vessel wall. The inhibitory peptides were produced in *E. coli* BL21 cells, purified using Ni^{2+} chromatography and, following their intravenous injection (0.25–$0.5\,mg\,kg^{-1}$), were rapidly taken up by the endothelial cells. This led to an inhibition of exocytosis, as well as an increase in the bleeding time, from 5 min in control mice to more than 20 min in TAT-NSF peptide-treated mice. When the authors examined the bioavailability of the peptides, they showed the peptide blood levels to fall rapidly during the first 5 min after injection, but then to remain stable for the next 60 min. There was no effect on the bleeding time if the peptides were injected intraperitoneally, however. Although other reports have suggested that the intraperitoneal route leads to the uptake of CPP-linked proteins in the bloodstream and in all tissues [141], it seems that every transducible peptide would have its own properties with regards to cellular entry and distribution within the body.

The administration of CPP-linked peptides *in vivo* is hampered by the fact that the protein transduction process has no cell type preference, and peptides are taken up by many cells in the body. This most likely contributes to the rapid clearance and also causes a strong dilution effect. It must be assumed, therefore, that only small amounts of protein will actually reach their target cells, and that treatment will probably require the administration of high dose levels. Additionally, this will lead to an uptake of peptides into normal cells, with the possible cause of adverse side effects. In an effort to direct peptide uptake to tumor cells, Tan *et al.* constructed a peptide fusion capable of binding to tumor cells overexpressing the ErbB2 receptor [195]. For these studies, the length of the TAT sequence was shortened in order to reduce immunogenicity, and the sequence was also altered in such a way as to reduce nonspecific uptake. To this construct a targeting moiety was added. The modified Tat (p3) was fused to a 12-amino acid ErbB2 peptide mimetic, which bound to the ErbB2 receptor with high affinity [196]. A fusion peptide, composed of a pYXXL sequence as described above, was also added to block Stat3 signaling in the tumor cells; this peptide was chemically synthesized and biotinylated for detection. Mice were transplanted with breast cancer-derived MDA-MB-435 cells transfected with or without an ErbB2 expression vector. Following the establishment of tumors in the fat pad, the mice were injected intraperitoneally with 150 nmol of the peptide, three times weekly. The monitoring of tumor growth revealed a clear 50% reduction in size after 30 days of treatment.

8.9
Concluding Remarks

Many crucial aspects must be considered when therapeutic peptides that target intracellular proteins are being developed. The first–perhaps most critical–step is the choice of target protein, which should be central and preferably limiting in its function for a particular disease or a physiological malfunction. The target should also play a non-redundant role in the etiology or maintenance of the diseased cells, and it should be of no particular importance in the cellular processes of normal cells. Such a differential importance might reduce the adverse side effects of inhibitors.

When the target has been identified, a peptide must be selected that lends itself to the inhibition of that target. Peptide aptamers and antibodies with specific target recognition sequences can be selected against almost any protein or protein domain. *Designed peptides* derived from natural interaction partners usually bind to a single domain in the target protein, and exhibit a limited functional interference. Furthermore, structural analysis is required, and such domains may have additional functions in the cell. *Bioactive peptides* act only on a distinct set of target molecules, with their availability depending on the discovery and characterization of these substances found in materials such as venoms. The best generally applicable strategy to identify a specific interacting peptide rests on the screening of random peptide libraries.

The development and application of *therapeutic peptides* requires the selection of appropriate production and purification strategies. This is absolutely crucial in order to obtain peptides with a useful 3-D structure and for later applications of the peptides *in vivo*. A variety of expression systems based on bacteria, yeasts, insect or mammalian cells, transgenic animals and plants are available to produce therapeutic peptides. The most effective system must be determined for each protein separately, and depends on the structural features of the peptide, its purpose, and the required amounts.

One field with fascinating conceptual and technological perspectives is the development of therapeutic peptides capable of targeting intracellular structures, although for this area to succeed intense investigations will need to be conducted into many biotechnological aspects. Here, attention will focus on increasing *in vivo* stability, preventing immunogenicity and, most importantly, identifying possibilities for targeted delivery to special organs or cell-types. The data obtained to date clearly show that intracellularly acting therapeutic peptides have great potential, as they offer a solid basis for scientific progress and, hopefully, for the development of useful drugs in the near future.

References

1 Leader, B., Baca, Q.J. and Golan, D.E. (2008) Protein therapeutics: a summary and pharmacological classification. *Nat. Rev. Drug Discov.*, **7**, 21–39.

2 Enback, J. and Laakkonen, P. (2007) Tumour-homing peptides: tools for targeting, imaging and destruction. *Biochem. Soc. Trans.*, **35**, 780–3.

3 Qi, X., Inagaki, K., Sobel, R.A. and Mochly-Rosen, D. (2008) Sustained pharmacological inhibition of deltaPKC protects against hypertensive encephalopathy through prevention of blood-brain barrier breakdown in rats. *J. Clin. Invest.*, **118**, 173–82.

4 Chen, L., Hahn, H., Wu, G., Chen, C.H., Liron, T., Schechtman, D., Cavallaro, G., Banci, L. *et al.* (2001) Opposing cardioprotective actions and parallel hypertrophic effects of delta PKC and epsilon PKC. *Proc. Natl Acad. Sci. USA*, **98**, 11114–19.

5 Peti, W. and Page, R. (2007) Strategies to maximize heterologous protein expression in *Escherichia coli* with minimal cost. *Protein Exp. Purif.*, **51**, 1–10.

6 Kurokawa, Y., Yanagi, H. and Yura, T. (2000) Overexpression of protein disulfide isomerase DsbC stabilizes multiple-disulfide-bonded recombinant protein produced and transported to the periplasm in *Escherichia coli*. *Appl. Environ. Microbiol.*, **66**, 3960–5.

7 Westers, L., Westers, H. and Quax, W.J. (2004) *Bacillus subtilis* as cell factory for pharmaceutical proteins: a biotechnological approach to optimize the host organism. *Biochim. Biophys. Acta*, **1694**, 299–310.

8 Morello, E., Bermudez-Humaran, L.G., Llull, D., Sole, V., Miraglio, N., Langella, P. and Poquet, I. (2008) *Lactococcus lactis*, an efficient cell factory for recombinant protein production and secretion. *J. Mol. Microbiol. Biotechnol.*, **14**, 48–58.

9 van der Vossen, J.M., Kodde, J., Haandrikman, A.J., Venema, G. and Kok, J. (1992) Characterization of transcription initiation and termination signals of the proteinase genes of *Lactococcus lactis* Wg2 and enhancement of proteolysis in L. lactis. *Appl. Environ. Microbiol.*, **58**, 3142–9.

10 Kuipers, O.P., de Ruyter, P.G., Kleerebezem, M. and de Vos, W.M. (1997) Controlled overproduction of proteins by lactic acid bacteria. *Trends Biotechnol.*, **15**, 135–40.

11 Madsen, S.M., Arnau, J., Vrang, A., Givskov, M. and Israelsen, H. (1999) Molecular characterization of the pH-inducible and growth phase-dependent promoter P170 of *Lactococcus lactis*. *Mol. Microbiol.*, **32**, 75–87.

12 Llull, D. and Poquet, I. (2004) New expression system tightly controlled by zinc availability in *Lactococcus lactis*. *Appl. Environ. Microbiol.*, **70**, 5398–406.

13 Vera, A., Gonzalez-Montalban, N., Aris, A. and Villaverde, A. (2007) The conformational quality of insoluble recombinant proteins is enhanced at low growth temperatures. *Biotechnol. Bioeng.*, **96**, 1101–6.

14 Niiranen, L., Espelid, S., Karlsen, C.R., Mustonen, M., Paulsen, S.M., Heikinheimo, P. and Willassen, N.P. (2007) Comparative expression study to increase the solubility of cold adapted *Vibrio* proteins in *Escherichia coli*. *Protein Exp. Purif.*, **52**, 210–18.

15 Vasina, J.A. and Baneyx, F. (1996) Recombinant protein expression at low temperatures under the transcriptional control of the major *Escherichia coli* cold shock promoter cspA. *Appl. Environ. Microbiol.*, **62**, 1444–7.

16 Losen, M., Frolich, B., Pohl, M. and Buchs, J. (2004) Effect of oxygen limitation and medium composition on *Escherichia coli* fermentation in shake-flask cultures. *Biotechnol. Prog.*, **20**, 1062–8.

17 Nakamura, Y., Gojobori, T. and Ikemura, T. (2000) Codon usage tabulated from international DNA sequence databases: status for the year 2000. *Nucleic Acids Res.*, **28**, 292.

18 Bessette, P.H., Aslund, F., Beckwith, J. and Georgiou, G. (1999) Efficient folding of proteins with multiple disulfide bonds in the *Escherichia coli* cytoplasm. *Proc. Natl Acad. Sci. USA*, **96**, 13703–8.

19 Jurado, P., de Lorenzo, V. and Fernandez, L.A. (2006) Thioredoxin fusions increase folding of single chain Fv antibodies in the cytoplasm of *Escherichia coli*: evidence that chaperone activity is the prime effect of thioredoxin. *J. Mol. Biol.*, **357**, 49–61.

20 Bolla, J.M., Lazdunski, C., Inouye, M. and Pages, J.M. (1987) Export and secretion of overproduced OmpA-beta-lactamase in *Escherichia coli*. *FEBS Lett.*, **224**, 213–18.

21 Neumann-Haefelin, C., Schafer, U., Muller, M. and Koch, H.G. (2000) SRP-dependent co-translational targeting and SecA-dependent translocation analyzed as individual steps in the export of a bacterial protein. *EMBO J.*, **19**, 6419–26.

22 Yue, B.G., Ajuh, P., Akusjarvi, G., Lamond, A.I. and Kreivi, J.P. (2000) Functional coexpression of serine

protein kinase SRPK1 and its substrate ASF/SF2 in *Escherichia coli*. *Nucleic Acids Res.*, **28**, E14.

23 Mironova, R., Niwa, T., Hayashi, H., Dimitrova, R. and Ivanov, I. (2001) Evidence for non-enzymatic glycosylation in *Escherichia coli*. *Mol. Microbiol.*, **39**, 1061–8.

24 Zhang, Z., Gildersleeve, J., Yang, Y.Y., Xu, R., Loo, J.A., Uryu, S., Wong, C.H. and Schultz, P.G. (2004) A new strategy for the synthesis of glycoproteins. *Science*, **303**, 371–3.

25 Faber, K.N., Harder, W., Ab, G. and Veenhuis, M. (1995) Review: methylotrophic yeasts as factories for the production of foreign proteins. *Yeast*, **11**, 1331–44.

26 Faber, K.N., Westra, S., Waterham, H.R., Keizer-Gunnink, I., Harder, W. and Veenhuis, G.A. (1996) Foreign gene expression in *Hansenula polymorpha*. A system for the synthesis of small functional peptides. *Appl. Microbiol. Biotechnol.*, **45**, 72–9.

27 Shen, S., Sulter, G., Jeffries, T.W. and Cregg, J.M. (1998) A strong nitrogen source-regulated promoter for controlled expression of foreign genes in the yeast *Pichia pastoris*. *Gene*, **216**, 93–102.

28 Resina, D., Serrano, A., Valero, F. and Ferrer, P. (2004) Expression of a *Rhizopus oryzae* lipase in *Pichia pastoris* under control of the nitrogen source-regulated formaldehyde dehydrogenase promoter. *J. Biotechnol.*, **109**, 103–13.

29 Sears, I.B., O'Connor, J., Rossanese, O.W. and Glick, B.S. (1998) A versatile set of vectors for constitutive and regulated gene expression in *Pichia pastoris*. *Yeast*, **14**, 783–90.

30 Zhang, A.L., Zhang, T.Y., Luo, J.X., Chen, S.C., Guan, W.J., Fu, C.Y., Peng, S.Q. and Li, H.L. (2007) Constitutive expression of human angiostatin in *Pichia pastoris* by high-density cell culture. *J. Ind. Microbiol. Biotechnol.*, **34**, 117–22.

31 Segev, N., Mulholland, J. and Botstein, D. (1988) The yeast GTP-binding YPT1 protein and a mammalian counterpart are associated with the secretion machinery. *Cell*, **52**, 915–24.

32 Liu, H., Tan, X., Russell, K.A., Veenhuis, M. and Cregg, J.M. (1995) PER3, a gene required for peroxisome biogenesis in *Pichia pastoris*, encodes a peroxisomal membrane protein involved in protein import. *J. Biol. Chem.*, **270**, 10940–51.

33 Kobayashi, K., Kuwae, S., Ohya, T., Ohda, T., Ohyama, M. and Tomomitsu, K. (2000) Addition of oleic acid increases expression of recombinant human serum albumin by the AOX2 promoter in *Pichia pastoris*. *J. Biosci. Bioeng.*, **89**, 479–84.

34 Hong, F., Meinander, N.Q. and Jonsson, L.J. (2002) Fermentation strategies for improved heterologous expression of laccase in *Pichia pastoris*. *Biotechnol. Bioeng.*, **79**, 438–49.

35 Vassileva, A., Chugh, D.A., Swaminathan, S. and Khanna, N. (2001) Expression of hepatitis B surface antigen in the methylotrophic yeast *Pichia pastoris* using the GAP promoter. *J. Biotechnol.*, **88**, 21–35.

36 Clare, J.J., Rayment, F.B., Ballantine, S.P., Sreekrishna, K. and Romanos, M.A. (1991) High-level expression of tetanus toxin fragment C in *Pichia pastoris* strains containing multiple tandem integrations of the gene. *Biotechnology (NY)*, **9**, 455–60.

37 Charlwood, J., Bryant, D., Skehel, J.M. and Camilleri, P. (2001) Analysis of N-linked oligosaccharides: progress towards the characterisation of glycoprotein-linked carbohydrates. *Biomol. Eng.*, **18**, 229–40.

38 Miura, M., Hirose, M., Miwa, T., Kuwae, S. and Ohi, H. (2004) Cloning and characterization in *Pichia pastoris* of PNO1 gene required for phosphomannosylation of N-linked oligosaccharides. *Gene*, **324**, 129–37.

39 Bobrowicz, P., Davidson, R.C., Li, H., Potgieter, T.I., Nett, J.H., Hamilton, S.R., Stadheim, T.A., Miele, R.G. *et al.* (2004) Engineering of an artificial glycosylation pathway blocked in core oligosaccharide assembly in the yeast *Pichia pastoris*: production of complex humanized glycoproteins with terminal galactose. *Glycobiology*, **14**, 757–66.

40 Macauley-Patrick, S., Fazenda, M.L., McNeil, B. and Harvey, L.M. (2005) Heterologous protein production using the *Pichia pastoris* expression system. *Yeast*, **22**, 249–70.

41 Cereghino, J.L. and Cregg, J.M. (2000) Heterologous protein expression in the methylotrophic yeast *Pichia pastoris*. *FEMS Microbiol. Rev.*, **24**, 45–66.

42 Kost, T.A. and Condreay, J.P. (1999) Recombinant baculoviruses as expression vectors for insect and mammalian cells. *Curr. Opin. Biotechnol.*, **10**, 428–33.

43 Luckow, V.A. and Summers, M.D. (1988) Signals important for high-level expression of foreign genes in *Autographa californica* nuclear polyhedrosis virus expression vectors. *Virology*, **167**, 56–71.

44 Harrison, R.L. and Jarvis, D.L. (2006) Protein N-glycosylation in the baculovirus-insect cell expression system and engineering of insect cells to produce "mammalianized" recombinant glycoproteins. *Adv. Virus Res.*, **68**, 159–91.

45 Kost, T.A., Condreay, J.P. and Jarvis, D.L. (2005) Baculovirus as versatile vectors for protein expression in insect and mammalian cells. *Nat. Biotechnol.*, **23**, 567–75.

46 Ho, Y., Lo, H.R., Lee, T.C., Wu, C.P. and Chao, Y.C. (2004) Enhancement of correct protein folding in vivo by a non-lytic baculovirus. *Biochem. J.*, **382**, 695–702.

47 Sano, K., Maeda, K., Oki, M. and Maeda, Y. (2002) Enhancement of protein expression in insect cells by a lobster tropomyosin cDNA leader sequence. *FEBS Lett.*, **532**, 143–6.

48 Yokoyama, N., Hirata, M., Ohtsuka, K., Nishiyama, Y., Fujii, K., Fujita, M., Kuzushima, K., Kiyono, T. *et al.* (2000) Co-expression of human chaperone Hsp70 and Hsdj or Hsp40 co-factor increases solubility of overexpressed target proteins in insect cells. *Biochim. Biophys. Acta*, **1493**, 119–24.

49 Hofmann, C., Sandig, V., Jennings, G., Rudolph, M., Schlag, P. and Strauss, M. (1995) Efficient gene transfer into human hepatocytes by baculovirus vectors. *Proc. Natl Acad. Sci. USA*, **92**, 10099–103.

50 Fornwald, J.A., Lu, Q., Wang, D. and Ames, R.S. (2007) Gene expression in mammalian cells using BacMam, a modified baculovirus system. *Methods Mol. Biol.*, **388**, 95–114.

51 Kost, T.A. and Condreay, J.P. (2002) Recombinant baculoviruses as mammalian cell gene-delivery vectors. *Trends Biotechnol.*, **20**, 173–80.

52 Condreay, J.P., Witherspoon, S.M., Clay, W.C. and Kost, T.A. (1999) Transient and stable gene expression in mammalian cells transduced with a recombinant baculovirus vector. *Proc. Natl Acad. Sci. USA*, **96**, 127–32.

53 Ellis, L., Levitan, A., Cobb, M.H. and Ramos, P. (1988) Efficient expression in insect cells of a soluble, active human insulin receptor protein-tyrosine kinase domain by use of a baculovirus vector. *J. Virol.*, **62**, 1634–9.

54 Hsu, C.S., Ho, Y.C., Wang, K.C. and Hu, Y.C. (2004) Investigation of optimal transduction conditions for baculovirus-mediated gene delivery into mammalian cells. *Biotechnol. Bioeng.*, **88**, 42–51.

55 Kochendoerfer, G.G. and Kent, S.B. (1999) Chemical protein synthesis. *Curr. Opin. Chem. Biol.*, **3**, 665–71.

56 Dawson, P.E. and Kent, S.B. (2000) Synthesis of native proteins by chemical ligation. *Annu. Rev. Biochem.*, **69**, 923–60.

57 Shekhtman, A. (2005) Protein chemical ligation as an invaluable tool for structural NMR. *Protein Pept. Lett.*, **12**, 765–8.

58 Kochendoerfer, G.G. (2005) Site-specific polymer modification of therapeutic proteins. *Curr. Opin. Chem. Biol.*, **9**, 555–60.

59 Xu, M.Q. and Evans, T.C., Jr (2001) Intein-mediated ligation and cyclization of expressed proteins. *Methods*, **24**, 257–77.

60 Graddis, T.J., Remmele, R.L., Jr and McGrew J.T. (2002) Designing proteins that work using recombinant technologies. *Curr. Pharm. Biotechnol.*, **3**, 285–97.

61 Guo, Z. and Shao, N. (2005) Glycopeptide and glycoprotein synthesis involving unprotected carbohydrate building blocks. *Med. Res. Rev.*, **25**, 655–78.

62 Bailey, S.M., Blum, P.H. and Meagher, M.M. (1995) Improved homogenization of recombinant *Escherichia coli* following pretreatment with guanidine hydrochloride. *Biotechnol. Prog.*, **11**, 533–9.

63 Jungbauer, A. and Kaar, W. (2007) Current status of technical protein refolding. *J. Biotechnol.*, **128**, 587–96.

64 Misawa, S. and Kumagai, I. (1999) Refolding of therapeutic proteins produced in *Escherichia coli* as inclusion bodies. *Biopolymers*, **51**, 297–307.

65 Swietnicki, W. (2006) Folding aggregated proteins into functionally active forms. *Curr. Opin. Biotechnol.*, **17**, 367–72.

66 Batas, B., Schiraldi, C. and Chaudhuri, J.B. (1999) Inclusion body purification and protein refolding using microfiltration and size exclusion chromatography. *J. Biotechnol.*, **68**, 149–58.

67 Schlegl, R., Iberer, G., Machold, C., Necina, R. and Jungbauer, A. (2003) Continuous matrix-assisted refolding of proteins. *J. Chromatogr. A*, **1009**, 119–32.

68 Stempfer, G., Holl-Neugebauer, B., Kopetzki, E. and Rudolph, R. (1996) A fusion protein designed for noncovalent immobilization: stability, enzymatic activity, and use in an enzyme reactor. *Nat. Biotechnol.*, **14**, 481–4.

69 Gong, B., Wang, L., Wang, C. and Geng, X. (2004) Preparation of hydrophobic interaction chromatographic packings based on monodisperse poly(glycidylmethacrylate-co-ethylenedimethacrylate) beads and their application. *J. Chromatogr. A*, **1022**, 33–9.

70 Lee, S.H., Carpenter, J.F., Chang, B.S., Randolph, T.W. and Kim, Y.S. (2006) Effects of solutes on solubilization and refolding of proteins from inclusion bodies with high hydrostatic pressure. *Protein Sci.*, **15**, 304–13.

71 Tsumoto, K., Ejima, D., Kita, Y. and Arakawa, T. (2005) Review: why is arginine effective in suppressing aggregation? *Protein Pept. Lett.*, **12**, 613–19.

72 Bulaj, G. (2005) Formation of disulfide bonds in proteins and peptides. *Biotechnol. Adv.*, **23**, 87–92.

73 Davidson, A.R. and Sauer, R.T. (1994) Folded proteins occur frequently in libraries of random amino acid sequences. *Proc. Natl Acad. Sci. USA*, **91**, 2146–50.

74 Ladner, R.C. (1995) Constrained peptides as binding entities. *Trends Biotechnol.*, **13**, 426–30.

75 O'Neil, K.T., Hoess, R.H., Jackson, S.A., Ramachandran, N.S., Mousa, S.A. and DeGrado, W.F. (1992) Identification of novel peptide antagonists for GPIIb/IIIa from a conformationally constrained phage peptide library. *Proteins*, **14**, 509–15.

76 Adessi, C. and Soto, C. (2002) Converting a peptide into a drug: strategies to improve stability and bioavailability. *Curr. Med. Chem.*, **9**, 963–78.

77 Mattock, H., Lane, D.P. and Warbrick, E. (2001) Inhibition of cell proliferation by the PCNA-binding region of p21 expressed as a GFP miniprotein. *Exp. Cell Res.*, **265**, 234–41.

78 Hitoshi, Y., Gururaja, T., Pearsall, D.M., Lang, W., Sharma, P., Huang, B., Catalano, S.M., McLaughlin, J. *et al.* (2003) Cellular localization and antiproliferative effect of peptides discovered from a functional screen of a retrovirally delivered random peptide library. *Chem. Biol.*, **10**, 975–87.

79 Borghouts, C., Kunz, C., Delis, N. and Groner, B. (2008) Monomeric recombinant peptide aptamers are required for efficient intracellular uptake and target inhibition. *Mol. Cancer Res.*, **6**, 267–81.

80 Geyer, C.R. and Brent, R. (2000) Selection of genetic agents from random peptide aptamer expression libraries. *Methods Enzymol.*, **328**, 171–208.

81 Skerra, A. (2001) "Anticalins": a new class of engineered ligand-binding proteins with antibody-like properties. *J. Biotechnol.*, **74**, 257–75.

82 Gram, H., Marconi, L.A., Barbas, C.F., 3rd, Collet, T.A., Lerner, R.A. and Kang, A.S. (1992) In vitro selection and affinity maturation of antibodies from a naive combinatorial immunoglobulin library. *Proc. Natl Acad. Sci. USA*, **89**, 3576–80.

83 Hamers-Casterman, C., Atarhouch, T., Muyldermans, S., Robinson, G., Hamers, C., Songa, E.B., Bendahman, N. and Hamers, R. (1993) Naturally occurring antibodies devoid of light chains. *Nature*, **363**, 446–8.

84 Huston, J.S., Levinson, D., Mudgett-Hunter, M., Tai, M.S., Novotny, J., Margolies, M.N., Ridge, R.J., Bruccoleri, R.E. *et al.* (1988) Protein engineering of antibody binding sites: recovery of specific activity in an anti-digoxin single-chain Fv analogue produced in *Escherichia coli. Proc. Natl Acad. Sci. USA*, **85**, 5879–83.

85 Koide, A., Bailey, C.W., Huang, X. and Koide, S. (1998) The fibronectin type III domain as a scaffold for novel binding proteins. *J. Mol. Biol.*, **284**, 1141–51.

86 Martin, F., Toniatti, C., Salvati, A.L., Venturini, S., Ciliberto, G., Cortese, R. and Sollazzo, M. (1994) The affinity-selection of a minibody polypeptide inhibitor of human interleukin-6. *EMBO J.*, **13**, 5303–9.

87 Nuttall, S.D., Rousch, M.J., Irving, R.A., Hufton, S.E., Hoogenboom, H.R. and Hudson, P.J. (1999) Design and expression of soluble CTLA-4 variable domain as a scaffold for the display of functional polypeptides. *Proteins*, **36**, 217–27.

88 Pessi, A., Bianchi, E., Crameri, A., Venturini, S., Tramontano, A. and Sollazzo, M. (1993) A designed metal-binding protein with a novel fold. *Nature*, **362**, 367–9.

89 Dennis, M.S. and Lazarus, R.A. (1994) Kunitz domain inhibitors of tissue factor-factor VIIa. I. Potent inhibitors selected from libraries by phage display. *J. Biol. Chem.*, **269**, 22129–36.

90 Markland, W., Ley, A.C., Lee, S.W. and Ladner, R.C. (1996) Iterative optimization of high-affinity proteases inhibitors using phage display. 1. Plasmin. *Biochemistry*, **35**, 8045–57.

91 McConnell, S.J. and Hoess, R.H. (1995) Tendamistat as a scaffold for conformationally constrained phage peptide libraries. *J. Mol. Biol.*, **250**, 460–70.

92 Roberts, B.L., Markland, W., Ley, A.C., Kent, R.B., White, D.W., Guterman, S.K. and Ladner, R.C. (1992) Directed evolution of a protein: selection of potent neutrophil elastase inhibitors displayed on M13 fusion phage. *Proc. Natl Acad. Sci. USA*, **89**, 2429–33.

93 Rottgen, P. and Collins, J. (1995) A human pancreatic secretory trypsin inhibitor presenting a hypervariable highly constrained epitope via monovalent phagemid display. *Gene*, **164**, 243–50.

94 Wang, C.I., Yang, Q. and Craik, C.S. (1995) Isolation of a high affinity inhibitor of urokinase-type plasminogen activator by phage display of ecotin. *J. Biol. Chem.*, **270**, 12250–6.

95 Woodman, R., Yeh, J.T., Laurenson, S. and Ko Ferrigno, P. (2005) Design and validation of a neutral protein scaffold for the presentation of peptide aptamers. *J. Mol. Biol.*, **352**, 1118–33.

96 Christmann, A., Walter, K., Wentzel, A., Kratzner, R. and Kolmar, H. (1999) The cystine knot of a squash-type protease inhibitor as a structural scaffold for *Escherichia coli* cell surface display of conformationally constrained peptides. *Protein Eng.*, **12**, 797–806.

97 Smith, G.P., Patel, S.U., Windass, J.D., Thornton, J.M., Winter, G. and Griffiths, A.D. (1998) Small binding proteins selected from a combinatorial repertoire of knottins displayed on phage. *J. Mol. Biol.*, **277**, 317–32.

98 Vita, C., Roumestand, C., Toma, F. and Menez, A. (1995) Scorpion toxins as natural scaffolds for protein engineering. *Proc. Natl Acad. Sci. USA*, **92**, 6404–8.

99 Woodward, S.R., Cruz, L.J., Olivera, B.M. and Hillyard, D.R. (1990) Constant and hypervariable regions in conotoxin propeptides. *EMBO J.*, **9**, 1015–20.

100 Norman, T.C., Smith, D.L., Sorger, P.K., Drees, B.L., O'Rourke, S.M., Hughes, T.R., Roberts, C.J., Friend, S.H. *et al.* (1999) Genetic selection of peptide

inhibitors of biological pathways. *Science*, **285**, 591–5.

101 Widersten, M. and Mannervik, B. (1995) Glutathione transferases with novel active sites isolated by phage display from a library of random mutants. *J. Mol. Biol.*, **250**, 115–22.

102 LaVallie, E.R., DiBlasio, E.A., Kovacic, S., Grant, K.L., Schendel, P.F. and McCoy, J.M. (1993) A thioredoxin gene fusion expression system that circumvents inclusion body formation in the *E. coli* cytoplasm. *Biotechnology (NY)*, **11**, 187–93.

103 Quemeneur, E., Moutiez, M., Charbonnier, J.B. and Menez, A. (1998) Engineering cyclophilin into a proline-specific endopeptidase. *Nature*, **391**, 301–4.

104 Nixon, A.E., Firestine, S.M., Salinas, F.G. and Benkovic, S.J. (1999) Rational design of a scytalone dehydratase-like enzyme using a structurally homologous protein scaffold. *Proc. Natl Acad. Sci. USA*, **96**, 3568–71.

105 Altamirano, M.M., Blackburn, J.M., Aguayo, C. and Fersht, A.R. (2000) Directed evolution of new catalytic activity using the alpha/beta-barrel scaffold. *Nature*, **403**, 617–22.

106 Ku, J. and Schultz, P.G. (1995) Alternate protein frameworks for molecular recognition. *Proc. Natl Acad. Sci. USA*, **92**, 6552–6.

107 Nord, K., Nilsson, J., Nilsson, B., Uhlen, M. and Nygren, P.A. (1995) A combinatorial library of an alpha-helical bacterial receptor domain. *Protein Eng.*, **8**, 601–8.

108 Handel, T.M., Williams, S.A. and DeGrado, W.F. (1993) Metal ion-dependent modulation of the dynamics of a designed protein. *Science*, **261**, 879–85.

109 Muller, H.N. and Skerra, A. (1994) Grafting of a high-affinity Zn(II)-binding site on the beta-barrel of retinol-binding protein results in enhanced folding stability and enables simplified purification. *Biochemistry*, **33**, 14126–35.

110 Binz, H.K., Stumpp, M.T., Forrer, P., Amstutz, P. and Pluckthun, A. (2003) Designing repeat proteins: well-expressed, soluble and stable proteins from combinatorial libraries of consensus ankyrin repeat proteins. *J. Mol. Biol.*, **332**, 489–503.

111 Stumpp, M.T., Forrer, P., Binz, H.K. and Pluckthun, A. (2003) Designing repeat proteins: modular leucine-rich repeat protein libraries based on the mammalian ribonuclease inhibitor family. *J. Mol. Biol.*, **332**, 471–87.

112 Gururaja, T.L., Narasimhamurthy, S., Payan, D.G. and Anderson, D.C. (2000) A novel artificial loop scaffold for the noncovalent constraint of peptides. *Chem. Biol.*, **7**, 515–27.

113 Myszka, D.G. and Chaiken, I.M. (1994) Design and characterization of an intramolecular antiparallel coiled coil peptide. *Biochemistry*, **33**, 2363–72.

114 Abedi, M.R., Caponigro, G. and Kamb, A. (1998) Green fluorescent protein as a scaffold for intracellular presentation of peptides. *Nucleic Acids Res.*, **26**, 623–30.

115 Cheng, X., Boyer, J.L. and Juliano, R.L. (1997) Selection of peptides that functionally replace a zinc finger in the Sp1 transcription factor by using a yeast combinatorial library. *Proc. Natl Acad. Sci. USA*, **94**, 14120–5.

116 Binkowski, B.F., Miller, R.A. and Belshaw, P.J. (2005) Ligand-regulated peptides: a general approach for modulating protein-peptide interactions with small molecules. *Chem. Biol.*, **12**, 847–55.

117 Binz, H.K., Amstutz, P. and Pluckthun, A. (2005) Engineering novel binding proteins from nonimmunoglobulin domains. *Nat. Biotechnol.*, **23**, 1257–68.

118 Borghouts, C., Kunz, C. and Groner, B. (2005) Current strategies for the development of peptide-based anti-cancer therapeutics. *J. Pept. Sci.*, **11**, 713–26.

119 Hosse, R.J., Rothe, A. and Power, B.E. (2006) A new generation of protein display scaffolds for molecular recognition. *Protein Sci.*, **15**, 14–27.

120 Foerg, C. and Merkle, H.P. (2008) On the biomedical promise of cell penetrating peptides: limits versus prospects. *J. Pharm. Sci.*, **97**, 144–62.

121 Nygren, P.A. and Skerra, A. (2004) Binding proteins from alternative scaffolds. *J. Immunol. Methods*, **290**, 3–28.

122 Skerra, A. (2000) Engineered protein scaffolds for molecular recognition. *J. Mol. Recognit.*, **13**, 167–87.

123 Mae, M. and Langel, U. (2006) Cell-penetrating peptides as vectors for peptide, protein and oligonucleotide delivery. *Curr. Opin. Pharmacol.*, **6**, 509–14.

124 Lipinski, C.A., Lombardo, F., Dominy, B.W. and Feeney, P.J. (2001) Experimental and computational approaches to estimate solubility and permeability in drug discovery and development settings. *Adv. Drug Deliv. Rev.*, **46**, 3–26.

125 Luedtke, N.W., Carmichael, P. and Tor, Y. (2003) Cellular uptake of aminoglycosides, guanidinoglycosides, and poly-arginine. *J. Am. Chem. Soc.*, **125**, 12374–5.

126 Wagstaff, K.M. and Jans, D.A. (2006) Protein transduction: cell penetrating peptides and their therapeutic applications. *Curr. Med. Chem.*, **13**, 1371–87.

127 Derossi, D., Joliot, A.H., Chassaing, G. and Prochiantz, A. (1994) The third helix of the Antennapedia homeodomain translocates through biological membranes. *J. Biol. Chem.*, **269**, 10444–50.

128 Fawell, S., Seery, J., Daikh, Y., Moore, C., Chen, L.L., Pepinsky, B. and Barsoum, J. (1994) Tat-mediated delivery of heterologous proteins into cells. *Proc. Natl Acad. Sci. USA*, **91**, 664–8.

129 Derossi, D., Calvet, S., Trembleau, A., Brunissen, A., Chassaing, G. and Prochiantz, A. (1996) Cell internalization of the third helix of the Antennapedia homeodomain is receptor-independent. *J. Biol. Chem.*, **271**, 18188–93.

130 Futaki, S., Suzuki, T., Ohashi, W., Yagami, T., Tanaka, S., Ueda, K. and Sugiura, Y. (2001) Arginine-rich peptides. An abundant source of membrane-permeable peptides having potential as carriers for intracellular protein delivery. *J. Biol. Chem.*, **276**, 5836–40.

131 Leifert, J.A. and Whitton, J.L. (2003) "Translocatory proteins" and "protein transduction domains": a critical analysis of their biological effects and the underlying mechanisms. *Mol. Ther.*, **8**, 13–20.

132 Silhol, M., Tyagi, M., Giacca, M., Lebleu, B. and Vives, E. (2002) Different mechanisms for cellular internalization of the HIV-1 Tat-derived cell penetrating peptide and recombinant proteins fused to Tat. *Eur. J. Biochem.*, **269**, 494–501.

133 Vives, E., Brodin, P. and Lebleu, B. (1997) A truncated HIV-1 Tat protein basic domain rapidly translocates through the plasma membrane and accumulates in the cell nucleus. *J. Biol. Chem.*, **272**, 16010–17.

134 Suzuki, T., Futaki, S., Niwa, M., Tanaka, S., Ueda, K. and Sugiura, Y. (2002) Possible existence of common internalization mechanisms among arginine-rich peptides. *J. Biol. Chem.*, **277**, 2437–43.

135 Green, I., Christison, R., Voyce, C.J., Bundell, K.R. and Lindsay, M.A. (2003) Protein transduction domains: are they delivering? *Trends Pharmacol. Sci.*, **24**, 213–15.

136 Kaplan, I.M., Wadia, J.S. and Dowdy, S.F. (2005) Cationic TAT peptide transduction domain enters cells by macropinocytosis. *J. Control. Release*, **102**, 247–53.

137 Lundberg, M. and Johansson, M. (2002) Positively charged DNA-binding proteins cause apparent cell membrane translocation. *Biochem. Biophys. Res. Commun.*, **291**, 367–71.

138 Lundberg, M., Wikstrom, S. and Johansson, M. (2003) Cell surface adherence and endocytosis of protein transduction domains. *Mol. Ther.*, **8**, 143–50.

139 Vives, E. (2003) Cellular uptake of the Tat peptide: an endocytosis mechanism following ionic interactions. *J. Mol. Recognit.*, **16**, 265–71.

140 Wadia, J.S., Stan, R.V. and Dowdy, S.F. (2004) Transducible TAT-HA fusogenic peptide enhances escape of TAT-fusion proteins after lipid raft macropinocytosis. *Nat. Med.*, **10**, 310–15.

141 Schwarze, S.R., Ho, A., Vocero-Akbani, A. and Dowdy, S.F. (1999) In vivo protein transduction: delivery of a biologically active protein into the mouse. *Science*, **285**, 1569–72.

142 Tyagi, M., Rusnati, M., Presta, M. and Giacca, M. (2001) Internalization of HIV-1 tat requires cell surface heparan sulfate proteoglycans. *J. Biol. Chem.*, **276**, 3254–61.

143 Steinman, R.M. and Swanson, J. (1995) The endocytic activity of dendritic cells. *J. Exp. Med.*, **182**, 283–8.

144 Swanson, J.A. and Watts, C. (1995) Macropinocytosis. *Trends Cell. Biol.*, **5**, 424–8.

145 Mishra, S. and Joshi, P.G. (2007) Lipid raft heterogeneity: an enigma. *J. Neurochem.*, **103** (Suppl. 1), 135–42.

146 Sengupta, P., Baird, B. and Holowka, D. (2007) Lipid rafts, fluid/fluid phase separation, and their relevance to plasma membrane structure and function. *Semin. Cell Dev. Biol.*, **18**, 583–90.

147 Lewis, R.J. (2000) Ion channel toxins and therapeutics: from cone snail venoms to ciguatera. *Ther. Drug Monit.*, **22**, 61–4.

148 Joseph, R., Pahari, S., Hodgson, W.C. and Kini, R.M. (2004) Hypotensive agents from snake venoms. *Curr. Drug Targets Cardiovasc. Haematol. Disord.*, **4**, 437–59.

149 Mortari, M.R., Cunha, A.O., Ferreira, L.B. and dos Santos, W.F. (2007) Neurotoxins from invertebrates as anticonvulsants: from basic research to therapeutic application. *Pharmacol. Ther.*, **114**, 171–83.

150 Miljanich, G.P. (2004) Ziconotide: neuronal calcium channel blocker for treating severe chronic pain. *Curr. Med. Chem.*, **11**, 3029–40.

151 Klotz, U. (2006) Ziconotide – a novel neuron-specific calcium channel blocker for the intrathecal treatment of severe chronic pain – a short review. *Int. J. Clin. Pharmacol. Ther.*, **44**, 478–83.

152 Nabors, L.B. (2004) Targeted molecular therapy for malignant gliomas. *Curr. Treat. Options Oncol.*, **5**, 519–26.

153 Mamelak, A.N. and Jacoby, D.B. (2007) Targeted delivery of antitumoral therapy to glioma and other malignancies with synthetic chlorotoxin (TM-601). *Expert Opin. Drug Deliv.*, **4**, 175–86.

154 Schneider, J.J., Unholzer, A., Schaller, M., Schafer-Korting, M. and Korting, H.C. (2005) Human defensins. *J. Mol. Med.*, **83**, 587–95.

155 Raj, P.A. and Dentino, A.R. (2002) Current status of defensins and their role in innate and adaptive immunity. *FEMS Microbiol. Lett.*, **206**, 9–18.

156 Sahl, H.G., Pag, U., Bonness, S., Wagner, S., Antcheva, N. and Tossi, A. (2005) Mammalian defensins: structures and mechanism of antibiotic activity. *J. Leukoc. Biol.*, **77**, 466–75.

157 Thomma, B.P., Cammue, B.P. and Thevissen, K. (2003) Mode of action of plant defensins suggests therapeutic potential. *Curr. Drug Targets Infect. Disord.*, **3**, 1–8.

158 Lehmann, J., Retz, M., Sidhu, S.S., Suttmann, H., Sell, M., Paulsen, F., Harder, J., Unteregger, G. *et al.* (2006) Antitumor activity of the antimicrobial peptide magainin II against bladder cancer cell lines. *Eur. Urol.*, **50**, 141–7.

159 Soballe, P.W., Maloy, W.L., Myrga, M.L., Jacob, L.S. and Herlyn, M. (1995) Experimental local therapy of human melanoma with lytic magainin peptides. *Int. J. Cancer*, **60**, 280–4.

160 Papo, N. and Shai, Y. (2005) Host defense peptides as new weapons in cancer treatment. *Cell. Mol. Life Sci.*, **62**, 784–90.

161 Kokryakov, V.N., Harwig, S.S., Panyutich, E.A., Shevchenko, A.A., Aleshina, G.M., Shamova, O.V., Korneva, H.A. and Lehrer, R.I. (1993) Protegrins: leukocyte antimicrobial peptides that combine features of corticostatic defensins and tachyplesins. *FEBS Lett.*, **327**, 231–6.

162 Mygind, P.H., Fischer, R.L., Schnorr, K.M., Hansen, M.T., Sonksen, C.P., Ludvigsen, S., Raventos, D., Buskov, S. *et al.* (2005) Plectasin is a peptide antibiotic with therapeutic potential from a saprophytic fungus. *Nature*, **437**, 975–80.

163 Bickle, M.B., Dusserre, E., Moncorge, O., Bottin, H. and Colas, P. (2006) Selection and characterization of large

collections of peptide aptamers through optimized yeast two-hybrid procedures. *Nat. Protoc.*, **1**, 1066–91.

164 Borghouts, C., Kunz, C. and Groner, B. (2008) Peptide aptamer libraries. *Comb. Chem. High Throughput Screen.*, **11**, 135–45.

165 Borghouts, C., Kunz, C. and Groner, B. (2005) Peptide aptamers: recent developments for cancer therapy. *Expert Opin. Biol. Ther.*, **5**, 783–97.

166 Hoppe-Seyler, F., Crnkovic-Mertens, I., Tomai, E. and Butz, K. (2004) Peptide aptamers: specific inhibitors of protein function. *Curr. Mol. Med.*, **4**, 529–38.

167 Colas, P., Cohen, B., Jessen, T., Grishina, I., McCoy, J. and Brent, R. (1996) Genetic selection of peptide aptamers that recognize and inhibit cyclin-dependent kinase 2. *Nature*, **380**, 548–50.

168 Harada, H., Kizaka-Kondoh, S. and Hiraoka, M. (2006) Antitumor protein therapy; application of the protein transduction domain to the development of a protein drug for cancer treatment. *Breast Cancer*, **13**, 16–26.

169 Nagel-Wolfrum, K., Buerger, C., Wittig, I., Butz, K., Hoppe-Seyler, F. and Groner, B. (2004) The interaction of specific peptide aptamers with the DNA binding domain and the dimerization domain of the transcription factor Stat3 inhibits transactivation and induces apoptosis in tumor cells. *Mol. Cancer Res.*, **2**, 170–82.

170 Kunz, C., Borghouts, C., Buerger, C. and Groner, B. (2006) Peptide aptamers with binding specificity for the intracellular domain of the ErbB2 receptor interfere with AKT signaling and sensitize breast cancer cells to Taxol. *Mol. Cancer Res.*, **4**, 983–98.

171 Martel, V., Filhol, O., Colas, P. and Cochet, C. (2006) p53-dependent inhibition of mammalian cell survival by a genetically selected peptide aptamer that targets the regulatory subunit of protein kinase CK2. *Oncogene*, **25**, 7343–53.

172 Nouvion, A.L., Thibaut, J., Lohez, O.D., Venet, S., Colas, P., Gillet, G. and Lalle, P. (2007) Modulation of Nr-13 antideath activity by peptide aptamers. *Oncogene*, **26**, 701–10.

173 Tamm, I., Trepel, M., Cardo-Vila, M., Sun, Y., Welsh, K., Cabezas, E., Swatterthwait, A., Arap, W. *et al.* (2003) Peptides targeting caspase inhibitors. *J. Biol. Chem.*, **278**, 14401–5.

174 Xu, C.W. and Luo, Z. (2002) Inactivation of Ras function by allele-specific peptide aptamers. *Oncogene*, **21**, 5753–7.

175 Butz, K., Denk, C., Ullmann, A., Scheffner, M. and Hoppe-Seyler, F. (2000) Induction of apoptosis in human papillomaviruspositive cancer cells by peptide aptamers targeting the viral E6 oncoprotein. *Proc. Natl Acad. Sci. USA*, **97**, 6693–7.

176 Nauenburg, S., Zwerschke, W. and Jansen-Durr, P. (2001) Induction of apoptosis in cervical carcinoma cells by peptide aptamers that bind to the HPV-16 E7 oncoprotein. *FASEB J.*, **15**, 592–4.

177 Armon-Omer, A., Levin, A., Hayouka, Z., Butz, K., Hoppe-Seyler, F., Loya, S., Hizi, A., Friedler, A. *et al.* (2008) Correlation between shiftide activity and HIV-1 integrase inhibition by a peptide selected from a combinatorial library. *J. Mol. Biol.*, **376**, 971–82.

178 Butz, K., Denk, C., Fitscher, B., Crnkovic-Mertens, I., Ullmann, A., Schroder, C.H. and Hoppe-Seyler, F. (2001) Peptide aptamers targeting the hepatitis B virus core protein: a new class of molecules with antiviral activity. *Oncogene*, **20**, 6579–86.

179 Chène, P. (2003) Inhibiting the p53-MDM2 interaction: an important target for cancer therapy. *Nat. Rev. Cancer*, **3**, 102–9.

180 Chene, P. (2006) Drugs targeting protein-protein interactions. *ChemMedChem*, **1**, 400–11.

181 Yuan, W., Craig, S., Si, Z., Farzan, M. and Sodroski, J. (2004) CD4-induced T-20 binding to human immunodeficiency virus type 1 gp120 blocks interaction with the CXCR4 coreceptor. *J. Virol.*, **78**, 5448–57.

182 Ren, Z., Cabell, L.A., Schaefer, T.S. and McMurray, J.S. (2003) Identification of a high-affinity phosphopeptide inhibitor of

Stat3. *Bioorg. Med. Chem. Lett.*, **13**, 633–6.

183 Zhao, B.M. and Hoffmann, F.M. (2006) Inhibition of transforming growth factor-beta1-induced signaling and epithelial-to-mesenchymal transition by the Smad-binding peptide aptamer Trx-SARA. *Mol. Biol. Cell*, **17**, 3819–31.

184 Bray, G.L., Gomperts, E.D., Courter, S., Gruppo, R., Gordon, E.M., Manco-Johnson, M., Shapiro, A., Scheibel, E. *et al.* (1994) A multicenter study of recombinant factor VIII (recombinate): safety, efficacy, and inhibitor risk in previously untreated patients with hemophilia A. The Recombinate Study Group. *Blood*, **83**, 2428–35.

185 Rosado, J.L., Solomons, N.W., Lisker, R. and Bourges, H. (1984) Enzyme replacement therapy for primary adult lactase deficiency. Effective reduction of lactose malabsorption and milk intolerance by direct addition of beta-galactosidase to milk at mealtime. *Gastroenterology*, **87**, 1072–82.

186 Out, H.J., Driessen, S.G., Mannaerts, B.M. and Coelingh Bennink, H.J. (1997) Recombinant follicle-stimulating hormone (follitropin beta, Puregon) yields higher pregnancy rates in in vitro fertilization than urinary gonadotropins. *Fertil. Steril.*, **68**, 138–42.

187 Shoham, Z. and Insler, V. (1996) Recombinant technique and gonadotropins production: new era in reproductive medicine. *Fertil. Steril.*, **66**, 187–201.

188 Ghigo, E., Aimaretti, G., Gianotti, L., Bellone, J., Arvat, E. and Camanni, F. (1996) New approach to the diagnosis of growth hormone deficiency in adults. *Eur. J. Endocrinol.*, **134**, 352–6.

189 Norman, P. (2006) Mecasermin Tercica. *Curr. Opin. Invest. Drugs*, **7**, 371–80.

190 Mai, J.C., Mi, Z., Kim, S.H., Ng, B. and Robbins, P.D. (2001) A proapoptotic peptide for the treatment of solid tumors. *Cancer Res.*, **61**, 7709–12.

191 Harada, H., Hiraoka, M. and Kizaka-Kondoh, S. (2002) Antitumor effect of TAT-oxygen-dependent degradation-caspase-3 fusion protein specifically stabilized and activated in hypoxic tumor cells. *Cancer Res.*, **62**, 2013–18.

192 Snyder, E.L., Meade, B.R., Saenz, C.C. and Dowdy, S.F. (2004) Treatment of terminal peritoneal carcinomatosis by a transducible p53-activating peptide. *PLoS Biol.*, **2**, E36.

193 Hupp, T.R., Sparks, A. and Lane, D.P. (1995) Small peptides activate the latent sequence-specific DNA binding function of p53. *Cell*, **83**, 237–45.

194 Matsushita, K., Morrell, C.N. and Lowenstein, C.J. (2005) A novel class of fusion polypeptides inhibits exocytosis. *Mol. Pharmacol.*, **67**, 1137–44.

195 Tan, M., Lan, K.H., Yao, J., Lu, C.H., Sun, M., Neal, C.L., Lu, J. and Yu, D. (2006) Selective inhibition of ErbB2-overexpressing breast cancer in vivo by a novel TAT-based ErbB2-targeting signal transducers and activators of transcription 3-blocking peptide. *Cancer Res.*, **66**, 3764–72.

196 Park, B.W., Zhang, H.T., Wu, C., Berezov, A., Zhang, X., Dua, R., Wang, Q., Kao, G. *et al.* (2000) Rationally designed anti-HER2/neu peptide mimetic disables P185HER2/neu tyrosine kinases in vitro and in vivo. *Nat. Biotechnol.*, **18**, 194–8.

9
Peptide Arrays on Solid Supports: A Tool for the Identification of Peptide Ligands

Mike Schutkowski, Alexandra Thiele, and Joachim Koch

9.1
Introduction

It has been predicted that about five macromolecular interaction partners exist for any given cellular protein. This number illustrates the importance of protein–protein and protein–nucleic acid interactions, and has important implications for the mechanisms of disease processes. A major task for the development of novel leads and therapeutics is the identification of molecules which bind specifically and with high affinity to disease-related protein targets.

The majority of conventional drugs fall into two classes: (i) designed, small-molecular-weight chemical compounds; and (ii) whole proteins (e.g., antibodies), which modulate the functions of target proteins. High-throughput screening (HTS) procedures are mainly employed by pharmaceutical companies for the selection of lead compounds. For this, large chemical compound libraries of stable, small-molecular-weight molecules are used as a source for the selection of drug leads for both intracellular and extracellular targets. These molecules are subsequently optimized for favorable pharmacokinetic properties. However, in many cases the selection of potent small molecules which interact specifically with particular protein domains and inhibit predetermined protein functions fails, and the development of an alternative strategy is required.

Most cellular protein contacts are mediated by binding of small regions of the proteins to each other (e.g., paratope/epitope recognition of antibodies) or by specialized protein interaction domains (e.g., SH2, SH3, WW, PDZ). These domains are usually constituted by short linear peptide sequences. Moreover, many peptides have important biological functions in their own right, for example as neurotransmitters in the brain, as host defense molecules and part of the innate immune response, and as potent inhibitors of enzymes. This versatility of peptide functions can possibly further utilized in the field of drug discovery and drug development, and peptide-based drugs represent an emerging class of therapeutics. Usually, these so-called "peptidomimetics" are 5–30 amino acids in length, and often specifically modified to maintain prolonged functionality within the body. Although,

Peptides as Drugs. Discovery and Development. Edited by Bernd Groner
Copyright © 2009 WILEY-VCH Verlag GmbH & Co. KGaA, Weinheim
ISBN: 978-3-527-32205-3

these compounds require intravenous administration, they have distinct advantages (i) specific binding to targets which are difficult to address with other classes of molecules; (ii) low toxicity and few adverse side effects; (iii) their chemical synthesis allows for safe and reproducible production; and (iv) the small size and low complexity of peptides enable the development of stabilized variants.

In order to identify peptides, which can bind to proteins or nucleic acids, peptide arrays generated by parallel synthesis on cellulose membrane supports (SPOT method) represent an efficient screening platform [1–3]. These molecules can then serve as leads for the further development of peptidomimetics. Secondary modifications (e.g., phosphorylation) can be introduced during and after synthesis [4], which is often an advantageous feature. Although the conventionally used assay format is not miniaturized in a "lab-on-a-chip" fashion, it allows for parallel manual, semi- or fully automated synthesis of peptide arrays with 100–1000 individual peptide spots on a membrane of about $100\,cm^2$ [5, 6]. These peptide arrays are especially useful to investigate a particular group of interacting proteins. They can also be used to aid in the design of ligand variant analysis by mutagenesis and to test computer predictions of interaction networks. Novel array formats are arranged on microscope glass slides, laser printer-supported spotting systems or compact disc-based carriers allow for much larger screens due to higher spot density and automation of the entire screening process.

In this chapter we will describe the manufacture and applications of SPOT arrays in basic and applied life sciences. In particular, we will address the identification of peptide ligands as leads for drug development.

9.2
Synthesis of Peptide Arrays

9.2.1
Fmoc-Based Synthesis of Peptides on Cellulose Membranes

Robert Bruce Merrifield established the chemical synthesis of peptides on solid supports [7]. For his ground-breaking achievements he was awarded the Nobel Prize in Chemistry in 1984. Based on these principles, Ronald Frank and co-workers developed the SPOT method, which allows for the parallel synthesis of oligopeptide arrays on cellulose membranes [1]. Although initially developed as a manual procedure, the companies Jerini and Abimed (now Intavis) fostered the automation of peptide array synthesis of the SPOT method. Peptide synthesis is carried out using 9-fluorenyl-methoxycarbonyl (Fmoc)-protection chemistry according to Merrifield (Figure 9.1; for detailed protocols, see also Refs [5, 8]). Here, the activated amino acid building blocks (e.g. pentafluorophenyl esters (-OPfp)) are protected by an Fmoc group at their N-terminus to prevent multiple couplings per extension cycle at the growing peptide chain. Notably, OPfp-esters are frequently used; however, the amino acids can also be activated with hydroxybenzotriazole (HOBt) and diisopropyl carbodiimide (DIC).

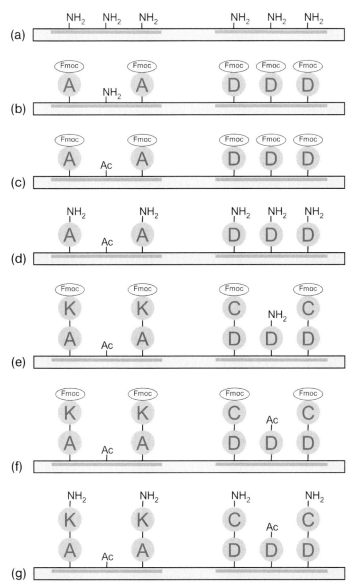

Figure 9.1 Schematic representation of Fmoc peptide synthesis. (a) Activated cellulose membrane with free amino groups; (b) Coupling of the first Fmoc-protected amino acid; (c) Acetylation (Ac) of free amino groups on the cellulose membrane; (d) Fmoc deprotection to generate free amino groups for the next coupling step; (e) Coupling of the second amino acid; (f) Acetylation of non-elongated peptide chains; (g) Fmoc deprotection. The procedure is continued until the desired length of the peptides is reached. After removal of all amino acid side-chain protection groups, the synthesis of the peptide array is completed.

Additional side-chain protection groups at the amino acids (e.g., trityl- (Trt), *tert*-butyl- (*t*Bu), *tert*-butyl-oxy- (O*t*Bu) or 2,2,4,6,7-pentamethyldihydrobenzofuran-5-sulfonyl-groups (Pbf) ensure the formation of defined linear peptides rather than branched molecules. The coupling of each amino acid is followed by N-terminal acetylation of non-elongated peptides. After acetylation, these peptides are excluded from further synthesis, thus preventing the generation of permutations of a given peptide. Notably, those peptides which are (*n-x*)-products (so-called "truncated sequences") of a given peptide can contain a full binding site for a ligand or no binding site. False-positive specificities could be generated if peptides were to comprise sequences in which an amino acid is missing within the binding region (so-called "deletion sequences"). In a second step, the Fmoc-protection group is removed from the elongated peptides by chemical cleavage with piperidine to allow for coupling of another amino acid in the next round of elongation.

Although, typically, peptide arrays comprise peptides of 6–18 amino acids in length, longer peptides have also been reported [9]. The fraction of full-length peptides decreases with increasing chain length due to an imperfect coupling efficiency of the amino acids [10]. As a consequence, the spot size – that is, the amount of starting material – should be increased for the synthesis of longer peptides in order to stay within the detection limits of the subsequent binding assays. On completion of the synthesis, all side chain protection groups are chemically cleaved – typically with trifluoroacetic acid (TFA) in the presence of scavenger cocktails – leaving the covalent bond to the cellulose intact. The peptide arrays can then be used directly for interaction studies.

9.2.2
Fabrication of CelluSpots

In many cases, SPOT arrays can only be used for a single incubation with target interaction partner. Assays such as the identification of enzyme substrates lead to irreversible modifications of the peptides. Moreover, some peptide–ligand complexes resist the regeneration procedure and the ligands cannot be removed quantitatively from the surface. Although this could be circumvented by the use of a larger number of arrays, the production of multiple copies of conventional peptide SPOT arrays with identical quality is both time-consuming and expensive, with each membrane being synthesized individually. Furthermore, parallel incubations for large screening experiments are not feasible with conventional SPOT arrays and, due to their size and porous nature, the required sample volumes are rather large. This hampers interaction studies with proteins of low quantity. All of these aspects are critical for the application of SPOT arrays in HTS settings.

Recently, CelluSpots – a new format of peptide arrays – was developed to overcome these limitations. Here, peptide synthesis is performed by Fmoc chemistry as described above on modified cellulose membranes. After dissolving the cellulose matrix, the peptides remain covalently bound to the dissolved cellulose-polymers, which can be respotted with conventional techniques onto coated microscope slides.

In this way, approximately 800 individual spots can be placed routinely on a standard microscope glass slide. After evaporation of the solvent, the spots remain attached to the glass support during incubation with ligand. By using this procedure, several hundred identical copies of a particular peptide array can be generated.

9.2.3
Generation of Peptide Arrays with a Laser Printer

In order to increase the spot density on peptide arrays, Breitling and colleagues established a color laser printer-based spotting method [11]. Besides increasing the spot density, the major advance of the method is the fast, minute-scale application of the amino acids when compared to conventional, syringe-based dispensing devices. The activated amino acids, which are provided from 20 independent toner cartridges, are embedded in *N,N*-diphenyl formamide, which is solid at room temperature and serves as the toner-particle matrix. After "printing" of the amino acids onto glass slides the solvent is liquid, and coupling of the Fmoc-protected amino acid building blocks to free amino groups of growing peptide chains is possible. Acetylation and Fmoc deprotection are used to prepare for the next coupling cycle, and side chain deprotection after synthesis can be performed as described above. Although a spot density of 400 spots per cm^2 has been described, the technical specifications should allow for more than 10 000 spots per cm^2.

9.2.4
Generation of Peptide Arrays on a Compact Disc Device

In order to generate a fully automated system for SPOT synthesis at high speed, Frank and colleagues have developed a "Bio Disc-Synthesizer", which is capable of dispensing activated amino acids in 2500 defined spots onto a rotating CD-ROM-sized disc within several minutes [12]. The acetylation and Fmoc deprotection steps to prepare for the next coupling cycle and the side chain deprotection after synthesis are also automated. The design of the disc material allows for direct mass spectrometric analysis of ligands captured at the surface, and is therefore of additional advantage. The authors have demonstrated the possibility of synthesizing peptide nucleic acid (PNA) libraries on the disc, which subsequently could be analyzed by using MALDI-TOF mass spectrometry on the same support. It should be noted that other fully automated synthesizers are commercially available (Intavis, MultiSynTech). However, application of the amino acids is time-consuming with these robots (several hours), and the individual monomer solutions must be dispensed by a plunger-driven pipetting needle.

9.2.5
Generation of Peptide Arrays by Chemoselective Immobilization

The immobilization of presynthesized peptide derivatives is the method of choice for long peptide sequences, which normally must be purified to obtain high-quality products. Chemoselective immobilization reactions are of particular interest for the preparation of peptide microarrays, because the orientation of the displayed peptides is controlled.

One intrinsic advantage of chemoselective reactions via N-terminal reactivity tags is the introduction of a purification step. If capping steps are used during peptide assembly, the resulting target peptide derivative is contaminated only by acetylated truncated sequences, and does not contain any deletion sequences. This assumes that the acetylation efficiency is 100% for every step. The final introduction of the chemical moiety, which allows chemoselective immobilization at the N-terminus of the peptide, will result in crude peptides exclusively comprising the target peptide equipped with the reactivity tag. The printing of such crude peptides to appropriately modified surfaces yields a covalent bond between the full-length target peptide derivative and the surface. Truncated and acetylated sequences are not immobilized and can be removed during post-printing processing. The resulting peptide microarrays display purified peptides which are free from deletion sequences, because of the capping steps during synthesis. They also do not contain any truncated sequences, because of the chemoselective immobilization via their N-terminal modification.

An aldehyde function at the surface of glass slides in combination with amino-oxy-acetyl moieties in the peptides [13–18] or cysteinyl-residues [13, 19, 20] were used for the preparation of peptide microarrays. The reaction between cysteine residues and surface-bound maleimide groups was used for preparation of peptide microarrays for kinase [21–26] and protease profiling [27]. Native chemical ligation, as introduced by Dawson *et al.* [28], was used to immobilize cysteine-containing peptides to thioester-modified glass slides [29–31]. A Diels–Alder reaction between benzoquinone groups on self-assembled monolayers and cyclopentadiene–peptide conjugates led to an efficient covalent attachment of kinase substrate peptides [32]. The formation of amide bonds by Staudinger ligation between azide-modified phosphopeptides and appropriate, phosphine-displaying glass surfaces were used for the preparation of phosphopeptide microarrays enabling profiling of protein tyrosine phosphatase activities [33]. A regioselective immobilization of poly(desoxythymidine)-modified kinase substrates onto differently coated glass slides was reported for experiments involving protein kinase A (PKA) and c-Src [34]. Photocleavable, acrylamide-labeled, cysteine-containing kinase substrates were incorporated into peptide–acrylamide copolymer hydrogel surfaces and v-Abl- or c-Abl-mediated phosphorylation was detected by MALDI-TOF/TOF, subsequent to laser-induced cleavage at the β-(2-nitrophenyl)-β-alanine residue [35]. There are several additional chemical procedures used for the chemoselective immobilization of peptides onto different surfaces. These were comprehensively reviewed in Ref. [36], and comprise – for example – the formation of covalent bonds by the reaction of salicylhydroxamic acids with 1,3-phenydiboronic acid derivatives [37–39], alkyne-modified biomolecules with sulfonylazides [40], or semicarbazides with aldehydes [41–45].

9.3
Applications of Peptide Arrays

Peptide arrays can be used in a variety of applications, ranging from simple binding experiments to high-throughput assays with complex mixtures of ligands. Since the SPOT method can be performed as either a manual or an automated procedure, it can be employed by many laboratories to analyze particular interaction pairs. Moreover, several companies offer custom peptide array synthesis. Despite the method itself being established more than 15 years ago, new applications continue to emerge; an overview and some examples are provided in the following sections (Figure 9.2).

9.3.1
Generation of Small Amounts of Soluble Peptide Libraries

SPOT arrays represent a fast and cheap tool to generate analytical quantities of a large set of peptides in parallel. These peptides can either be used bound to the cellulose matrix, or they can be obtained as soluble peptides after cleavage from the membrane. Peptide cleavage requires a cleavable linker coupled to the solid support prior to coupling of the first amino acid. The Fmoc-protected Rink linker [46] and Fmoc-protected photolabile linker [47] are the most commonly used versions, although other linkers have also been described [48]. The photolabile linker

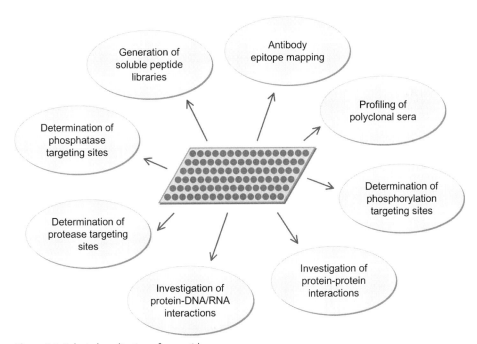

Figure 9.2 Selected applications for peptide arrays.

is favored, as it is resistant to the TFA treatment which is used to cleave off all side-chain protection groups after peptide synthesis. Therefore, remnants of the chemicals used for side-chain deprotection can be removed prior to photocleavage of the linker with UV light at 365 nm. Although photocleavage might damage some peptides, the resultant peptides are of high purity. Alternatively, peptides can be cleaved from the membrane by aminolysis or hydrolysis of the C-terminal ester bond using ammonia gas [49, 50] or aqueous triethylamine solution [14, 15, 17], respectively. The typical yields of peptides recovered by these procedures are between 0.4 and 0.6 µmol of peptide per cm² [5].

9.3.2
Epitope Mapping of Monoclonal Antibodies

The best established and most widely used application of peptide arrays is the mapping of antibody epitopes. For this purpose, the SPOT technique is used to synthesize arrays comprised of overlapping peptides (typically 15mers) which cover the entire protein or the relevant domains of interest. For binding studies, the arrays are incubated with antibody solutions in a manner similar to an immunoblot. Studies were performed to map the epitopes of antibodies in polyclonal sera [51–53], of monoclonal antibodies (mAbs) [54–58], and of recombinant antibody fragments [58–61]. Most of the identified epitopes comprise linear sequences shorter than ten amino acids. However, there are many examples where conformational epitopes occur; that is, the actual epitope is formed by a three-dimensional (3-D) arrangement of sequences, and it is not colinearly represented in the primary amino acid sequence [62–64]. Sufficient affinity of the antibody paratope to the individual epitope elements is a prerequisite for the identification of these complex epitopes, and even weak interactions with dissociation constants in the range of 10^{-3} to $10^{-4}M$ remain detectable [65, 66] in the array experiments. In the case of assembled epitopes, the availability of a 3-D structure of the target protein is useful, and helps to validate that the partial epitopes are localized in close proximity at the accessible protein surface. Moreover, special computer software is available to map linear peptide sequences on the 3-D structure of a protein [67, 68]. It should be noted that an identified sequence stretch buried within the protein structure might either be an artifact due to unspecific binding, or explained by different conformations of the protein in the native and crystallized state. As an example, conformational epitopes can be located in rather simple 3-D structures such as α-helices. In most cases, the determination of these is less challenging than for the more complex conformational epitopes, which are assembled from sequence stretches far apart on primary sequence, as 15mer peptides will form α-helices on the cellulose membrane [61, 69, 70].

In some cases a more detailed characterization of the epitope sequence and its interaction with the paratope is needed. This requires the identification of a sequence, which contains the antibody epitope, the minimal epitope, as well as the contacting amino acids. They can be determined on peptide arrays of N- and C-terminally truncated variants of the parental peptide, and variants in which successive exchanges of all amino acid positions have been performed [71]. As a representative example, a complex systematic epitope mapping study of a phosphotyrosine-specific antibody on microarrays is shown in Figure 9.3.

9.3.3
Investigation of Antibody Epitopes in Polyclonal Sera

Polyclonal sera contain antibodies of different specificities, and can bind for example to different separate or overlapping epitopes of a particular antigen. The

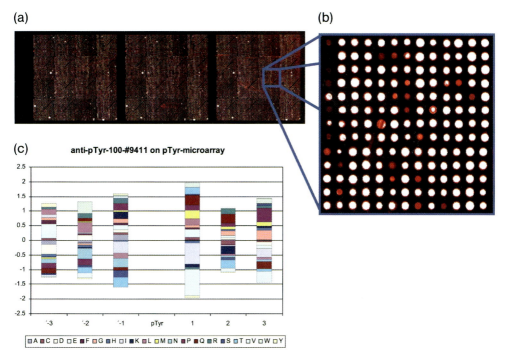

Figure 9.3 Profiling of an anti-phosphotyrosine antibody. (a) Fluorescence image of a peptide microarray displaying 6262 phosphotyrosine-containing peptides derived from annotated human protein phosphorylation sites together with background controls and fluorescent landmarks. Three identical subarrays result in 3 × 6262 = 18 786 data points. The microarray was incubated with a phosphotyrosine-specific antibody, followed by a fluorescently labeled secondary antibody; (b) The enlarged image shows strong signals (white color equal to the saturated signal at the used laser settings) and weak signals (red color); (c) The statistical analysis of detected strong binding phosphotyrosine-epitopes. The probability of each amino acid residue relative to the phosphotyrosine moiety is compared to the probability of each residue relative to phosphotyrosine in all displayed peptides. If a residue is preferred among the 5665 strongly binding phosphopeptides, the value is positive and proportional to preference. If a residue is disfavored at a given position, the values will be negative. The color code for amino acid residues is shown at the bottom of the graph. Amino acid residues with branched side chains (e.g., Val, Ile) that are C-terminal to the phosphotyrosine residue yield binders with low affinities. Notably, a peptide sequence composed of only disfavored residues (corresponding to negative values) will most likely result in a peptide which is no longer recognized as an epitope by that particular antibody.

recognition of different binding sites can either indicate the presence of different antibody populations within the serum sample, or be a consequence of cross-reactivity of a particular antibody. These scenarios are important in the development of antibody-mediated autoimmune diseases. SPOT arrays allow for the affinity purification of polyclonal antibodies on adjacent or immunologically related epitopes. Subsequently, the binding characteristics of these antibodies can be analyzed in competition assays with soluble peptides of the different recognized epitopes in a 96-well format by using enzyme-linked immunosorbent assay (ELISA) [52, 72, 73]. In addition, this procedure can be used not only for the mapping of antibody epitopes but also for the small-scale affinity purification and investigation of any other interaction partners in solution.

9.3.4
Investigation of Protein–Protein Interactions

9.3.4.1 General Considerations

A large proportion of folded proteins interact via the surfaces of exposed hydrophobic or hydrophilic amino acid side chains. This is similar to antibodies, which recognize conformational epitopes. The amino acids are assembled in the same surface area, but are not necessarily colinear on the primary sequence level. In order to characterize the interaction interface of two proteins, the identification of all contact sites is essential. To address this question, the SPOT technology can be used to screen an array of overlapping peptides covering the sequence of a target protein interaction domain with a soluble ligand protein. Both, linear as well as assembled/conformational binding sites have been identified [74–82]. Bound proteins can be detected by means of standard reagents, for example horseradish peroxidase (HRP)-conjugated primary or secondary antibodies or a streptavidin–HRP conjugate in the case of a biotinylated ligand [83]. Furthermore, radioactively labeled ligands, obtained by *in vitro* translation, or electrotransfer of bound ligands to nitrocellulose, can be employed for subsequent detection. This increases the signal-to-background ratio and minimizes the interference of the detection system, for example steric hindrance due to bound antibody, with the interaction. Notably, spot arrays can be repeatedly incubated with the same ligand, always followed by electrotransfer of the bound ligand to the same nitrocellulose membrane prior to the detection procedure. Regardless of the method used, the analysis of protein–protein interactions is challenging as most such interactions are much weaker (μM range) than paratope–epitope interactions of antibodies (nM–pM range). Therefore, interaction studies require optimization with regards to blocking conditions, buffer composition (e.g., salt, ionic strength, pH), incubation time and temperature, as well as the detection system, to minimize unspecific binding without affecting the actual interaction. Although these procedures might be tedious, they are of paramount importance in order to achieve reliable results. The need to search for the correct incubation conditions might complicate HTS approaches (as discussed below). Notably, information on the 3-D structure of at least one of the two interacting partners can be very helpful for confirming the accessibility of the interaction surface and distinguishing any potential screening artifacts from an assembled docking site.

A variety of proteins interact by the specific recognition of post-translational modifications. Among these are phosphorylation, sulfation, acetylation, glycosylation, ubiquitinylation, sumoylation, and methylation. Often, these modifications are recognized by specialized protein interaction domains (e.g., SH2, SH3, WW, PDZ, Chromo, Bromo domains) within a defined sequence context. The *in vitro* affinities of these interactions lie in the micromolar range and, as many of these protein–protein interactions are mediated by domain binding to a linear binding site, peptide arrays have proven very useful in their investigation [78, 84–86].

The reversible phosphorylation of serine, threonine, and tyrosine residues plays a crucial role in the downstream signaling of cell-surface receptors, the coordination of the cell cycle, and the regulation of protein activities, for example transcription factors. Many of these phosphorylated proteins are components of signaling cascades, and comprise binding modules for target sequences and kinase domains. In a cascade-like fashion, these activities can phosphorylate further downstream effectors and thus can branch out or amplify signaling events. The deregulation of phosphorylation cascades is associated with severe disease. To gain insight into these complex signaling pathways, investigations into the interactions of individual proteins involved are of major importance [87].

9.3.4.2 Identification of Enzyme Substrates

Measuring the activity of enzymes that modify peptides involves either the addition of chemical moieties to displayed peptides (kinases, acetyl transferases, glycosyltransferases, ADP-ribosyl transferases, etc.) or the release of a part of the immobilized peptide derivative (proteases, phosphatases, demethylases, etc.). In principle, all enzymes modifying peptides or proteins can be applied to screen peptide arrays.

In order to analyze the phosphorylation of peptides by a specific kinase on peptide arrays, three different types of assay are available (Figure 9.4).

The incorporated phosphate moiety can be modified, for example through the use of the radioisotopes ^{32}P or ^{33}P [15, 17, 18, 88, 89], followed by phosphoimaging or photographic emulsions that deposit silver grains directly onto the glass surface [97], by thiophosphate [98] which can be detected electrochemically using gold nanoparticles [98], by biotinylated phosphate derivatives [91, 92], or by ferrocene-labeled phosphate [90] which can be detected electrochemically. Alternatively, the attached phosphate residue can be recognized by phosphospecific reagents (protein domains, antibodies [15, 16, 30, 31, 93], or chelating molecules [21, 22, 25, 26, 94, 99–101]) which are labeled directly or can be visualized by indirect methods such as surface plasmon resonance (SPR) [21, 22, 25, 32], resonance light scattering [92, 102], and MALDI-TOF mass spectrometry [103, 104]). Additionally, kinase-mediated phosphorylation can be detected, subsequent to chemical modification of the resulting phosphopeptide. Shults *et al.* [96] reported the carbodiimide-mediated, selective formation of a covalent bond between a fluorescent dye derivative and the phosphate moiety, while Akita *et al.* [95] used β-elimination to

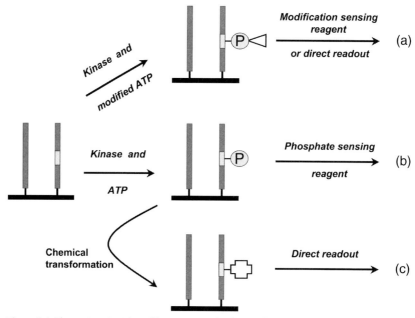

Figure 9.4 The main principles of kinase assays on peptide microarrays. (a) Kinase-mediated transfer of modified phosphate residues from γ-labeled-ATP to surface-bound peptides results in labeled phosphopeptides which can be detected by phosphoimaging, electrochemically or with surface plasmon resonance/fluorescence if radioisotopically labeled ATP [15, 17, 18, 88, 89], ferrocene-labeled ATP [90] or biotinylated ATP [91, 92] in combination with streptavidin are used; (b) Kinase-mediated phosphate transfer yields bound phosphopeptides which will capture phosphospecific reagents, such as phosphospecific antibodies [15, 16, 30, 32, 93] or fluorescent dyes such as ProQ-Diamond [94]. Bound phosphate-sensing molecules can be detected directly by fluorescence imaging if the molecule itself is fluorescently labeled, or indirectly by incubation with secondary reagents which interact specifically with a phosphate-sensing moiety; (c) Bound phosphopeptides generated by kinase action can be transformed by a selective chemical reaction into peptide derivatives which react chemoselectively with fluorescently labeled reagents [95, 96]. The fluorescence signals generated can be read by fluorescence imaging. Mixed forms of these assay principles were reported, such as the enzymatic introduction of thiophosphate moieties, which were chemoselectively transformed via Michael addition into biotinylated phosphopeptides.

selectively transform cellulose-surface-bound phosphopeptides into dehydroalanine-containing peptides which could be labeled with reactive fluorescent dyes. A representative example of a kinase screening performed on peptide microarrays in the presence of γ-^{33}P-ATP is shown in Figure 9.5.

Several types of library were used for kinase profiling on peptide arrays. Identification of the actual amino acid residue which serves as an acceptor of the phosphate group is achieved by scans of overlapping peptides derived from the entire sequence of the substrate protein in question [18]. Alternatively, libraries of peptides covering only the sequence around potential phosphoacceptor residues have been used [105, 106]. Similarly, the sequences of experimentally identified phos-

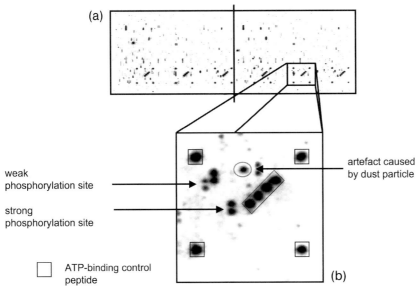

Figure 9.5 Results of kinase screening using peptide microarrays. (a) Phosphoimage of a peptide microarray, displaying overlapping peptides in quadruplicates covering all human cyclophilins, subsequent to incubation with protein kinase Cα kinase in the presence of γ-^{33}P-ATP. The black spots represent peptide spots which are labeled by the incorporation of ^{33}P-phosphate moieties. The vertical, solid line separates the two identical subarrays; (b) Enlarged region within one subarray. ATP binding control spots (eight identical peptide spots which are known to capture ATP from the assay solution) are visible at the edges of the square and as a diagonal line (marked with squares). The diagonal line of control spots enables proper orientation of the phosphoimage. Additionally, strong and weak phosphorylation sites are visible as pairs of spots which are arranged side by side. This arrangement enables the easy identification of artifacts which would result in single spots only.

phorylation sites, found in databases and the literature, were comprehensively evaluated on peptide arrays [14–16, 18, 23, 24, 77, 89, 107–115]. An extension to the knowledge-based libraries' concept is provided by the introduction of post-translational modifications into the peptide sequences. Phosphorylation, methylation, or acetylation within the peptide sequences can affect the substrate specificity. This more adequately mimics the cellular environment in which these modifications occur as initial priming events for subsequent kinase reactions. Such modifications can be introduced enzymatically after chemical synthesis of the unmodified peptides on the chips [18], or chemically by using modified building blocks for the peptide synthesis on the chips [18]. On-chip-chemistry using chemoselective chemical reactions can also be used; this was achieved by the selective acetylation of lysine side chains in microarray-bound peptides [100].

For the *de novo* detection of kinase substrates, both combinatorial approaches and randomly generated libraries of individual peptides have proved to be useful. As a characteristic feature, combinatorial libraries display one or more defined amino acid at a particular position and a number of randomized amino acids at others [30, 116–121]. Only one particular amino acid is introduced at the defined positions, whilst a mixture of amino acids is introduced at the randomized positions. This results in a mixture of different sequences in each single spot. Once the amino acids that are amenable for phosphorylation by a given kinase have been identified at the defined positions, the remaining randomized positions must be deconvoluted using follow-up combinations. Combinatorial libraries were successfully used with cellulose membranes as the solid support. However, the equal representation of each single sequence of a peptide mixture is not guaranteed when using peptide microarrays on glass slides, because of the low concentration of each individual peptide per spot [30].

The impressive miniaturization of peptide libraries possible on planar surfaces, such as glass slides, enables the application of randomly generated libraries of single peptides that cover a significant (although not complete) part of the potential sequence space. Such randomly generated libraries for kinase substrate identification and kinase profiling have a defined phosphoacceptor residue and random sequences in the flanking areas [17]. In contrast to combinatorial libraries. each spot represents one single sequence. If information on the consensus sequence for the substrates of a kinase is available, the random libraries can be biased by introducing certain amino acids at defined positions derived from the consensus sequences. Randomly generated libraries show a higher sequence diversity compared to knowledge-based libraries, which are biased towards known kinase substrates. However, this can be an advantage when searching for selective substrates for closely related enzymes.

The *substrate characteristics* – that is, the key interaction residues – can be deduced from all these library types by using statistical analysis, provided that the number of identified substrates is high enough [15, 17, 116, 117, 120–122]. Alternatively, different library types based on single substrate sequences, such as alanine scans, deletion [30] and so-called "substitutional libraries", which represent combinations of all possible amino acid scans in one experiment [14, 114, 123, 124], permit comprehensive substrate characterization.

The dephosphorylation of proteins by specific phosphatases is used to switch off signaling cascades. This represents a means of downregulating a pathway and generating transient signals. In a subsequent round of stimulation, a target protein can be rephosphorylated to participate in another round of signaling. Dephosphorylation can exert two principal effects: (i) it might inactivate the intrinsic activity of a target protein; or (ii) it might mask a phosphorylation-dependent binding site for an interaction partner (e.g., SH2-domain-containing protein). Both effects lead to a rapid attenuation of the activating signal due to disruption of the cascade.

In general, each assay which is suited for kinase profiling on peptide (micro) arrays can also be adapted for the analysis of the phosphatase-mediated release of phosphate moieties from phosphopeptides. For this purpose, surface-bound phosphopeptides can be generated either enzymatically [93] or chemically [93, 125–129]. Phosphatase action can be detected on (micro)array bound phosphopeptides by the decrease of a signal generated by the binding of phosphotyrosine antibodies [93, 125, 126] or phosphospecific dyes [129, 130].

Proteases play a major role in protein maturation and degradation. Hence, the identification of protease substrates and protease substrate specificities is essential for an understanding of important cellular processes. Several assay principles have been developed to measure protease activity on peptide arrays. The assays measure increased signal intensity upon substrate cleavage, which can result from a quantitation of the released proteolytic fragments [131–135] or the fragments retained on the surface [136, 137].

In order to measure the release of proteolytic fragments, individual peptide spots from peptide arrays with a terminal fluorescent label are transferred to 96-well plates and incubated with protease samples. Release of the fluorescent label into the solvent can be quantified using a fluorescence plate reader, in a time-dependent manner, which allows kinetic measurements to be made [132]. Another sophisticated procedure involves the synthesis of peptides on cellulose membranes with an antibody epitope tag comprising a biotinylated lysine residue at their N-terminus. Protease-mediated cleavage releases the N-terminal part of a substrate peptide, including the epitope tag and the biotin moiety. This fragment can be affinity-blotted onto a streptavidin-coated PVDF membrane and detected via an enzyme-conjugated antibody [138]. A similar procedure was used by Kozlov *et al.* [139] in combination with DNA-encoded substrates and DNA-microarrays as a sorting device. Cleavage site peptides flanked by biotin on one side and a penta-histidine tag/DNA tag on the other side, were incubated with different proteases or cell lysates. Streptavidin-coated magnetic beads were used to remove non-cleaved peptides and biotinylated cleavage fragments, such that the remaining members of the library represented His-tagged DNA encoded fragments of cleaved substrates. These could be detected and deconvoluted using anti-penta-histidine antibodies and fluorescence imaging, subsequent to hybridization onto appropriate DNA microarrays [139]. Surface-bound proteolytic fragments can be detected through an increase in signal using internally fluorescence quenched peptides [136, 137] or peptide derivatives containing a substituted fluorogenic group C-terminal to the scissile bond [140]. Alternatively, proteolytic activity can be followed by monitoring removal of the detection moieties from the displayed peptide and a loss of signal. Biotinylated peptides synthesized on cellulose membranes were used to detect the protease cleavage sites [4].

Recently, Langedijk and colleagues [141] have established an interaction screen in order to analyze the specificity and selectivity of the small-ubiquitin like modifiers' (SUMO) target sites. Reminiscent of ubiquitylation, the sumoylation of target proteins is involved in the regulation of a variety of cellular processes. By sumoylation of peptide arrays, the authors were able to characterize the consensus motif for lysine-specific sumoylation sites and the contribution of flanking amino acids to the selectivity and specificity of the modification. Moreover, the substrate specificities of lysine methyltransferases [80, 142], peptidyl-prolyl *cis/trans* isomerases [143, 144], glycosyltransferases [145, 146], ADP-ribosyltransferases [147], hydrolases [140], and esterases [148] have been profiled using peptide (micro)arrays.

9.3.5
Mapping of Protein–Nucleic Acid Interactions

Many cellular processes, including DNA condensation, transcription, translation, DNA/RNA stabilization, DNA/RNA degradation and restriction, depend on specific interactions of proteins with nucleic acids. As an example, SPOT arrays have been used to identify the DNA-binding domains of the restriction endonuclease *Eco*RII [149]. Overlapping peptide arrays derived from the *Eco*RII sequence were probed with radioactively labeled substrate DNA. Visualization of the bound DNA with a phosphoimager then led to the identification of two DNA binding regions within *Eco*RII of approximately 20 amino acids.

Protein–RNA interactions are more difficult to map, because RNA molecules are rather unstable. However, the elucidation of these interactions is crucial for many cellular processes. They are also essential for the development of antiviral therapies, as many pathogenic viruses contain RNA genomes. In order to interfere with the packaging of HIV genomes, as a potential therapeutic approach, a screening and detection system was recently developed for peptide–RNA interactions based on the SPOT method [150] (Figure 9.6). The highly structured RNA packaging signal Ψ of the human immunodeficiency virus (HIV-1) comprises approximately 120 nucleotides, consists of four stem loops (SLs), and is localized at the 5′ untranslated region (UTR) of the HIV-1 genome. Interaction of the Ψ-RNA structure with the nucleocapsid NCp7 of the HIV-1 Gagpol precursor protein during virus assembly, results in the specific encapsidation of viral RNA genomes, but not cellular RNAs, into nascent virus particles [151]. As a robust detection system, *in vitro*-transcribed Ψ-RNA or control RNA was hybridized with an HRP-conjugated oligonucleotide complementary to the 5′ end of the RNA. Arrays of 6mer peptides flanked by glycine-serine linkers were incubated with the Ψ-RNA/DNA-HRP-hybrid, and bound RNA was visualized using chemiluminescence imaging. Finally, membranes could be reused after a stripping procedure which included an RNAse digestion step. As a result, it was possible to identify a peptide sequence which bound specifically and with high affinity to the Ψ-RNA, and to show antiviral activity by interference with packaging of HIV-1 genomes *in vivo* [150].

9.3.6
Screening for Antimicrobial Peptides

The innate immune system employs peptides which are toxic to bacteria to defend the body against invading pathogens. However, this concept can also be exploited for the discovery and development of novel therapeutics against, for example, antibiotic-resistant pathogenic microorganisms such as *Staphylococcus aureus*, *Klebsiella pneumoniae* or *Pseudomonas aeruginosa*. For this, SPOT arrays were employed in *in vivo* screens for antimicrobial peptides [152, 153]. In order to select cationic antimicrobial peptides as leads for the generation of novel antimicrobials, bacteria were transformed with the *luxCDABE* (luciferase) gene cassette, which

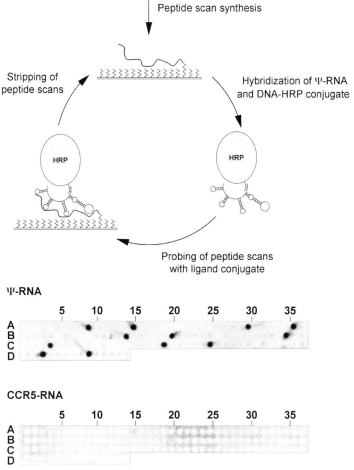

Figure 9.6 HIV-1 Ψ-RNA binding to peptide arrays. Arrays of permutations of the peptide HWWPWW were probed with Ψ-RNA and CCR5-RNA (negative control). Bound RNA was visualized by chemiluminescence imaging. Modified with permission from Ref. [150]; © Wiley-VCH Verlag GmbH & Co. KGaA.

causes the bacteria to luminesce. A decrease in the bacterial energy level, triggered by for example the antimicrobial activity of a particular peptide, can be detected and quantified as a reduction in luminescence. The authors have released peptides from immobilized libraries and transferred the soluble peptides to 96-well plates, in serial dilutions. Live bacteria were incubated with the peptides and monitored for reduced luminescence, indicative of the therapeutic potential of the peptide.

9.3.7
Identification, Characterization, and Optimization of Peptidic Ligands

Peptide arrays have been applied to identify peptide ligands for a particular protein or other binding partners. As the initial hits are usually suboptimal with respect to affinity, specificity or stability, substitutional analysis represents an ideal tool to optimize these properties. It is possible to gain, simultaneously, additional information about any structure–activity relationships, and this was carried out for the optimization of the Strep-tag II interacting with streptavidin [154], and also for the identification and optimization of peptides binding blood coagulation factor VIII (FVIII). This peptide can be used as an affinity ligand in the purification of FVIII, which is administered to treat patients with hemophilia A [155].

Unnatural amino acids – especially D-amino acids – can be incorporated into peptides in order to stabilize them against proteolytic degradation, although it is difficult to predict which amino acids can be substituted without altering the peptide's biological properties. To address this point, Kramer *et al.* [156] described a stepwise systematic analysis in which all-L-amino acids in an epitope were replaced with all-D-amino acids. A complete array-based D-amino acid substitution analysis was performed in the first transformation cycle. One peptide (containing one D-amino acid) with the same binding activity was selected and used for the next transformation cycle and the conversion of a second position into a D-amino acid. Finally, all-D-peptides with completely different side-chain functionalities which retained antibody binding specificity and affinity were identified. A similar procedure was described to optimize a vascular endothelial growth factor (VEGF) -inhibiting peptide derived from the VEGF receptor II sequence [157], whereby amino acids in four positions were replaced by D-amino acids [158]. Wildemann *et al.* [144] described a systematic approach for the optimization of peptidic substrates/inhibitor for peptidyl prolyl *cis/trans* isomerase Pin1 using peptide arrays on cellulose membranes. Thousands of (phospho)-peptides, each containing several nonproteinogenic amino acid residues, were synthesized using the SPOT technique and screened for binding to either the Pin1-isomerase domain alone or the full-length Pin1, composed of the isomerase domain and a WW-domain. This approach yielded inhibitor molecules with affinities in the low nanomolar range which were selective for the two different domains.

9.3.8
Identification of Metal Ion-Selective Peptides

Combinatorial peptide libraries on cellulose membranes were utilized to study the interaction of peptides with different metal ions. This included the chromogenic detection of Ni^{2+}, Pb^{2+} and Ag^+ ions by reduction to the colloidal state, as well as assays with radioactive isotopes – that is, $^{45}Ca^{2+}$, $^{55}Fe^{3+}$ and technetium-99m ions [159–161]. Of particular interest is the identification of technetium-99m binding hexapeptides using an 8000-membered combinatorial peptide library array of the type $O_1XO_2XO_3X$, where X represents a mixture of amino acids and O represents a defined residue [162]. These peptides were intended for tumor imaging applications upon genetic fusion to an anti-carcinoembryonic antigen antibody. The binding of Pb^{2+} and As^{3+} to four different dansyl-labeled peptides displayed on peptide microarrays was shown [163, 164]. The binding of metal ions was monitored by fluorescence changes.

9.4
Challenges in High-Throughput Screening (HTS)

Peptide arrays immobilized on solid supports allow the automated HTS of large "interactomes" (for a review, see Ref. [148]). Although multiple measurements of the same sample are feasible for statistically significant and reproducible datasets, these platforms face a variety of challenges:

- HTS generates an enormous amount of data, especially when entire proteomes are probed. Besides data storage and data management, which often require non-standard solutions, the major issue is how the information relating to a particular interaction can be extracted from the bulk measurement.

- Although a particular interaction might be highly reproducible under conditions found on the chip, it might not be relevant *in vivo*. This could occur for several reasons:

  ○ The two interaction partners are present in separate cellular compartments.

  ○ The interaction sites are not available for interactions because they are not exposed on the protein surface due to a particular conformation *in vivo*, or due to interference by another interacting protein.

  ○ Secondary modifications of particular amino acids *in vivo* might inactivate the binding site.

  ○ The cellular compartments where the proteins reside might exhibit pH and ionic strength conditions which prevent interaction. Therefore, data obtained from interaction screening requires careful validation in a cellular context. As these data are mostly unavailable from publications, and automation is difficult to adapt to this task, these studies are time-consuming and require a skilled bench scientist.

- The identification of all *in vivo* interaction partners of a query protein might not be achieved on chip because:

  ○ Two proteins interact transiently or with an affinity below the detection limit determined by the experimental conditions of the array.

  ○ The detection system for the ligand, for example a labeled antibody, interferes with the binding interface.

  ○ An additional factor/interaction partner is required for stable interaction.

- The instrumentation for HTS and the screen itself is expensive, thus limiting global approaches to specialized research centers and companies. In this regard, proceeding miniaturization of the arrays will further reduce the costs per individual query. However, the fidelity of the screen is inversely correlated with the reaction volume as the physical constraints in the nanoscopic world are technically difficult to handle.

In addition to these limitations, a variety of other parameters must be considered during investigations of the binding properties of an individual protein. When antibody epitope mapping studies are conducted, the general incubation conditions might be similar for many samples. The analysis of other protein–protein interactions might require individual adaptations of the protocol, and in this regard the choice of blocking reagent to saturate unspecific binding sites is critical. If the stringency of blocking is too low, then the background signals will create too many irrelevant hits. However, if the stringency of blocking is too high, this might prevent the actual interaction. Frequently used blocking solutions are adapted from those used for immunoblotting, and are based on non-ionic detergents such as Tween-20 or Triton X-100, the milk casein proteins (usually obtained in the form of skimmed milk powder), bovine serum albumin or whole sera of different species, for example human or horse [165, 166]. In many cases, mixtures of the compounds listed above are used and supplemented with gelatin or sucrose to increase the viscosity of the solution. For optimal results different conditions must be tested which, again, increases the load of data which must ultimately be evaluated.

9.5
Future Perspectives

In order to elucidate complex protein–protein and protein–nucleic acid interaction networks, SPOT arrays have proven to be a cheap, reliable and a convenient tool. Moreover, as the method allows not only for manual but also automated synthesis, it can be employed by many laboratories. Although, the method itself was established more than 15 years ago, new applications continue to emerge. For example, only recently Honda and colleagues [167] used peptide arrays to identify cell-adhesive peptides that could enhance cell growth as a tissue engineering scaffold. Here, the peptide arrays were probed with live cells, and the interacting spots identified by means of calcein violet AM ester, a cell-permeable substrate which is converted to a polyanionic fluorescent dye (calcein violet, excitation/emission 400/452 nm) by ubiquitous intracellular esterases. This development might allow for the systematic screening of receptor–ligand and cell–cell interactions at the plasma membrane. Likewise, Frank and colleagues [168] reported the use of peptide arrays as a panning surface in phage display. Further improvements of this technique should allow for the rapid parallel selection of recombinant antibodies or interaction partners from phage libraries. Although the available platforms are complementary, peptide microarrays produced by the immobilization of peptides on glass surfaces have several advantages when compared to the classical SPOT membranes. Notably, they allow the reduction of sample volume due to miniaturization and the easy production of copies of synthesized libraries. This assay format will continue to attract research teams from different disciplines, and stimulate the development of novel applications.

Acknowledgments

The Georg-Speyer-Haus is supported by the Bundesministerium für Gesundheit (BfG) and the Hessisches Ministerium für Wissenschaft und Kunst (HMWK). The authors thank Dr. Manuel Grez for his critical reading of the manuscript and helpful discussions.

Abbreviations

CDR(s)	complementarity-determining region(s)
ELISA	enzyme-linked immunosorbent assay
Fmoc	9-fluorenyl-methoxycarbonyl
HIV	human immunodeficiency virus
HRP	horseradish peroxidase
HTS	high-throughput screening
mAb	monoclonal antibody
PKA	protein kinase A
PNA	peptide nucleic acid

References

1 Frank, R. (1992) Spot-synthesis: an easy technique for the positionally addressable, parallel chemical synthesis on a membrane support. *Tetrahedron*, **48** (42), 9217–32.

2 Koch, J. and Mahler, M. (2002) *Peptide Arrays on Membrane Supports*, Springer, Berlin, Heidelberg.

3 Kramer, A. and Schneider-Mergener, J. (1998) Synthesis and screening of peptide libraries on continuous cellulose membrane supports. *Methods Mol. Biol.*, 87, 25–39.

4 Winkler, D.F. and McGeer, P.L. (2008) Protein labeling and biotinylation of peptides during spot synthesis using biotin p-nitrophenyl ester (biotin-ONp). *Proteomics*, **8** (5), 961–7.

5 Hilpert, K., Winkler, D.F. and Hancock, R.E. (2007) Peptide arrays on cellulose support: SPOT synthesis, a time and cost efficient method for synthesis of large numbers of peptides in a parallel and addressable fashion. *Nat. Protoc.*, **2** (6), 1333–49.

6 Zander, N. (2004) New planar substrates for the in situ synthesis of peptide arrays. *Mol. Divers.*, **8** (3), 189–95.

7 Merrifield, R.B. (1963) Solid phase peptide synthesis. I. The synthesis of a tetrapeptide. *J. Am. Chem. Soc.*, **85**, 2149–54.

8 Koch, J. and Mahler, M. (eds) (2002) *Peptide Arrays on Membrane Supports*, Springer, Berlin, Heidelberg.

9 Toepert, F., Knaute, T., Guffler, S., Pires, J.R., Matzdorf, T., Oschkinat, H. and Schneider-Mergener, J. (2003) Combining SPOT synthesis and native peptide ligation to create large arrays of WW protein domains. *Angew. Chem. Int. Ed. Engl.*, **42** (10), 1136–40.

10 Fields, G.B. and Noble, R.L. (1990) Solid phase peptide synthesis utilizing 9-fluorenylmethoxycarbonyl amino acids. *Int. J. Pept. Protein Res.*, **35** (3), 161–214.

11 Stadler, V., Felgenhauer, T., Beyer, M., Fernandez, S., Leibe, K., Güttler, S., Gröning, M., König, K., Torralba, G., Hausmann, M., Lindenstruth, V., Nesterov, A., Block, I., Pipkorn, R., Poustka, A., Bischoff, F.R. and Breitling, F. (2008) Combinatorial synthesis of peptide arrays with a laser printer. *Angew. Chem. Int. Ed. Engl.*, **47**, 1–5.

12 Dikmans, A.J., Morr, M., Zander, N., Adler, F., Türk, G. and Frank, R. (2004) A new compact disc format of high density array synthesis applied to peptide nucleic acids and in situ MALDI analysis. *Mol. Divers.*, **8** (3), 197–207.

13 Falsey, J.R., Renil, M., Park, S., Li, S. and Lam, K.S. (2001) Peptide and small molecule microarray for high throughput cell adhesion and functional assays. *Bioconjug. Chem.*, **12** (3), 346–53.

14 Lizcano, J.M., Deak, M., Morrice, N., Kieloch, A., Hastie, C.J., Dong, L., Schutkowski, M., Reimer, U. and Alessi, D.R. (2002) Molecular basis for the substrate specificity of NIMA-related kinase-6 (NEK6). Evidence that NEK6 does not phosphorylate the hydrophobic motif of ribosomal S6 protein kinase and serum- and glucocorticoid-induced protein kinase in vivo. *J. Biol. Chem.*, **277** (31), 27839–49.

15 Panse, S., Dong, L., Burian, A., Carus, R., Schutkowski, M., Reimer, U. and Schneider-Mergener, J. (2004) Profiling of generic anti-phosphopeptide antibodies and kinases with peptide microarrays using radioactive and fluorescence-based assays. *Mol. Divers.*, **8** (3), 291–9.

16 Reimer, U., Reineke, U. and Schneider-Mergener, J. (2002) Peptide arrays: from macro to micro. *Curr. Opin. Biotechnol.*, **13** (4), 315–20.

17 Rychlewski, L., Kschischo, M., Dong, L., Schutkowski, M. and Reimer, U. (2004) Target specificity analysis of the Abl kinase using peptide microarray data. *J. Mol. Biol.*, **336** (2), 307–11.

18 Schutkowski, M., Reimer, U., Panse, S., Dong, L., Lizcano, J.M., Alessi, D.R. and Schneider-Mergener, J. (2004) High-content peptide microarrays for deciphering kinase specificity and biology. *Angew. Chem. Int. Ed. Engl.*, **43** (20), 2671–4.

19 Inoue, Y., Mori, T., Yamanouchi, G., Han, X., Sonoda, T., Niidome, T. and Katayama, Y. (2008) Surface plasmon resonance imaging measurements of caspase reactions on peptide microarrays. *Anal. Biochem.*, **375** (1), 147–9.

20 Lesaicherre, M.L., Uttamchandani, M., Chen, G.Y. and Yao, S.Q. (2002) Developing site-specific immobilization strategies of peptides in a microarray. *Bioorg. Med. Chem. Lett.*, **12** (16), 2079–83.

21 Inamori, K., Kyo, M., Matsukawa, K., Inoue, Y., Sonoda, T., Tatematsu, K., Tanizawa, K., Mori, T. and Katayama, Y. (2008) Optimal surface chemistry for peptide immobilization in on-chip phosphorylation analysis. *Anal. Chem.*, **80** (3), 643–50.

22 Inamori, K., Kyo, M., Nishiya, Y., Inoue, Y., Sonoda, T., Kinoshita, E., Koike, T. and Katayama, Y. (2005) Detection and quantification of on-chip phosphorylated peptides by surface plasmon resonance imaging techniques using a phosphate capture molecule. *Anal. Chem.*, **77** (13), 3979–85.

23 Lemeer, S., Jopling, C., Naji, F., Ruijtenbeek, R., Slijper, M., Heck, A.J. and den Hertog, J. (2007) Protein-tyrosine kinase activity profiling in knock down zebrafish embryos. *PLoS ONE*, **2** (7), e581.

24 Lemeer, S., Ruijtenbeek, R., Pinkse, M.W., Jopling, C., Heck, A.J., den Hertog, J. and Slijper, M. (2007) Endogenous phosphotyrosine signaling in zebrafish embryos. *Mol. Cell. Proteomics*, **6** (12), 2088–99.

25 Mori, T., Inamori, K., Inoue, Y., Han, X., Yamanouchi, G., Niidome, T. and Katayama, Y. (2008) Evaluation of protein kinase activities of cell lysates using peptide microarrays based on surface plasmon resonance imaging. *Anal. Biochem.*, **375** (2), 223–31.

26 Shigaki, S., Yamaji, T., Han, X., Yamanouchi, G., Sonoda, T., Okitsu, O., Mori, T., Niidome, T. and Katayama, Y. (2007) A peptide microarray for the detection of protein kinase activity in cell lysate. *Anal. Sci.*, **23** (3), 271–5.

27 Han, A., Sonoda, T., Kang, J.H., Murata, M., Niidome, T. and Katayam, Y. (2006) Development of a fluorescence peptide chip for the detection of caspase activity. *Comb. Chem. High Throughput Screen.*, **9** (1), 21–5.

28 Dawson, P.E., Muir, T.W., Clark-Lewis, I. and Kent, S.B. (1994) Synthesis of proteins by native chemical ligation. *Science*, **266** (5186), 776–9.

29 Lesaicherre, M.L., Uttamchandani, M., Chen, G.Y. and Yao, S.Q. (2002) Antibody-based fluorescence detection of kinase activity on a peptide array. *Bioorg. Med. Chem. Lett.*, **12** (16), 2085–8.

30 Uttamchandani, M., Chan, E.W., Chen, G.Y. and Yao, S.Q. (2003) Combinatorial peptide microarrays for the rapid determination of kinase specificity. *Bioorg. Med. Chem. Lett.*, **13** (18), 2997–3000.

31 Uttamchandani, M., Chen, G.Y., Lesaicherre, M.L. and Yao, S.Q. (2004) Site-specific peptide immobilization strategies for the rapid detection of kinase activity on microarrays. *Methods Mol. Biol.*, **264**, 191–204.

32 Houseman, B.T., Huh, J.H., Kron, S.J. and Mrksich, M. (2002) Peptide chips for the quantitative evaluation of protein kinase activity. *Nat. Biotechnol.*, **20** (3), 270–4.

33 Kohn, M., Wacker, R., Peters, C., Schroder, H., Soulere, L., Breinbauer, R., Niemeyer, C.M. and Waldmann, H. (2003) Staudinger ligation: a new immobilization strategy for the preparation of small-molecule arrays.

Angew. Chem. Int. Ed. Engl., **42** (47), 5830–4.

34 Kimura, N., Okegawa, T., Yamazaki, K. and Matsuoka, K. (2007) Site-specific, covalent attachment of poly(dT)-modified peptides to solid surfaces for microarrays. *Bioconjug. Chem.*, **18** (6), 1778–85.

35 Parker, L.L., Brueggemeier, S.B., Rhee, W.J., Wu, D., Kent, S.B., Kron, S.J. and Palecek, S.P. (2006) Photocleavable peptide hydrogel arrays for MALDI-TOF analysis of kinase activity. *Analyst*, **131** (10), 1097–104.

36 Reineke, U., Schneider-Mergener, J. and Schutkowski, M. (2004) Peptide arrays in proteomics and drug discovery, in *Micro/Nano Technology for Genomics and Proteomics* (eds M. Ozkan and M. Heller), Springer, Berlin, Heidelberg, pp. 161–282.

37 Lynch, M., Mosher, C., Huff, J., Nettikadan, S., Johnson, J. and Henderson, E. (2004) Functional protein nanoarrays for biomarker profiling. *Proteomics*, **4** (6), 1695–702.

38 Stolowitz, M.L., Ahlem, C., Hughes, K.A., Kaiser, R.J., Kesicki, E.A., Li, G., Lund, K.P., Torkelson, S.M. and Wiley, J.P. (2001) Phenylboronic acid-salicylhydroxamic acid bioconjugates. 1. A novel boronic acid complex for protein immobilization. *Bioconjug. Chem.*, **12** (2), 229–39.

39 Wiley, J.P., Hughes, K.A., Kaiser, R.J., Kesicki, E.A., Lund, K.P. and Stolowitz, M.L. (2001) Phenylboronic acid-salicylhydroxamic acid bioconjugates. 2. Polyvalent immobilization of protein ligands for affinity chromatography. *Bioconjug. Chem.*, **12** (2), 240–50.

40 Govindaraju, T., Jonkheijm, P., Gogolin, L., Schroeder, H., Becker, C.F., Niemeyer, C.M. and Waldmann, H. (2008) Surface immobilization of biomolecules by click sulfonamide reaction. *Chem. Commun. (Camb.)*, **32**, 3723–5.

41 Carion, O., Souplet, V., Olivier, C., Maillet, C., Medard, N., El-Mahdi, O., Durand, J.O. and Melnyk, O. (2007) Chemical micropatterning of polycarbonate for site-specific peptide immobilization and biomolecular

interactions. *Chembiochem*, **8** (3), 315–22.

42 Coffinier, Y., Olivier, C., Perzyna, A., Grandidier, B., Wallart, X., Durand, J.O., Melnyk, O. and Stievenard, D. (2005) Semicarbazide-functionalized Si(111) surfaces for the site-specific immobilization of peptides. *Langmuir*, **21** (4), 1489–96.

43 Coffinier, Y., Szunerits, S., Jama, C., Desmet, R., Melnyk, O., Marcus, B., Gengembre, L., Payen, E., Delabouglise, D. and Boukherroub, R. (2007) Peptide immobilization on amine-terminated boron-doped diamond surfaces. *Langmuir*, **23** (8), 4494–7.

44 Melnyk, O., Duburcq, X., Olivier, C., Urbes, F., Auriault, C. and Gras-Masse, H. (2002) Peptide arrays for highly sensitive and specific antibody-binding fluorescence assays. *Bioconjug. Chem.*, **13** (4), 713–20.

45 Olivier, C., Perzyna, A., Coffinier, Y., Grandidier, B., Stievenard, D., Melnyk, O. and Durand, J.O. (2006) Detecting the chemoselective ligation of peptides to silicon with the use of cobalt-carbonyl labels. *Langmuir*, **22** (16), 7059–65.

46 Bernatowicz, M.S., Daniels, S.B. and Köster, H. (1989) A comparison of acid labile linkage agents for the synthesis of peptide C-terminal amides. *Tetrahedron Lett.*, **30** (35), 4645–8.

47 Holmes, C.P. and Jones, D.G. (1995) Reagents for combinatorial organic synthesis: development of a new o-nitrobenzyl photolabile linker for solid-phase synthesis. *J. Org. Chem.*, **60** (8), 2318–19.

48 Bray, A.M., Maeji, N.J. and Geysen, H.M. (1990) The simultaneous multiple production of solution phase peptides; assessment of the Geysen method of simultaneous peptide synthesis. *Tetrahedron Lett.*, **31** (40), 5811–14.

49 Bray, A.M., Maeji, N.J., Jhingran, A.G. and Velerio, R.M. (1991) Gas phase cleavage of peptides from a solid support with ammonia vapour. Application in simultaneous multiple peptide synthesis. *Tetrahedron Lett.*, **32** (43), 6163–6.

50 Bray, A.M., Velerio, R.M. and Maeji, N.J. (1993) Cleavage of resin-bound peptide esters with ammonia vapour. Simultaneous multiple synthesis of peptide amides. *Tetrahedron Lett.*, **34** (27), 4411–14.

51 Kessenbrock, K., Fritzler, M.J., Groves, M., Eissfeller, P., von Muhlen, C.A., Höpfl, P. and Mahler, M. (2007) Diverse humoral autoimmunity to the ribosomal P proteins in systemic lupus erythematosus and hepatitis C virus infection. *J. Mol. Med.*, **85** (9), 953–9.

52 Mahler, M., Mierau, R., Schlumberger, W. and Blüthner, M. (2001) A population of autoantibodies against a centromere-associated protein A major epitope motif cross-reacts with related cryptic epitopes on other nuclear autoantigens and on the Epstein-Barr nuclear antigen 1. *J. Mol. Med.*, **79** (12), 722–31.

53 Soutullo, A., Santi, M.N., Perin, J.C., Beltramini, L.M., Borel, I.M., Frank, R. and Tonarelli, G.G. (2007) Systematic epitope analysis of the p26 EIAV core protein. *J. Mol. Recognit.*, **20** (4), 227–37.

54 Dunn, C., O'Dowd, A. and Randall, R.E. (1999) Fine mapping of the binding sites of monoclonal antibodies raised against the Pk tag. *J. Immunol. Methods*, **224** (1-2), 141–50.

55 Kalaycioglu, A.T., Russell, P.H. and Howard, C.R. (2007) Selection of mimotopes of Bovine Viral Diarrhoea Virus using a solid-phase peptide library. *Vaccine*, **25** (41), 7081–6.

56 Oggero, M., Frank, R., Etcheverrigaray, M. and Kratje, R. (2004) Defining the antigenic structure of human GM-CSF and its implications for receptor interaction and therapeutic treatments. *Mol. Divers.*, **8** (3), 257–69.

57 Reineke, U., Ivascu, C., Schlief, M., Landgraf, C., Gericke, S., Zahn, G., Herzel, H., Volkmer-Engert, R. and Schneider-Mergener, J. (2002) Identification of distinct antibody epitopes and mimotopes from a peptide array of 5520 randomly generated sequences. *J. Immunol. Methods*, **267** (1), 37–51.

58 Zander, H., Reineke, U., Schneider-Mergener, J. and Skerra, A. (2007) Epitope mapping of the neuronal growth inhibitor Nogo-A for the Nogo receptor and the cognate monoclonal antibody IN-1 by means of the SPOT technique. *J. Mol. Recognit.*, **20** (3), 185–96.

59 Choulier, L., Laune, D., Orfanoudakis, G., Wlad, H., Janson, J., Granier, C. and Altschuh, D. (2001) Delineation of a linear epitope by multiple peptide synthesis and phage display. *J. Immunol. Methods*, **249** (1-2), 253–64.

60 Hawlisch, H., Frank, R., Hennecke, M., Baensch, M., Sohns, B., Arseniev, L., Bautsch, W., Kola, A., Klos, A. and Kohl, J. (1998) Site-directed C3a receptor antibodies from phage display libraries. *J. Immunol.*, **160** (6), 2947–58.

61 Liu, Z., Song, D., Kramer, A., Martin, A.C., Dandekar, T., Schneider-Mergener, J., Bautz, E.K. and Dübel, S. (1999) Fine mapping of the antigen-antibody interaction of scFv215, a recombinant antibody inhibiting RNA polymerase II from *Drosophila melanogaster*. *J. Mol. Recognit.*, **12** (2), 103–11.

62 Bresson, D., Laune, D., Chardes, T., Charreire, J., Bes, C., Bouanani, M. and Peraldi-Roux, S. (2004) Evidence for two discontinuous regions on the thyrotropin receptor involved in the binding of the monoclonal antibody 34A. *Hum. Antibodies*, **13** (4), 119–29.

63 Gao, B. and Esnouf, M.P. (1996) Multiple interactive residues of recognition: elucidation of discontinuous epitopes with linear peptides. *J. Immunol.*, **157** (1), 183–8.

64 Reineke, U., Schneider-Mergener, J., Glaser, R.W., Stigler, R.D., Seifert, M., Volk, H.D. and Sabat, R. (1999) Evidence for conformationally different states of interleukin-10: binding of a neutralizing antibody enhances accessibility of a hidden epitope. *J. Mol. Recognit.*, **12** (4), 242–8.

65 Kramer, A., Reineke, U., Dong, L., Hoffmann, B., Hoffmüller, U., Winkler, D., Volkmer-Engert, R. and Schneider-Mergener, J. (1999) Spot synthesis: observations and optimizations. *J. Pept. Res.*, **54** (4), 319–27.

66 Reineke, U., Sabat, R., Kramer, A., Stigler, R.D., Seifert, M., Michel, T., Volk, H.D. and Schneider-Mergener, J.

(1996) Mapping protein-protein contact sites using cellulose-bound peptide scans. *Mol. Divers.*, **1** (3), 141–8.

67 Huang, J., Gutteridge, A., Honda, W. and Kanehisa, M. (2006) MIMOX: a web tool for phage display based epitope mapping. *BMC Bioinformatics*, **7**, 451.

68 Schreiber, A., Humbert, M., Benz, A. and Dietrich, U. (2005) 3D-Epitope-Explorer (3DEX): localization of conformational epitopes within three-dimensional structures of proteins. *J. Comput. Chem.*, **26** (9), 879–87.

69 Blüthner, M., Mahler, M., Müller, D.B., Dunzl, H. and Bautz, F.A. (2000) Identification of an alpha-helical epitope region on the PM/Scl-100 autoantigen with structural homology to a region on the heterochromatin p25beta autoantigen using immobilized overlapping synthetic peptides. *J. Mol. Med.*, **78** (1), 47–54.

70 Kneissel, S., Queitsch, I., Petersen, G., Behrsing, O., Micheel, B. and Dübel, S. (1999) Epitope structures recognised by antibodies against the major coat protein (g8p) of filamentous bacteriophage fd (Inoviridae). *J. Mol. Biol.*, **288** (1), 21–8.

71 Plewnia, G., Schulze, K., Hunte, C., Tampé, R. and Koch, J. (2007) Modulation of the antigenic peptide transporter TAP by recombinant antibodies binding to the last five residues of TAP1. *J. Mol. Biol.*, **369** (1), 95–107.

72 Mahler, M., Mierau, R. and Blüthner, M. (2000) Fine-specificity of the anti-CENP-A B-cell autoimmune response. *J. Mol. Med.*, **78** (8), 460–7.

73 Valle, M., Munoz, M., Kremer, L., Valpuesta, J.M., Martinez, A.C., Carrascosa, J.L. and Albar, J.P. (1999) Selection of antibody probes to correlate protein sequence domains with their structural distribution. *Protein Sci.*, **8** (4), 883–9.

74 Groves, M.R., Mant, A., Kuhn, A., Koch, J., Dübel, S., Robinson, C. and Sinning, I. (2001) Functional characterization of recombinant chloroplast signal recognition particle. *J. Biol. Chem.*, **276** (30), 27778–86.

75 Huang, W., Beharry, Z., Zhang, Z. and Palzkill, T. (2003) A broad-spectrum peptide inhibitor of beta-lactamase identified using phage display and peptide arrays. *Protein Eng.*, **16** (11), 853–60.

76 Kesti, T., Ruppelt, A., Wang, J.H., Liss, M., Wagner, R., Tasken, K. and Saksela, K. (2007) Reciprocal regulation of SH3 and SH2 domain binding via tyrosine phosphorylation of a common site in CD3epsilon. *J. Immunol.*, **179** (2), 878–85.

77 Lajoix, A.D., Gross, R., Aknin, C., Dietz, S., Granier, C. and Laune, D. (2004) Cellulose membrane supported peptide arrays for deciphering protein-protein interaction sites: the case of PIN, a protein with multiple natural partners. *Mol. Divers.*, **8** (3), 281–90.

78 Landgraf, C., Panni, S., Montecchi-Palazzi, L., Castagnoli, L., Schneider-Mergener, J., Volkmer-Engert, R. and Cesareni, G. (2004) Protein interaction networks by proteome peptide scanning. *PLoS Biol.*, **2** (1), E14.

79 Lentze, N. and Narberhaus, F. (2004) Detection of oligomerisation and substrate recognition sites of small heat shock proteins by peptide arrays. *Biochem. Biophys. Res. Commun.*, **325** (2), 401–7.

80 Rathert, P., Zhang, X., Freund, C., Cheng, X. and Jeltsch, A. (2008) Analysis of the substrate specificity of the Dim-5 histone lysine methyltransferase using peptide arrays. *Chem. Biol.*, **15** (1), 5–11.

81 Reineke, U., Sabat, R., Misselwitz, R., Welfle, H., Volk, H.D. and Schneider-Mergener, J. (1999) A synthetic mimic of a discontinuous binding site on interleukin-10. *Nat. Biotechnol.*, **17** (3), 271–5.

82 Xu, T.R., Baillie, G.S., Bhari, N., Houslay, T.M., Pitt, A.M., Adams, D.R., Kolch, W., Houslay, M.D. and Milligan, G. (2008) Mutations of beta-arrestin 2 that limit self-association also interfere with interactions with the beta2-adrenoceptor and the ERK1/2 MAPKs: implications for beta2-adrenoceptor signalling via the ERK1/2 MAPKs. *Biochem. J.*, **413** (1), 51–60.

83 Dürauer, A., Kopecky, E., Berger, E., Seifert, M., Hahn, R. and Jungbauer, A. (2006) Evaluation of a sensitive detection method for peptide arrays prepared by SPOT synthesis. *J. Biochem. Biophys. Methods*, **66** (1-3), 45–57.

84 Boisguerin, P., Leben, R., Ay, B., Radziwill, G., Moelling, K., Dong, L. and Volkmer-Engert, R. (2004) An improved method for the synthesis of cellulose membrane-bound peptides with free C termini is useful for PDZ domain binding studies. *Chem. Biol.*, **11** (4), 449–59.

85 Tomassi, L., Costantini, A., Corallino, S., Santonico, E., Carducci, M., Cesareni, G. and Castagnoli, L. (2008) The central proline rich region of POB1/REPS2 plays a regulatory role in epidermal growth factor receptor endocytosis by binding to 14-3-3 and SH3 domain-containing proteins. *BMC Biochem.*, **9**, 21.

86 Wiedemann, U., Boisguerin, P., Leben, R., Leitner, D., Krause, G., Moelling, K., Volkmer-Engert, R. and Oschkinat, H. (2004) Quantification of PDZ domain specificity, prediction of ligand affinity and rational design of super-binding peptides. *J. Mol. Biol.*, **343** (3), 703–18.

87 Martinelli, S., Torreri, P., Tinti, M., Stella, L., Bocchinfuso, G., Flex, E., Grottesi, A., Ceccarini, M., Palleschi, A., Cesareni, G., Castagnoli, L., Petrucci, T.C., Gelb, B.D. and Tartaglia, M. (2008) Diverse driving forces underlie the invariant occurrence of the T42A, E139D, I282V and T468M SHP2 amino acid substitutions causing Noonan and LEOPARD syndromes. *Hum. Mol. Genet.*, **17** (13), 2018–29.

88 Collins, M.O., Yu, L., Coba, M.P., Husi, H., Campuzano, I., Blackstock, W.P., Choudhary, J.S. and Grant, S.G. (2005) Proteomic analysis of in vivo phosphorylated synaptic proteins. *J. Biol. Chem.*, **280** (7), 5972–82.

89 Mah, A.S., Elia, A.E., Devgan, G., Ptacek, J., Schutkowski, M., Snyder, M., Yaffe, M.B. and Deshaies, R.J. (2005) Substrate specificity analysis of protein kinase complex Dbf2-Mob1 by peptide library and proteome array screening. *BMC Biochem.*, **6**, 22.

90 Song, H., Kerman, K. and Kraatz, H.B. (2008) Electrochemical detection of kinase-catalyzed phosphorylation using ferrocene-conjugated ATP. *Chem. Commun. (Camb.)*, **4**, 502–4.

91 Green, K.D. and Pflum, M.K. (2007) Kinase-catalyzed biotinylation for phosphoprotein detection. *J. Am. Chem. Soc.*, **129** (1), 10–11.

92 Sun, L., Liu, D. and Wang, Z. (2007) Microarray-based kinase inhibition assay by gold nanoparticle probes. *Anal. Chem.*, **79** (2), 773–7.

93 Espanel, X., Walchli, S., Ruckle, T., Harrenga, A., Huguenin-Reggiani, M. and Hooft van Huijsduijnen, R. (2003) Mapping of synergistic components of weakly interacting protein-protein motifs using arrays of paired peptides. *J. Biol. Chem.*, **278** (17), 15162–7.

94 Martin, K., Steinberg, T.H., Cooley, L.A., Gee, K.R., Beechem, J.M. and Patton, W.F. (2003) Quantitative analysis of protein phosphorylation status and protein kinase activity on microarrays using a novel fluorescent phosphorylation sensor dye. *Proteomics*, **3** (7), 1244–55.

95 Akita, S., Umezawa, N., Kato, N. and Higuchi, T. (2008) Array-based fluorescence assay for serine/threonine kinases using specific chemical reaction. *Bioorg. Med. Chem. Lett.*, **16** (16), 7788–94.

96 Shults, M.D., Kozlov, I.A., Nelson, N., Kermani, B.G., Melnyk, P.C., Shevchenko, V., Srinivasan, A., Musmacker, J., Hachmann, J.P., Barker, D.L., Lebl, M. and Zhao, C. (2007) A multiplexed protein kinase assay. *Chembiochem*, **8** (8), 933–42.

97 MacBeath, G. and Schreiber, S.L. (2000) Printing proteins as microarrays for high-throughput function determination. *Science*, **289** (5485), 1760–3.

98 Kerman, K. and Kraatz, H.B. (2007) Electrochemical detection of kinase-catalyzed thiophosphorylation using gold nanoparticles. *Chem. Commun. (Camb.)*, **47**, 5019–21.

99 Rupcich, N., Green, J.R. and Brennan, J.D. (2005) Nanovolume kinase inhibition assay using a sol-gel-derived

100 Zerweck, J., Masch, A. and Schutkowski, M. (2008) Peptide microarrays for profiling of modification state specific antibodies, in *Methods in Molecular Biology, Epitope Mapping Protocols*, 2nd edn (eds U. Reineke and M. Schutkowski), Morris Humana Press Inc., Cold Spring Harbor.

101 Zhu, Q., Hong, A., Sheng, N., Zhang, X., Matejko, A., Jun, K.Y., Srivannavit, O., Gulari, E., Gao, X. and Zhou, X. (2007) microParaflo biochip for nucleic acid and protein analysis. *Methods Mol. Biol.*, **382**, 287–312.

102 Wang, Z., Lee, J., Cossins, A.R. and Brust, M. (2005) Microarray-based detection of protein binding and functionality by gold nanoparticle probes. *Anal. Chem.*, **77** (17), 5770–4.

103 Min, D.H., Su, J. and Mrksich, M. (2004) Profiling kinase activities by using a peptide chip and mass spectrometry. *Angew. Chem. Int. Ed. Engl.*, **43** (44), 5973–7.

104 Su, J., Bringer, M.R., Ismagilov, R.F. and Mrksich, M. (2005) Combining microfluidic networks and peptide arrays for multi-enzyme assays. *J. Am. Chem. Soc.*, **127** (20), 7280–1.

105 Edlund, M., Wikstrom, K., Toomik, R., Ek, P. and Obrink, B. (1998) Characterization of protein kinase C-mediated phosphorylation of the short cytoplasmic domain isoform of C-CAM. *FEBS Lett.*, **425** (1), 166–70.

106 Szallasi, Z., Denning, M.F., Chang, E.Y., Rivera, J., Yuspa, S.H., Lehel, C., Olah, Z., Anderson, W.B. and Blumberg, P.M. (1995) Development of a rapid approach to identification of tyrosine phosphorylation sites: application to PKC delta phosphorylated upon activation of the high affinity receptor for IgE in rat basophilic leukemia cells. *Biochem. Biophys. Res. Commun.*, **214** (3), 888–94.

107 Diks, S.H., Kok, K., O'Toole, T., Hommes, D.W., van Dijken, P., Joore, J. and Peppelenbosch, M.P. (2004) Kinome profiling for studying lipopolysaccharide signal transduction in human peripheral blood mononuclear cells. *J. Biol. Chem.*, **279** (47), 49206–13.

108 Diks, S.H., Parikh, K., van der Sijde, M., Joore, J., Ritsema, T. and Peppelenbosch, M.P. (2007) Evidence for a minimal eukaryotic phosphoproteome? *PLoS ONE*, **2** (1), e777.

109 Hayashi, M., Fearns, C., Eliceiri, B., Yang, Y. and Lee, J.D. (2005) Big mitogen-activated protein kinase 1/ extracellular signal-regulated kinase 5 signaling pathway is essential for tumor-associated angiogenesis. *Cancer Res.*, **65** (17), 7699–706.

110 Lowenberg, M., Tuynman, J., Bilderbeek, J., Gaber, T., Buttgereit, F., van Deventer, S., Peppelenbosch, M. and Hommes, D. (2005) Rapid immunosuppressive effects of glucocorticoids mediated through Lck and Fyn. *Blood*, **106** (5), 1703–10.

111 Lowenberg, M., Tuynman, J., Scheffer, M., Verhaar, A., Vermeulen, L., van Deventer, S., Hommes, D. and Peppelenbosch, M. (2006) Kinome analysis reveals nongenomic glucocorticoid receptor-dependent inhibition of insulin signaling. *Endocrinology*, **147** (7), 3555–62.

112 Ritsema, T., Joore, J., van Workum, W. and Pieterse, C.M. (2007) Kinome profiling of Arabidopsis using arrays of kinase consensus substrates. *Plant Methods*, **3**, 3.

113 Stulemeijer, I.J., Stratmann, J.W. and Joosten, M.H. (2007) Tomato mitogen-activated protein kinases LeMPK1, LeMPK2, and LeMPK3 are activated during the Cf-4/Avr4-induced hypersensitive response and have distinct phosphorylation specificities. *Plant Physiol.*, **144** (3), 1481–94.

114 Toomik, R. and Ek, P. (1997) A potent and highly selective peptide substrate for protein kinase C assay. *Biochem. J.*, **322**, 455–60.

115 van Baal, J.W., Diks, S.H., Wanders, R.J., Rygiel, A.M., Milano, F., Joore, J., Bergman, J.J., Peppelenbosch, M.P. and Krishnadath, K.K. (2006) Comparison of kinome profiles of Barrett's esophagus with normal squamous esophagus and normal gastric cardia. *Cancer Res.*, **66** (24), 11605–12.

116 Dostmann, W.R., Nickl, C., Thiel, S., Tsigelny, I., Frank, R. and Tegge, W.J. (1999) Delineation of selective cyclic GMP-dependent protein kinase Ialpha substrate and inhibitor peptides based on combinatorial peptide libraries on paper. *Pharmacol. Ther.*, **82** (2-3), 373–87.

117 Dostmann, W.R., Tegge, W., Frank, R., Nickl, C.K., Taylor, M.S. and Brayden, J.E. (2002) Exploring the mechanisms of vascular smooth muscle tone with highly specific, membrane-permeable inhibitors of cyclic GMP-dependent protein kinase Ialpha. *Pharmacol. Ther.*, **93** (2-3), 203–15.

118 Luo, K., Zhou, P. and Lodish, H.F. (1995) The specificity of the transforming growth factor beta receptor kinases determined by a spatially addressable peptide library. *Proc. Natl Acad. Sci. USA*, **92** (25), 11761–5.

119 Mukhija, S., Germeroth, L., Schneider-Mergener, J. and Erni, B. (1998) Identification of peptides inhibiting enzyme I of the bacterial phosphotransferase system using combinatorial cellulose-bound peptide libraries. *Eur. J. Biochem.*, **254** (2), 433–8.

120 Rodriguez, M., Li, S.S., Harper, J.W. and Songyang, Z. (2004) An oriented peptide array library (OPAL) strategy to study protein-protein interactions. *J. Biol. Chem.*, **279** (10), 8802–7.

121 Tegge, W., Frank, R., Hofmann, F. and Dostmann, W.R. (1995) Determination of cyclic nucleotide-dependent protein kinase substrate specificity by the use of peptide libraries on cellulose paper. *Biochemistry*, **34** (33), 10569–77.

122 Dostmann, W.R., Taylor, M.S., Nickl, C.K., Brayden, J.E., Frank, R. and Tegge, W.J. (2000) Highly specific, membrane-permeant peptide blockers of cGMP-dependent protein kinase Ialpha inhibit NO-induced cerebral dilation. *Proc. Natl Acad. Sci. USA*, **97** (26), 14772–7.

123 Himpel, S., Tegge, W., Frank, R., Leder, S., Joost, H.G. and Becker, W. (2000) Specificity determinants of substrate recognition by the protein kinase DYRK1A. *J. Biol. Chem.*, **275** (4), 2431–8.

124 Loog, M., Toomik, R., Sak, K., Muszynska, G., Jarv, J. and Ek, P. (2000) Peptide phosphorylation by calcium-

dependent protein kinase from maize seedlings. *Eur. J. Biochem.*, **267** (2), 337–43.

125 Espanel, X. and Hooft van Huijsduijnen, R. (2005) Applying the SPOT peptide synthesis procedure to the study of protein tyrosine phosphatase substrate specificity: probing for the heavenly match in vitro. *Methods*, **35** (1), 64–72.

126 Espanel, X., Huguenin-Reggiani, M. and Hooft van Huijsduijnen, R. (2002) The SPOT technique as a tool for studying protein tyrosine phosphatase substrate specificities. *Protein Sci.*, **11** (10), 2326–34.

127 Kohn, M., Gutierrez-Rodriguez, M., Jonkheijm, P., Wetzel, S., Wacker, R., Schroeder, H., Prinz, H., Niemeyer, C.M., Breinbauer, R., Szedlacsek, S.E. and Waldmann, H. (2007) A microarray strategy for mapping the substrate specificity of protein tyrosine phosphatase. *Angew. Chem. Int. Ed. Engl.*, **46** (40), 7700–3.

128 Pasquali, C., Curchod, M.L., Walchli, S., Espanel, X., Guerrier, M., Arigoni, F., Strous, G. and Van Huijsduijnen, R.H. (2003) Identification of protein tyrosine phosphatases with specificity for the ligand-activated growth hormone receptor. *Mol. Endocrinol.*, **17** (11), 2228–39.

129 Sun, H., Lu, C.H., Uttamchandani, M., Xia, Y., Liou, Y.C. and Yao, S.Q. (2008) Peptide microarray for high-throughput determination of phosphatase specificity and biology. *Angew. Chem. Int. Ed. Engl.*, **47** (9), 1698–702.

130 Sun, H., Lu, C.H., Shi, H., Gao, L. and Yao, S.Q. (2008) Peptide microarrays for high-throughput studies of Ser/Thr phosphatases. *Nat. Protoc.*, **3** (9), 1485–93.

131 Duan, Y. and Laursen, R.A. (1994) Protease substrate specificity mapping using membrane-bound peptides. *Anal. Biochem.*, **216** (2), 431–8.

132 Janssen, S., Jakobsen, C.M., Rosen, D.M., Ricklis, R.M., Reineke, U., Christensen, S.B., Lilja, H. and Denmeade, S.R. (2004) Screening a combinatorial peptide library to develop a human glandular kallikrein 2-activated prodrug as targeted therapy for prostate cancer. *Mol. Cancer Ther.*, **3** (11), 1439–50.

133 Kaup, M., Dassler, K., Reineke, U., Weise, C., Tauber, R. and Fuchs, H. (2002) Processing of the human transferrin receptor at distinct positions within the stalk region by neutrophil elastase and cathepsin G. *Biol. Chem.*, **383** (6), 1011–20.

134 Naus, S., Reipschlager, S., Wildeboer, D., Lichtenthaler, S.F., Mitterreiter, S., Guan, Z., Moss, M.L. and Bartsch, J.W. (2006) Identification of candidate substrates for ectodomain shedding by the metalloprotease-disintegrin ADAM8. *Biol. Chem.*, **387** (3), 337–46.

135 Reineke, U., Kurzhals, D., Köhler, A., Blex, C., McCarthy, J.E.G., Li, P., Germeroth, L. and Schneider-Mergener, J. (2001) High throughput screening assay for the identification of protease substrates, in *Peptides 2000: Proceedings of the Twenty-Sixth European Peptide Symposium* (eds J. Martinez and J.A. Fehrentz), EDK, Paris, p. 721.

136 Dekker, N., Cox, R.C., Kramer, R.A. and Egmond, M.R. (2001) Substrate specificity of the integral membrane protease OmpT determined by spatially addressed peptide libraries. *Biochemistry*, **40** (6), 1694–701.

137 Reineke, U., Bhargava, S., Schutkowski, M., Landgraf, C., Germeroth, L., Fischer, G. and Schneider-Mergener, J. (1999) Spatial addressable fluorescence-quenched peptide libraries for the identification and characterisation of protease substrates, in *Peptides 1998* (eds S. Bajusz and F. Hudecz), Akademiai Kiado, Budapest, Ungarn, pp. 562–3.

138 Kramer, A., Afffedt, M., Volkmer-Engert, R. and Schneider-Mergener, J. (1999) A novel type of protease cleavage assay based on cellulose-bound libraries, in *Peptides 1998* (eds S. Bajusz and F. Hudecz), Akademiai Kiado, Budapest, Ungarn, pp. 546–7.

139 Kozlov, I.A., Melnyk, P.C., Hachmann, J.P., Srinivasan, A., Shults, M., Zhao, C., Musmacker, J., Nelson, N., Barker, D.L. and Lebl, M. (2008) A high-complexity, multiplexed solution-phase assay for profiling protease activity on

microarrays. *Comb. Chem. High Throughput Screen.*, **11** (1), 24–35.

140 Zhu, Q., Uttamchandani, M., Li, D., Lesaicherre, M.L. and Yao, S.Q. (2003) Enzymatic profiling system in a small-molecule microarray. *Org. Lett.*, **5** (8), 1257–60.

141 Schwamborn, K., Knipscheer, P., van Dijk, E., van Dijk, W.J., Sixma, T.K., Meloen, R.H. and Langedijk, J.P. (2008) SUMO assay with peptide arrays on solid support: insights into SUMO target sites. *J. Biochem.*, **144** (1), 39–49.

142 Rathert, P., Dhayalan, A., Murakami, M., Zhang, X., Tamas, R., Jurkowska, R., Komatsu, Y., Shinkai, Y., Cheng, X. and Jeltsch, A. (2008) Protein lysine methyltransferase G9a acts on non-histone targets. *Nat. Chem. Biol.*, **4** (6), 344–6.

143 Lu, P.J., Zhou, X.Z., Shen, M. and Lu, K.P. (1999) Function of WW domains as phosphoserine- or phosphothreonine-binding modules. *Science*, **283** (5406), 1325–8.

144 Wildemann, D., Erdmann, F., Alvarez, B.H., Stoller, G., Zhou, X.Z., Fanghanel, J., Schutkowski, M., Lu, K.P. and Fischer, G. (2006) Nanomolar inhibitors of the peptidyl prolyl cis/trans isomerase Pin1 from combinatorial peptide libraries. *J. Med. Chem.*, **49** (7), 2147–50.

145 Fazio, F., Bryan, M.C., Blixt, O., Paulson, J.C. and Wong, C.H. (2002) Synthesis of sugar arrays in microtiter plate. *J. Am. Chem. Soc.*, **124** (48), 14397–402.

146 Houseman, B.T. and Mrksich, M. (1999) The role of ligand density in the enzymatic glycosylation of carbohydrates presented on self-assembled monolayers of alkanethiolates on gold. *Angew. Chem. Int. Ed. Engl.*, **38** (6), 782–5.

147 von Olleschik-Elbheim, L., el Baya, A. and Schmidt, M.A. (1997) Membrane anchored synthetic peptides as a tool for structure-function analysis of pertussis toxin and its target proteins, in *ADP-Ribosylation in Animal Tissues: Structure and Biology of Mono(ADP Ribosyl) Transferases and Related Enzymes* (eds F. Koch-Nolte and F. Haag), Plenum Press, New York, pp. 87–91.

148 Zhu, H. and Snyder, M. (2003) Protein chip technology. *Curr. Opin. Chem. Biol.*, **7** (1), 55–63.

149 Reuter, M., Schneider-Mergener, J., Kupper, D., Meisel, A., Mackeldanz, P., Krüger, D.H. and Schroeder, C. (1999) Regions of endonuclease EcoRII involved in DNA target recognition identified by membrane-bound peptide repertoires. *J. Biol. Chem.*, **274** (8), 5213–21.

150 Dietz, J., Koch, J., Kaur, A., Raja, C., Stein, S., Grez, M., Pustowka, A., Mensch, S., Ferner, J., Möller, L., Bannert, N., Tampé, R., Divita, G., Mely, Y., Schwalbe, H. and Dietrich, U. (2008) Inhibition of HIV-1 by a peptide ligand of the genomic RNA packaging signal Psi. *ChemMedChem*, **3** (5), 749–55.

151 Pustowka, A., Dietz, J., Ferner, J., Baumann, M., Landersz, M., Königs, C., Schwalbe, H. and Dietrich, U. (2003) Identification of peptide ligands for target RNA structures derived from the HIV-1 packaging signal psi by screening phage-displayed peptide libraries. *Chembiochem*, **4** (10), 1093–7.

152 Hilpert, K., Elliott, M.R., Volkmer-Engert, R., Henklein, P., Donini, O., Zhou, Q., Winkler, D.F. and Hancock, R.E. (2006) Sequence requirements and an optimization strategy for short antimicrobial peptides. *Chem. Biol.*, **13** (10), 1101–7.

153 Hilpert, K. and Hancock, R.E. (2007) Use of luminescent bacteria for rapid screening and characterization of short cationic antimicrobial peptides synthesized on cellulose using peptide array technology. *Nat. Protoc.*, **2** (7), 1652–60.

154 Schmidt, T.G., Koepke, J., Frank, R. and Skerra, A. (1996) Molecular interaction between the Strep-tag affinity peptide and its cognate target, streptavidin. *J. Mol. Biol.*, **255** (5), 753–66.

155 Amatschek, K., Necina, R., Hahn, R., Schallaun, E., Schwinn, H., Josic, D. and Jungbauer, A. (2000) Affinity chromatography of human blood coagulation factor VIII on monoliths with peptides from a combinatorial library. *J. High Resolut. Chromatogr.*, **23** (1), 47–58.

156 Kramer, A., Stigler, R.D., Knaute, T., Hoffmann, B. and Schneider-Mergener, J. (1998) Stepwise transformation of a cholera toxin and a p24 (HIV-1) epitope into D-peptide analogs. *Protein Eng.*, **11** (10), 941–8.

157 Piossek, C., Schneider-Mergener, J., Schirner, M., Vakalopoulou, E., Germeroth, L. and Thierauch, K.H. (1999) Vascular endothelial growth factor (VEGF) receptor II-derived peptides inhibit VEGF. *J. Biol. Chem.*, **274** (9), 5612–19.

158 Piossek, C., Thierauch, K.H., Schneider-Mergener, J., Volkmer-Engert, R., Bachmann, M.F., Korff, T., Augustin, H.G. and Germeroth, L. (2003) Potent inhibition of angiogenesis by D,L-peptides derived from vascular endothelial growth factor receptor 2. *Thromb. Haemost.*, **90** (3), 501–10.

159 Kramer, A., Schuster, A., Reineke, U., Malin, R., Volkmer-Engert, R., Landgraf, C. and Schneider-Mergener, J. (1994) Combinatorial cellulose-bound peptide libraries: Screening tools for the identification of peptides that bind ligands with predefined specificity. *Methods: Companion Methods Enzymol.*, **6**, 388–95.

160 Kramer, A., Volkmer-Engert, R., Malin, R., Reineke, U. and Schneider-Mergener, J. (1993) Simultaneous synthesis of peptide libraries on single resin and continuous cellulose membrane supports: examples for the identification of protein, metal and DNA binding peptide mixtures. *J. Pept. Res.*, **6** (6), 314–19.

161 Schneider-Mergener, J., Kramer, A. and Reineke, U. (1996) Peptide libraries bound to continuous cellulose

membranes: tools to study molecular recognition, in *Combinatorial Libraries* (ed. R. Cortese), W. de Gruyter, Berlin, pp. 53–68.

162 Malin, R., Steinbrecher, A., Semmler, W., Noll, B., Johannsen, B., Frammel, C., Hohne, W. and Schneider-Mergener, J. (1995) Identification of technetium-99m binding peptides using cellulose-bound combinatorial peptide libraries. *J. Am. Chem. Soc.*, **117**, 11821–22.

163 Gao, X., Zhou, X. and Gulari, E. (2003) Light directed massively parallel on-chip synthesis of peptide arrays with t-Boc chemistry. *Proteomics*, **3** (11), 2135–41.

164 Komolpis, K., Srivannavit, O. and Gulari, E. (2002) Light-directed simultaneous synthesis of oligopeptides on microarray substrate using a photogenerated acid. *Biotechnol. Prog.*, **18** (3), 641–6.

165 Peterfi, Z. and Kocsis, B. (2000) Comparison of blocking agents for an ELISA for LPS. *J. Immunoassay Immunochem.*, **21** (4), 341–54.

166 Vogt, R.F., Jr, Phillips, D.L., Henderson, L.O., Whitfield, W. and Spierto, F.W. (1987) Quantitative differences among various proteins as blocking agents for ELISA microtiter plates. *J. Immunol. Methods*, **101** (1), 43–50.

167 Kato, R., Kaga, C., Kunimatsu, M., Kobayashi, T. and Honda, H. (2006) Peptide array-based interaction assay of solid-bound peptides and anchorage-dependant cells and its effectiveness in cell-adhesive peptide design. *J. Biosci. Bioeng.*, **101** (6), 485–95.

168 Bialek, K., Swistowski, A. and Frank, R. (2003) Epitope-targeted proteome analysis: towards a large-scale automated protein-protein-interaction mapping utilizing synthetic peptide arrays. *Anal. Bioanal. Chem.*, **376** (7), 1006–13.

Index

Page numbers in *italics* refer to Figures; those in **bold** to Tables.

Peptides as Drugs. Discovery and Development. Edited by Bernd Groner
Copyright © 2009 WILEY-VCH Verlag GmbH & Co. KGaA, Weinheim
ISBN: 978-3-527-32205-3